# Immunotherapy

*Guest Editors*

ISAAC YANG, MD
MICHAEL LIM, MD

# NEUROSURGERY CLINICS OF NORTH AMERICA

www.neurosurgery.theclinics.com

*Consulting Editors*
ANDREW T. PARSA, MD, PhD
PAUL C. McCORMICK, MD, MPH

January 2010 • Volume 21 • Number 1

SAUNDERS an imprint of ELSEVIER, Inc.

**W.B. SAUNDERS COMPANY**
*A Division of Elsevier Inc.*

1600 John F. Kennedy Blvd. ● Suite 1800 ● Philadelphia, PA 19103-2899

http://www.theclinics.com

NEUROSURGERY CLINICS OF NORTH AMERICA Volume 21, Number 1
January 2010 ISSN 1042-3680, ISBN-13: 978-1-4377-1839-3

Editor: Ruth Malwitz
Developmental Editor: Donald Mumford

*Neurosurgery Clinics of North America* (ISSN 1042-3680) is published quarterly by Elsevier Inc., 360 Park Avenue South, New York, NY 10010-1710. Months of issue are January, April, July, and October. Business and Editorial Offices: 1600 John F. Kennedy Blvd., Suite 1800, Philadelphia, PA 19103-2899. Customer Service Office: 11830 Westline Industrial Drive, St. Louis, MO 63146. Periodicals postage paid at New York, NY, and additional mailing offices. Subscription prices are $296.00 per year (US individuals), $447.00 per year (US institutions), $324.00 per year (Canadian individuals), $546.00 per year (Canadian institutions), $414.00 per year (international individuals), $546.00 per year (international institutions), $149.00 per year (US students), and $204.00 per year (international students). International air speed delivery is included in all *Clinics* subscription prices. All prices are subject to change without notice. **POSTMASTER:** Send address changes to *Neurosurgery Clinics of North America*, Elsevier Periodicals Customer Service, 11830 Westline Industrial Drive, St. Louis, MO 63146. **Customer Service: 1-800-654-2452 (US and Canada). From outside the US and Canada, call: 1-314-453-7041. Fax: 1-314-453-5170. E-mail: JournalsCustomerService-usa@elsevier.com (for print support) and journalsonlinesupport-usa@elsevier.com (for online support).**

*Reprints.* For copies of 100 or more, of articles in this publication, please contact the Commercial Reprints Department, Elsevier Inc., 360 Park Avenue South, New York, NY 10010-1710. Tel. (212) 633-3812; Fax: (212) 462-1935; E-mail: reprints@elsevier.com.

*Neurosurgery Clinics of North America* is covered in *MEDLINE/PubMed (Index Medicus), EMBASE/Excerpta Medica, and Current Contents/Clinical Medicine (CC/CM).*

Printed and bound by CPI Group (UK) Ltd, Croydon, CR0 4YY

Transferred to Digital Print 2011

# Contributors

## GUEST EDITORS

**ISAAC YANG, MD**
Chief Resident, Department of Neurological Surgery, University of California, San Francisco, California

**MICHAEL LIM, MD**
Assistant Professor of Neurosurgery, Department of Neurosurgery, Johns Hopkins Hospital, Baltimore, Maryland

## AUTHORS

**PANKAJ K. AGARWALLA, MSt**
Brain Tumor Immunotherapy Laboratory, Department of Neurosurgery, Massachusetts General Hospital/Harvard Medical School, Boston, Massachusetts

**EMILIA ALBESIANO, PhD**
Department of Oncology, The Sidney Kimmel Comprehensive Cancer Center, Johns Hopkins University School of Medicine, Baltimore, Maryland

**ZACHARY R. BARNARD, MS**
Department of Neurosurgery, Stephen E. and Catherine Pappas Center for Neuro-oncology, Massachusetts General Hospital, Boston, Massachusetts

**KEITH L. BLACK, MD**
Chairman, Department of Neurosurgery, Cedars-Sinai Medical Center; Director, Maxine Dunitz Neurosurgical Institute, Los Angeles, California

**NICHOLAS BUTOWSKI, MD**
Assistant Professor Neuro-Oncology Service, Department of Neurological Surgery, University of California San Francisco, San Francisco, California

**COURTNEY CRANE, PhD**
Department of Neurological Surgery, University of California at San Francisco, San Francisco, California

**WILLIAM T. CURRY Jr, MD**
Department of Neurosurgery, Stephen E. and Catherine Pappas Center for Neuro-oncology, Massachusetts General Hospital; Assistant Professor of Surgery, Department of Neurosurgery, Harvard Medical School, Boston, Massachusetts

**DALE DING, BS**
School of Medicine, Duke University, Durham, North Carolina

**SHANNA FANG, BS**
Department of Neurological Surgery, University of California at San Francisco, San Francisco, California

**JAMES L. FRAZIER, MD**
Department of Neurosurgery, The Johns Hopkins University School of Medicine, The Johns Hopkins Hospital, Baltimore, Maryland

**JAMES E. HAN, BA**
Department of Neurosurgery, The Johns Hopkins University School of Medicine, The Johns Hopkins Hospital, Baltimore, Maryland

**SEUNGGU J. HAN, BS**
Howard Hughes Fellow, Department of Neurological Surgery, University of California at San Francisco, San Francisco, California

**GRIFFITH R. HARSH IV, MD**
Professor, Department of Neurosurgery, Stanford University School of Medicine, Stanford, California

**AMY B. HEIMBERGER, MD**
Associate Professor, Department of
Neurosurgery, University of Texas, M.D.
Anderson Cancer Center, Houston, Texas

**NANCY G. HUH, MD**
Department of Neurological Surgery, University
of California at San Francisco, San Francisco,
California

**WILLIAM HUMPHRIES, MD**
Resident, Department of Neurosurgery, The
University of Texas M. D. Anderson Cancer
Center, Houston, Texas

**JIANFEI JI, PhD**
Research Scientist, Cedars-Sinai Medical
Center, Maxine Dunitz Neurosurgical Institute,
Los Angeles, California

**BRIAN JIAN, MD, PhD**
Department of Neurological Surgery, University
of California, San Francisco, San Francisco,
California

**CHARLES W. KANALY, MD**
Division of Neurosurgery, Department
of Surgery, Duke University Medical Center,
Durham, North Carolina

**ARI KANE, BA**
Howard Hughes Fellow, Department of
Neurological Surgery, University of California
at San Francisco, San Francisco, California

**GURVINDER KAUR, BS**
Department of Neurological Surgery, University
of California at San Francisco, San Francisco,
California

**WON KIM, MD**
Resident, UCLA Department of Neurosurgery,
David Geffen School of Medicine at UCLA,
Los Angeles, California

**MACIEJ S. LESNIAK, MD**
Director, Neurosurgical Oncology and
The University of Chicago Brain Tumor
Center, The University of Chicago, Chicago,
Illinois

**GORDON LI, MD**
Resident and Post-Doctoral Research Fellow,
Department of Neurosurgery, Stanford
University School of Medicine, Stanford,
California

**LINDA M. LIAU, MD, PhD**
Professor, UCLA Department of Neurosurgery,
David Geffen School of Medicine at UCLA,
Los Angeles, California

**MICHAEL LIM, MD**
Assistant Professor of Neurosurgery,
Department of Neurological Surgery, Johns
Hopkins University School of Medicine,
Baltimore, Maryland

**SIDDHARTHA MITRA, PhD**
Post-Doctoral Research Fellow, Department
of Neurosurgery, Stanford University School
of Medicine, Stanford, California

**ALESSANDRO OLIVI, MD**
Professor of Neurosurgery, Department
of Neurosurgery, The Johns Hopkins
University School of Medicine, The Johns
Hopkins Hospital, Baltimore, Maryland

**ANDREW T. PARSA, MD, PhD**
Department of Neurological Surgery, University
of California at San Francisco, San Francisco,
California

**CLEO E. ROLLE, PhD**
The University of Chicago Brain Tumor Center,
The University of Chicago, Chicago, Illinois

**JOHN H. SAMPSON, MD, PhD, MHSc**
Professor, Division of Neurosurgery,
Department of Surgery, The Preston Robert
Tisch Brain Tumor Center at Duke, Duke
University Medical Center, Durham, North
Carolina

**SADHAK SENGUPTA, PhD**
The University of Chicago Brain Tumor Center,
The University of Chicago, Chicago, Illinois

**ZACHARY A. SMITH, MD**
Department of Neurological Surgery, University
of California at Los Angeles, Los Angeles,
California

**ALLEN WAZIRI, MD**
Assistant Professor of Neurosurgery,
Department of Neurosurgery, University of
Colorado Health Sciences Center, Aurora,
Colorado

**JUN WEI, PhD**
Instructor, Department of Neurosurgery, The
University of Texas M. D. Anderson Cancer
Center, Houston, Texas

**ALBERT J. WONG, MD**
Professor, Department of Neurosurgery,
Stanford University School of Medicine,
Stanford, California

**ISAAC YANG, MD**
Chief Resident, Department of
Neurological Surgery, University of
California, San Francisco, San Francisco,
California

**JOHN S. YU, MD**
Director, Brain Tumor Center, Cedars-Sinai
Medical Center, Maxine Dunitz Neurosurgical
Institute, Los Angeles, California; Director,
Surgical Neuro-oncology; Neurosurgical
Director, Gamma Knife Center, Los Angeles,
California

# Contributors

**ALLEN WAZIRI, MD**
Assistant Professor of Neurosurgery, Department of Neurosurgery, University of Colorado Health Sciences Center, Aurora, Colorado

**JUN WU, PhD**
Instructor, Department of Neurosurgery, The University of Texas M. D. Anderson Cancer Center, Houston, Texas

**ALBERT J. WONG, MD**
Professor, Department of Neurosurgery, Stanford University School of Medicine, Stanford, California

**ISAAC YANG, MD**
Chief Resident, Department of Neurological Surgery, University of California, San Francisco, California

**JOHN S. YU, MD**
Director, Brain Tumor Center, Cedars-Sinai Medical Center, Maxine Dunitz Neurosurgical Institute, Los Angeles, California; Director, Surgical Neuro-oncology; Neurosurgical Director, Gamma Knife Center, Los Angeles, California

# Contents

The most common primary brain neoplasm is glioblastoma multiforme, which is associated with a dismal prognosis. Despite the recommended treatment regimen of aggressive surgical resection, radiation, and chemotherapy, the median survival remains approximately only 14 months. Due to these minimal improvements in survival of patients despite recent advances in conventional treatments, new modalities such as immunotherapy are being investigated and studied. A hurdle to developing effective immunotherapy is the immunosuppressive characteristics that are the hallmark of malignant gliomas. Effective therapeutic strategies will require overcoming these mechanisms, by augmenting tumor antigen presentation, perhaps in a setting isolated from the tumor microenvironment. The heterogeneity of potential glioma antigens warrants potential targeting of multiple tumor-specific antigens, and discovery and investigation of additional antigens. This article describes the current strategies and principles of immunotherapy for malignant gliomas.

Even though the central nervous system (CNS) was conventionally defined as "immunologically privileged", new discoveries have demonstrated the role of the immune system in neurologic disease and illness, including gliomas. Brain tumor immunotherapy is an exciting and revived area of research, in which neurosurgeons have taken a major position. Despite the ability to induce a tumor-specific systemic immune response, the challenge to effectively eradicate intracranial gliomas remains mainly because of tumor-induced immunoresistance. This article gives an overview of the immunologic responses that occur in the CNS and their potential role in brain tumors. The main cellular and molecular mechanisms that mediate tumor escape from natural immune surveillance are also covered in this article. Glioma cells have been shown to diminish the expression of danger signals necessary for immune activation and to increase the concentration of immunosuppressive factors in the tumor microenvironment, which results in T-cell anergy or apoptosis. Finally, the authors discuss most of the over-expressed oncogenic signaling pathways that cause tumor tolerance.

Abnormalities of cellular immunity are commonly seen in patients with glioblastoma (GBM), and the subsequent relative immunosuppression likely contributes to poor tumor-specific responses in affected individuals. Endogenous immune regulation is likely to limit the efficacy of a wide array of immunotherapeutic strategies, therefore mandating consideration in the continued development of novel treatments for

GBM. Various tumor-associated factors have been implicated as potential generators of the immunosuppressive effect. This article outlines relevant experimentation exploring the nature of immune defects in patients with GBM, including a critical discussion of tumor-secreted factors, cell-surface proteins, and more recently described populations of immunoregulatory leukocytes that have potential roles in the subversion of cellular immunity.

The central nervous system (CNS) has evolved as an immune-privileged site to protect its vital functions from damaging immune-mediated inflammation. There must be a CNS-adapted system of surveillance that continuously evaluates local changes in the nervous system and communicates to the peripheral immune system during an injury or a disease. Recent advances leading to a better understanding of the CNS disease processes has placed microglia, the CNS-based resident macrophages, at center stage in this system of active surveillance. Evidence points to microglia cells contributing to the immunosuppressive environment of gliomas and actually promoting tumor growth. Microglia accumulation exists in almost every CNS disease process, including CNS tumors. This article discusses the role of microglia in CNS immunity and highlights key advances made in glioma immunology.

Several immunostimulant approaches have been studied in the treatment of gliomas. The advent of recombinant DNA technology led to a nonspecific immunostimulation via systemic administration of cytokines. Recently, in attempts to more closely mimic their natural activity, cytokines have been delivered by implanting genetically transduced cells or by using in vivo gene transfer techniques. The latest efforts have focused on immunostimulatory agents that act directly on antigen-presenting cells and effector cells of the immune system via pattern recognition receptors. Combining these strategies with more than one mode of immunotherapy may provide better clinical results.

Despite advances in understanding the molecular mechanisms of brain cancer, the outcome of patients with malignant gliomas treated according to the current standard of care remains poor. Novel therapies are needed, and immunotherapy has emerged with great promise. The diffuse infiltration of malignant gliomas is a major challenge to effective treatment; immunotherapy has the advantage of accessing the entire brain with specificity for tumor cells. Therapeutic immune approaches include cytokine therapy, passive immunotherapy, and active immunotherapy. Cytokine therapy involves the administration of immunomodulatory cytokines to activate the immune system. Active immunotherapy is the generation or augmentation of an immune response, typically by vaccination against tumor antigens. Passive immunotherapy connotes either adoptive therapy, in which tumor-specific immune cells are expanded ex vivo and reintroduced into the patient, or passive antibody-mediated therapy. In this article, the authors discuss the preclinical and clinical studies that have used passive antibody-mediated immunotherapy, otherwise known as serotherapy, for the treatment of malignant gliomas.

Interferon-gamma (IFNγ) is a cytokine that acts on cell-surface receptors, activating transcription of genes that offer treatment potential by increasing tumor immunogenicity, disrupting proliferative mechanisms, and inhibiting tumor angiogenesis. However, abnormally low levels of IFNγ are produced by tumor cells and local T cells in the glioma microenvironment. Current investigations into the immunomodulating effects of IFNγ suggest that IFNγ has the potential to be used clinically in the treatment of brain tumors and as a promising adjunct to other immunotherapeutic modalities. Here the authors review the published literature that highlights the potential role of IFNγ in the treatment and immunotherapy of malignant gliomas.

Epidermal growth factor variant III (EGFRvIII) is the most common alteration of the epidermal growth factor (EGF) receptor found in human tumors. It is commonly expressed in glioblastoma multiforme (GBM), where it was initially identified. This constitutively active mutant receptor leads to unregulated growth, survival, invasion, and angiogenesis in cells that express it. EGFRvIII results from an in-frame deletion of exons 2 to 7 resulting in the fusion of exon 1 to exon 8 of the EGF receptor gene creating a novel glycine at the junction in the extracellular amino terminal domain. The juxtaposition of ordinarily distant amino acids in combination with the glycine that forms at the junction leads to a novel tumor-specific epitope that would make an ideal tumor-specific target. A peptide derived from the EGFRvIII junction can be used as a vaccine to prevent or induce the regression of tumors. This peptide vaccine has now proceeded to phase 1 and 2 clinical trials where it has been highly successful and is now undergoing investigation in a larger human clinical trial for patients who have newly diagnosed GBM. In this article, the authors discuss the preclinical data that led to the human trials and the exciting preliminary data from the clinical trials.

Glioblastoma multiforme is a malignant, relentless brain cancer with no known cure, and standard therapies leave significant room for the development of better, more effective treatments. Immunotherapy is a promising approach to the treatment of solid tumors that directs the patient's own immune system to destroy tumor cells. The most successful immunologically based cancer therapy to date involves the passive administration of monoclonal antibodies, but significant antitumor responses have also been generated with active vaccination strategies and cell-transfer therapies. This article summarizes the important components of the immune system, discusses the specific difficulty of immunologic privilege in the central nervous system, and reviews treatment approaches that are being attempted, with an emphasis on active immunotherapy using peptide vaccines.

Glioblastoma multiforme is the most common primary central nervous system tumor. The prognosis for these malignant brain tumors is poor, with a median survival of 14 months and a 5-year survival rate below 2%. Development of novel treatments is essential to improving survival and quality of life for these patients. Endogenous heat shock proteins have been implicated in mediation of both adaptive and innate immunity, and there is a rising interest in the use of this safe and multifaceted heat shock protein vaccine therapy as a promising treatment for human cancers, including glioblastoma multiforme.

The role of regulatory T cells (Tregs) in mediating immune suppression of antitumor immune responses is increasingly appreciated in patients with malignancies—especially within the malignant glioma patient population. This article discuss the role and prognostic significance of Tregs within glioma patients and delineates potential approaches for their inhibition that can be used alone or in combination with other immune therapeutics in clinical trials and in the clinical settings of recurrent or residual disease.

Over the past decade, dendritic cell–based immunotherapy for central nervous system tumors has progressed from preclinical rodent models and safety assessments to phase I/II clinical trials in over 200 patients, which have produced measurable immunologic responses and some prolonged survival rates. Many questions regarding the methods and molecular mechanisms behind this new treatment option, however, remain unanswered. Results from currently ongoing and future studies will help to elucidate which dendritic cell preparations, treatment protocols, and adjuvant therapeutic regimens will optimize the efficacy of dendritic cell vaccination. As clinical studies continue to report results on dendritic cell–mediated immunotherapy, it will be critical to continue refining treatment methods and developing new ways to augment this promising form of glioma treatment.

Glioma, especially high-grade glioblastoma multiforme (GBM), is the most common and aggressive type of brain tumor, accounting for about half of all the primary brain tumors. Despite continued advances in surgery, chemotherapy, and radiotherapy, the clinical outcomes remain dismal. The 2-year survival rate of GBM is less than 30%. Better understanding of GBM biology is needed to develop novel therapies. Recent studies have demonstrated the existence of a small subpopulation of cells with stemlike features called cancer stem cells (CSCs). These GBM CSCs are self renewable and highly tumorigenic. They not only are chemo-radio resistant but also often contain multidrug resistance genes and drug transporter genes. These characteristics enable GBM CSCs to survive standard cytotoxic therapies. Among GBM CSCs, CD133$^+$ cells are a well-defined population and are prospectively isolated by their cell-surface marker. Increasing data show that the presence of CD133$^+$ CSCs highly correlates with patient survival, making these cells an ideal immunotherapy target population. The authors have reviewed recent studies related with GBM CSCs (particularly CD133$^+$ CSCs) and the novel therapeutic strategies targeting these cells.

## Virally Mediated Immunotherapy for Brain Tumors          167

Pankaj K. Agarwalla, Zachary R. Barnard, and William T. Curry Jr

Brain tumors are a leading cause of mortality and morbidity in the United States. Malignant brain tumors occur in approximately 80,000 adults. Furthermore, the average 5-year survival rate for malignant brain tumors across all ages and races is approximately 30% and has remained relatively static over the past few decades, showing the need for continued research and progress in brain tumor therapy. Improved techniques in molecular biology have expanded understanding of tumor genetics and permitted viral engineering and the anticancer therapeutic use of viruses as directly cytotoxic agents and as gene vectors. Preclinical models have shown promising antitumor effects, and generation of clinical grade vectors is feasible. In parallel to these developments, better understanding of antitumor immunity has been accompanied by progress in cancer immunotherapy, the goal of which is to stimulate host rejection of a growing tumor. This article reviews the intersection between the use of viral therapy and immunotherapy in the treatment of malignant gliomas. Each approach shows great promise on its own and in combined or integrated forms.

## Distinguishing Glioma Recurrence from Treatment Effect After Radiochemotherapy and Immunotherapy          181

Isaac Yang, Nancy G. Huh, Zachary A. Smith, Seunggu J. Han, and Andrew T. Parsa

Recent advancements have made radiation and chemotherapy the standard of care for newly diagnosed glioblastomas. The use of these therapies has resulted in an increased diagnosis of pseudoprogression and radiation-induced necrosis. Standard MRI techniques are inadequate in differentiating tumor recurrence from posttreatment effects. Diagnosis of a posttreatment lesion as glioma recurrence rather than radiochemotherapy or immunotherapy treatment effect is critical. This increase in accuracy plays a role as newer immunotherapies incurring posttreatment effects on MRI emerge. Advancements with magnetic resonance spectroscopy, diffusion-weighted imaging, and functional positron emission tomography scans have shown promising capabilities. Further investigations are necessary to assess the imaging algorithms and accuracy of these modalities to differentiate true glioma recurrence from radiotherapy or immunotherapy treatment effect.

## Immunotherapy Combined with Chemotherapy in the Treatment of Tumors          187

James L. Frazier, James E. Han, Michael Lim, and Alessandro Olivi

This article provides a broad overview of the data, including laboratory and clinical studies, currently available on the combination of immunotherapy and chemotherapy for treating cancer. The various forms of immunotherapy combined with chemotherapy include monoclonal antibodies, adoptive lymphocyte transfer, or active specific immunotherapy, such as tumor proteins, irradiated tumor cells, tumor cell lysates, dendritic cells pulsed with peptides or lysates, or tumor antigens expressed in plasmids or viral vectors. This discussion is not limited to malignant brain tumors, because many of the studies have been conducted on various cancer types, thereby providing a comprehensive perspective that may encourage further studies that combine chemotherapy and immunotherapy for treating brain tumors.

## Monitoring Immune Responses After Glioma Vaccine Immunotherapy          195

Brian Jian, Isaac Yang, and Andrew T. Parsa

Immunotherapy provides the ideal candidate of therapeutic attack against malignant gliomas because it allows for targeting of cancer cells without the potential for nonspecific toxicity. This is important when glial tumor cells spread far through normal brain tissue. Current vaccine therapies are in clinical trials and are showing beneficial responses. Given that the inflammatory response may make serial radiographic imaging more difficult to interpret, newer methodologies of immuno-monitoring must be developed to assess the biologic efficacy of these immunotherapies. This article reviews methods of monitoring the immune system after vaccination against malignant gliomas. Improvements in immunomonitoring should lead to an increase in the efficiency of identifying viable avenues of therapeutic research, and assess the efficacy of those currently employed.

Glioblastoma multiforme (GBM) is the most common and lethal primary malignant brain tumor. The traditional treatments for GBM, including surgery, radiation, and chemotherapy, only modestly improve patient survival. Therefore, immunotherapy has emerged as a novel therapeutic modality. Immunotherapeutic strategies exploit the immune system's ability to recognize and mount a specific response against tumor cells, but not normal cells. Current immunotherapeutic approaches for glioma can be divided into 3 categories: immune priming (active immunotherapy), immuno-modulation (passive immunotherapy), and adoptive immunotherapy. Immune priming sensitizes the patient's immune cells to tumor antigens using various vaccination protocols. In the case of immunomodulation, strategies are aimed at reducing suppressive cytokines in the tumor microenvironment or using immune molecules to specifically target tumor cells. Adoptive immunotherapy involves harvesting the patient's immune cells, followed by ex vivo activation and expansion before reinfusion. This article provides an overview of the interactions between the central nervous system and the immune system, and discusses the challenges facing current immunotherapeutic strategies.

# Neurosurgery Clinics of North America

## RELATED INTEREST

*Immunology and Allergy Clinics of North America,* May 2009 (Volume 29, Issue 2)
**Psychoneuroimmunology**
Gregory G. Freund, MD, *Guest Editor*

## THE CLINICS ARE NOW AVAILABLE ONLINE!

Access your subscription at:
**www.theclinics.com**

# Neurosurgery Clinics of North America

# Preface

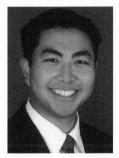 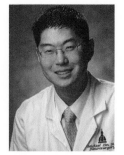

Isaac Yang, MD     Michael Lim, MD
*Guest Editors*

Malignant brain tumors are the most common and deadly primary brain tumor. Average survival from a malignant brain tumor is approximately 1 year, and, despite modern advancements with current therapies, survival has only minimally improved over the past two decades. Novel therapies need to be developed and investigated to advance the efficacy of brain tumor treatment. An important principle of developing new therapies is to maximize the antitumor effects while minimizing damage to normal brain tissue. Immunotherapy offers the anticancer precision of directed tumor-specific toxicity. In addition, immunotherapy offers the possibility of surveillance and durability. This therapeutic potential has made immunotherapy as a potential brain tumor treatment modality a rapidly expanding and investigated field.

Much work has been accomplished in the laboratory and in early clinical trials establishing the feasibility and potential efficacy of malignant brain tumor immunotherapy. Although most of the data for brain tumor immunotherapy and vaccines are from animal studies, current clinical trials are investigating the immune response, feasibility, and safety of brain tumor immunotherapy. Data thus far obtained from the clinical trials suggest that the therapies are efficacious and side effects of immunotherapy are mild. Hence, brain tumor immunotherapy holds promise not only as an effective anticancer effect through specific tailored and individualized therapies against malignant brain tumors but also for the real and tangible possibility of improved survival and quality of life.

This edition of *Neurosurgery Clinics of North America* represents an organized and thorough survey with critical analysis of the scientific and clinical studies focused on brain tumor immunotherapy from an assembly of leading researchers and expert clinicians. We hope this critical analysis of brain tumor immunotherapy and vaccines will provide clinicians and research scientists with a comprehensive and systematic overview of modern brain tumor immunotherapy to act as a resource and to stimulate future studies and investigations in this highly promising and exciting field.

Isaac Yang, MD
Department of Neurological Surgery
University of California, San Francisco
505 Parnassus Avenue, M779
San Francisco, CA 94143-0112, USA

Michael Lim, MD
Department of Neurosurgery
Johns Hopkins Hospital
Phipps Building Room 123
600 North Wolfe Street
Baltimore, MD 21287, USA

E-mail addresses:
yangi@neurosurg.ucsf.edu (I. Yang)
mlim3@jhmi.edu (M. Lim)

Neurosurg Clin N Am 21 (2010) xv
doi:10.1016/j.nec.2009.09.006
1042-3680/09/$ – see front matter

neurosurgery.theclinics.com

# Biologic Principles of Immunotherapy for Malignant Gliomas

Seunggu J. Han, BS[a], Gurvinder Kaur, BS[a],
Isaac Yang, MD[a,*], Michael Lim, MD[b]

**KEYWORDS**

- Immunotherapy • Glioma • Tumor-specific antigen
- Immunosuppression

The most common primary brain neoplasm is glioblastoma multiforme (GBM), which is associated with a dismal prognosis. Despite the recommended treatment regimen of aggressive surgical resection, radiation, and chemotherapy, the median survival remains approximately only 14 months.[1] Due to these minimal improvements in survival of patients despite recent advances in conventional treatments, new modalities such as immunotherapy are being investigated and studied.[2] In this article the current strategies and principles of immunotherapy for gliomas is described.

The central nervous system (CNS) historically has been considered an immune-privileged organ where immune activity is significantly silenced.[3] Several unique anatomic and physiologic characteristics limit immune surveillance and response functions in the brain,[4] such as: (1) the CNS lacks a lymphatic system; (2) the brain is shielded from the peripheral circulatory system by the blood-brain barrier (BBB), and thus is isolated from most peripheral immune cells, soluble factors, and plasma proteins; (3) the high levels of immunoregulatory cells and factors in the brain further mute immune functions; and (4) cells of the CNS at baseline express very low levels of major histocompatibility complex (MHC) molecules responsible for antigen presentation to immune effector cells.[5,6]

However, despite these factors minimizing CNS immune function, a highly adapted system of immune surveillance exists, and effective immune responses can occur in the CNS. Activity of both the complement system[7] and the antigen-antibody system, including functional B cells,[8,9] have been found within the CNS. During CNS insults, resident antigen-presenting cells (APC) of the CNS, microglia cells, undergo activation and upregulate both MHC and costimulatory molecules, and also contribute to both CD4+ and CD8+ specific T-cell responses.[10–12] A small number of lymphocytes are found in normal, healthy brain,[13] but both naïve lymphocytes[14] and activated T cells have the ability to cross the BBB.[13,15,16] Many different types of lymphocytes also infiltrate the CNS in the presence of a variety of CNS pathologies, including glioma.[17–20] However, the magnitude and potency of these immune responses in the CNS still remains to be clearly elucidated.[16]

## TUMOR-ASSOCIATED IMMUNOSUPPRESSION

Malignant brain tumors such as gliomas display an ability to evade and suppress the immune system.[21] Gliomas can evade the immune system at different levels of antigen recognition and immune activation.[22] First, by limiting effective signaling between glioma and immune cells, glioma cells evade immune detection. Many glioma cells express low levels of human leukocyte antigens (HLA) or express defective HLA.[6] A recent report by Facoetti and colleagues[23] described approximately 50% of 47 glioma

[a] Department of Neurological Surgery, University of California at San Francisco, 505 Parnassus Avenue, San Francisco, CA 94117, USA
[b] Department of Neurological Surgery, Johns Hopkins University School of Medicine, Phipps Building, Room 123, 600 N. Wolfe Street, Baltimore, MD 21287, USA
* Corresponding author.
*E-mail address:* yangi@neurosurg.ucsf.edu (I. Yang).

Neurosurg Clin N Am 21 (2010) 1–16
doi:10.1016/j.nec.2009.08.001
1042-3680/09/$ – see front matter © 2010 Elsevier Inc. All rights reserved.

samples displayed loss of the HLA type I antigen. Among these, 80% showed evidence of selective loss of HLA-A2 antigen. Of note, loss of HLA type I antigen was more common among higher grade tumors, suggesting a role of deficient antigen presentation in glioma progression.

Inhibition of antigen presentation by microglia and macrophages in the tumor microenvironment also contributes to the tumors' ability to escape immune detection. In vitro, the presence of glioma cells induces monocytes to reduce their phagocytic activity.[24] In addition, microglia found within glioma tissue appear to be deficient in proper antigen presentation for cytotoxic and helper T-cell activation.[25] Schartner and colleagues[26] demonstrated that MHC-II induction by stimulation was significantly less in microglia and infiltrating macrophages derived from gliomas than in those isolated from normal brain. The mechanism for this defective MHC-II response in tumor-associated microglia and macrophages remains unclear in regard to whether they result from a local immunosuppressive milieu, impaired signaling, or another unique inherent phenotype of tumor-associated microglia and macrophages. Stimulation of microglia in the presence of tumor cells reduces the secretion of proinflammatory cytokines, such as tumor necrosis factor (TNF)-$\alpha$, but also increases the secretion of the inhibitory cytokine interleukin (IL)-10.[27]

In the presence of glioma, T cells, specifically the CD4+ population, both in peripheral blood and in the tumor microenvironment, have depressed function.[28,29] Innate helper T cells (CD4+) display weak proliferative responses and dramatically lowered synthesis of the $T_H1$ cytokine IL-2.[30]

The degree of infiltrating lymphocytes found within gliomas has been found to correlate with patient survival.[31–33] However, other studies have failed to reproduce this finding.[34] Despite the presence of large numbers of glioma-infiltrating lymphocytes, the function and activity of these lymphocytes is difficult to predict. In fact, Hussain and Heimberger[35] demonstrated that the vast majority of CD8+ T cells found within gliomas are not activated. One hypothesis states that these are actually naïve T cells passively infiltrating the tumor across a compromised BBB caused by the tumor; alternatively, they may represent a population that once was active but has been subsequently rendered inactive by the host of immunosuppressive mechanisms found in the tumor microenvironment.

In patients with malignant glioma, a subpopulation of T lymphocytes termed T-regulatory cells (CD4+CD25+ cells; $T_{regs}$), which suppresses activity of effector T cells, is increased.[23,26,36–38] By downregulating the production of key cytokines, such as IL-2[39] and interferon (IFN)-$\gamma$[40,41] from target lymphocytes, they potently inhibit T-cell activation, proliferation, and differentiation.[39] $T_{regs}$ also induce lymphocytes to secrete predominantly $T_H2$ cytokines, such as IL-10,[42] and TGF-$\beta$2,[43] which in turn continues to propagate the regulatory phenotypes of T lymphocytes.[44] In vivo experiments have demonstrated significantly improved survival after depleting $T_{regs}$ in brains of mice harboring GL261 gliomas by injecting an antibody targeting against $T_{regs}$ (anti-CD25+ mAb).[45,46]

Secretion of various immune inhibitory cytokines and molecules by glioma cells also plays a large role in glioma-associated immunosuppression. IL-10 is also selectively secreted by invasive glioma.[47] Malignant glioma cells produces large amounts of prostaglandin E2,[48,49] which in turn inhibits IL-2 activation of lymphocytes.[50,51] High levels of expression of TGF-$\beta$2 are present in malignant glioma.[50,52] TGF-$\beta$2 mRNA is present in samples of human glioblastoma but not in normal adult brain.[52] TGF-$\beta$2 has previously been referred to as glioblastoma cell-derived T-cell suppressor factor (G-TsF) because of its potent immunosuppressive activity,[53] particularly in inhibition of cytotoxic T cells.[54,55] In addition, inhibition of signaling through the TGF-$\beta$2 pathway by antisense RNA in the C6 rat glioma model significantly prolonged survival,[56] and at times eradicated the tumor entirely.[57] These experiments are strongly supportive of the key role TGF-$\beta$2 plays in the immunosuppression that seems essential for the survival of glioblastoma cells.

In addition to the secreted immunosuppressive factors, expression of molecules that induce apoptosis of immune effectors, such as Fas ligand, galectin-1, and B7-H1, contribute to the immunosuppressive activity of gliomas.[58,59] Fas ligand (FasL, CD95L) and its receptor Fas (CD95) are important mediators of apoptosis in the immune system, particularly of CD8+ cytotoxic lymphocytes. High expression of FasL by human glioma cells naturally has been found to be associated with low levels of T-cell infiltration,[60] suggesting that FasL expression by tumor cells may contribute to T-cell depletion in tumors by increased T-cell apoptosis. However, the clinical significance of levels of FasL expression remains to be determined. Galectin-1 induces apoptosis in a variety of immune cell types through an alternative signaling pathway from Fas/FasL.[61] Overexpression of galectin-1 by gliomas likely also contributes to increased apoptosis of T cells by gliomas, serving as another method of evasion from antitumor activity of T lymphocytes. Higher levels of expression of galectin are found in higher grade astrocytomas.[62] B7-H1 is a potent immunosuppressive surface molecule that induces T-cell apoptosis by the PD-1 signaling pathway. A subset of gliomas with particularly strong immunoresistant phenotypes has high levels of B7-H1 expression on the surface.[59] In addition to the expression of apoptotic molecules targeted at T lymphocytes on glioma cells, microglia in presence of glioma have elevated levels of FasL and B7-H1.[63–65]

Iatrogenic factors may cause a systemic immunosuppression in patients with glioma. Corticosteroids given for tumor-associated edema may cause inhibition of cytokine production and sequestration of CD4+ T cells.[66] Recent evidence suggests, however, that at therapeutic doses corticosteroids may not interfere with immunotherapy.[67] Chemotherapeutic agents, such as temozolomide, for example, can cause lymphopenia, particularly of the CD4+ population,[68] which may compound immunotherapeutic modalities that depend on CD4+ T cell response. Other agents such as rapamycin inhibit production of the proliferative cytokine IL-2.[66]

## IMMUNOTHERAPY

Challenges in management of malignant gliomas have been rooted in inevitable recurrences of the tumor despite aggressive therapy. This challenge highlights the diffusely infiltrative nature of the tumor with evidence of microscopic disease that has already spread diffusely beyond the tumor mass at the time of clinical presentation.

The development of a successful mode of therapy requires systemic efficacy throughout the brain, with the ability to target tumor cells left behind after surgical resection and conventional adjuvant therapies. Such systemic therapy must also be highly specific for infiltrating tumor cells. Immunotherapy represents an attractive modality, with the potential to harness the potency, specificity, and memory of the immune system against infiltrating glioma cells.

Strategies in antiglioma immunotherapy broadly include cytokine therapy, passive immunotherapy, and active immunotherapy. Cytokine therapy is based on the concept that administration of immunomodulatory cytokines will activate the immune system. Passive immunotherapy includes serotherapy, in which monoclonal antibodies are given to aid immune recognition of tumor and deliver toxins to tumor cells, and adoptive therapy, which involves tumor-specific immune cells that are expanded ex vivo and reintroduced to the patient. Active immunotherapy involves generating or augmenting the patient's own immune response to tumor antigens, typically by administering tumor antigens or professional APCs.

### Cytokine Therapy

Cytokines have a potent capacity for immunomodulation, and immunotherapy with cytokines has been applied in oncology against a variety of tumors with variable success. In vitro experiments have established the efficacy of cytokines in eliciting antitumor activity of immune effector cells.[69] Different strategies for delivery of cytokines to the CNS have been explored, including injection/infusion of recombinant cytokines, vectors containing cytokine encoding genes, cells that secrete cytokines, or cytokines linked to toxins.

The first clinical trial using cytokine immunotherapy employed intratumoral IFN-α in addition to surgery and radiotherapy, and compared the trial group with a group who received surgical resection, radiation, and chemotherapy.[70] Although the investigators reported encouraging results, conclusions drawn regarding efficacy of IFN-α were limited due to flaws in study design.[21] Farkkila and colleagues[71] published the results of their trial using IFN-γ neoadjuvant and adjuvant to radiotherapy. Although the therapeutic regimen was well tolerated, there was no statistically significant difference in overall survival between the trial and control groups.[71] Studies that followed using systemic or intrathecal administration of IFN-α, IFN-γ, or IL-2 continued to find no significant improvement in survival while patients in the treatment arm encountered considerable toxicities.[72–74] Current approaches are looking to targeted delivery of cytokines to reduce systemic toxicity and increase the effective cytokine concentrations within the tumor.

Viral vectors have been used for local delivery of cytokines, with evidence of glioma-specific responses.[75–77] Strategies using intratumoral implantation of various cell types genetically modified to produce cytokines have produced more encouraging results. Injection of IL-2–secreting allogeneic fibroblasts into GL261 tumors in mice significantly delayed tumor development when injected before the tumor cells, and prolonged survival in mice with established tumors.[78–80] Neural stem/progenitor cells have many qualities that make them attractive candidates for carriers for delivery of cytokines. These cells self replicate, have prolonged survival, and migrate further than do viral vectors. Injection of neural stem/progenitor cells transfected to produce IL-2,[81] IL-4,[82]

IL-12,[83] and IL-23[84] into animals with established gliomas improved survival.

Alternative vehicles for intratumoral injection include liposomes and biopolymer microspheres. Injection of liposomes containing a plasmid with the IFN-β gene into GL261 gliomas in mice induced a robust activation of natural killer cells,[85] IFN-β expression by tumor cells, significant infiltration of cytotoxic T cells, a 16-fold reduction in mean tumor volume, and a complete response in 40% of animals.[86] These effects were much more robust than those seen with exogenous administration of IFN-β.[86] These infiltrative T cells as well as systemic T cells were isolated from treated mice, and were shown to have specific antitumor responses.[87] Biopolymer microspheres containing IL-2 are also effective in generating a specific response when injected into tumors of mice[88,89] and rats.[90]

Cytokines have also been used to deliver toxins such as Pseudomonas exotoxin. Malignant glioma cells[91,92] and medulloblastoma cells[93] express high levels of the IL-4 receptor (IL-4R) on their surface not found on normal brain cells. This overexpression has been used for selective delivery of toxins. Cytotoxic effects of Pseudomonas exotoxin conjugated to IL-4 against glioma and medulloblastoma cells have been demonstrated in culture.[92,93] In a clinical trial of intratumoral injection of IL-4–pseudomonas exotoxin for patients with high-grade glioma, 6 of 9 patients enrolled showed evidence of tumor necrosis, and there was no significant toxicity found in any patient.[94] Current clinical trials are continuing to evaluate this modality's efficacy and maximum tolerated dose.[95,96]

IL-13R is similarly overexpressed in malignant glioma, but not in normal brain cells.[97–99] IL-13 conjugated to Pseudomonas exotoxin also is well tolerated when given intratumorally for patients with recurrent, malignant glioma.[100–102] Recent efforts have focused on optimizing the specificity and strength of the interaction between IL-13 and IL-13R of glioma cells,[103] as well as novel modes of delivery of the interleukin-toxin.[104] Pseudomonas exotoxin conjugated to TGF-α has also resulted in improvement in survival of mice bearing tumor xenografts, with greater improvements seen in mice that express the epidermal growth factor receptor (EGFR).[105,106] In a phase 1 trial, 2 patients received intratumoral infusions of TGF-α conjugated to the Pseudomonas exotoxin, and showed radiographic response with relative safety.[107]

Overall, immunotherapy with cytokines has demonstrated relative safety, with variable efficacy. Thus, given the relative nonspecificity of cytokine therapy, it may ultimately prove most useful as an adjunct to other types of therapies, and potential use of cytokines as adjunct to chemotherapy, termed chemoimmunotherapy, is an active area of development.[90,108]

## Passive Immunotherapy

### Serotherapy

Passive immunotherapy includes serotherapy and adoptive immunotherapy. Serotherapy uses monoclonal antibodies to effect an antitumor response or to achieve very specific delivery of toxins, chemotherapy, or radiotherapy to the tumor cells. An important determinant of its success is the identification of "tumor antigens," specific antigens expressed on tumor cell surfaces but not on normal brain parenchyma. In human gliomas, antigens of interest have been those with quantitative differences between glioma and normal cells. Targeted glioma antigens have included tenascin, EGFR and its mutated form EGFRvIII, chondroitin sulfate, vascular endothelial growth factor (VEGF) receptor, neural cell adhesion molecule (NCAM),[109] and hepatocyte growth factor/scatter factor.[110]

Tenascin is an extracellular matrix protein that is strongly expressed in gliomas but not in normal brain. Tenascin is readily identified immunohistochemically by monoclonal antibody (mAb) 81C6.[111] Systemic administration of [131]I-conjugated 81C6 mAb to mice with human glioblastoma xenografts prolonged survival,[112,113] with evidence of localization of the radioisotope to the tumor.[114] Clinical trials of [131]I-conjugated 81C6 mAb given intrathecally have shown relative safety of the technique at low radiation doses, with dose-limiting neurotoxicity and hematologic toxicity at higher dose.[115–117] Several phase 1 and 2 trials studying [131]I-conjugated 81C6 mAb injected into the surgical resection cavity in humans with glioblastoma have shown improved survival in patients with malignant gliomas relative to those receiving traditional therapies.[115,118–123]

Similar to tenascin, EGFR is specifically overexpressed by glioma cells, and signaling through EGFR is believed to play a key role in survival, proliferation, and progression of gliomas. In a clinical trial by Kalofonos and colleagues,[124] patients with high-grade gliomas with evidence of localization of markers linked to anti-EGFR mAb to tumor radiographically were treated with [131]I-conjugated mAb to EGFR injected intravenously or infused into the internal carotid artery.[125] Six of 10 treated patients showed clinical response lasting 6 months to 3 years, with no major toxicity.[125] In another trial, increasing doses of murine anti-EGFR mAb, EMD55900 (mAb 425) was given in a single intravenous injection to 30 patients with malignant gliomas.[126] In 73% of patients, there was evidence of significant binding of EMD55900 to the tumor.[126] Similar binding was observed by Crombet and colleagues.[127] In a phase 1/2 study in which patients were given repeated infusions of EMD55900, toxicity was minimal, but no significant therapeutic benefit was found, as 46% of patients had progressed at 3 months.[128] Yet another trial using EMD55900 was stopped due to high levels of toxicity of inflammatory reactions.[129] Another phase 1/2 trial used a humanized anti-EGFR antibody, h-R3, designed to inhibit the kinase activity of the receptor for patients with malignant glioma, and demonstrated no high-grade toxicity and overall 37.9% response rate with stable disease in 41.4% patients at median follow-up of 29 months.[130] Several other phase 1, 2, and 3 trials have been conducted using EMD55900 conjugated to $^{125}$I.[131–134] These trials have demonstrated that the conjugated mAb effectively localizes to the GBM and is well tolerated. A phase 2 trial in which patients received radiolabeled mAb following standard surgical resection and radiation therapy demonstrated a median survival of 15.6 months.[133] A similar study reported median survival of 13.5 months.[134] Phase 3 trials are currently ongoing.[131]

EGFRvIII is a constitutively active mutant form of EGFR, and as a tumor antigen that likely has a large role in tumorigenicity, is an attractive target for serotherapy.[135] Y10, a mAb developed against a murine homologue of EGFRvIII, can generate antibody-dependent cell-mediated cytotoxicity in vitro.[136] In vivo, a single dose of Y10, injected intratumorally into an intracranial murine B16 melanoma transfected to produce EGFRvIII, prolonged survival by 286%.[136] This mechanism of this effect was Fc receptor-dependent.[136] Systemic injections of the anti-EGFRvIII mAb 806 into mice with U87 glioma xenografts significantly reduced tumor volume and increased survival.[137]

Antibodies can provide specific targeted delivery of chemotherapeutics or toxins as well. Mamot and colleagues[138] used fragments of mAbs binding both EGFR and EGFRvIII conjugated to immunoliposomes containing the cytotoxic drugs doxorubicin, vinorelbine, and methotrexate, and observed delivery of these drugs to glioblastoma cells in vitro. These investigators observed intracellular accumulation in glioma cells of the drug at high rates, beginning at 15 minutes.[138] The toxicity to the tumor cells was also higher when immunoliposomal formulation was given, compared with the same drugs given without the liposomes.[138] The same group followed this study with experiments in xenograft models, showing superior efficacy in slowing tumor growth of EGFR-targeted immunoliposomes containing cetuximab.[139] Antibodies have also been conjugated to several different toxins, with varying results.[140] The specificity of delivery of therapeutic agents by mAb to tumor-specific antigens holds great potential for limiting therapeutic toxicity in immunotherapy against gliomas.

### Adoptive immunotherapy

Adoptive immunotherapy augments the antitumor response with the reintroduction of immune effector cells that have been isolated from patients and expanded ex vivo. Expansion of cells ex vivo permits amplification under controlled conditions isolated from the immunosuppressive tumor microenvironment. Most adoptive immunotherapeutic strategies have used harvested lymphocytes stimulated with IL-2, without the presence of specific antigens. This process creates lymphokine-activated killer cells (LAKs). Others have used tumor-infiltrating lymphocytes, neural stem cells (discussed earlier), tumor-draining lymph node T cells, and non-MHC-restricted, cytotoxic T-cell leukemic cell lines.

Jacobs and colleagues[141] reported the first clinical trial studying immunotherapy with LAKs. LAKs and IL-2 were infused directly into the tumor bed of patients with malignant glioma, with minimal toxicity,[142] and mean progression-free survival in this small cohort was 25 weeks.[143]

Other trials using this technique found a small benefit in patient survival, but demonstrated dose-limiting neural toxicity related to cerebral edema, due to IL-2.[144–146] A recent study by Dillman and colleagues[147] reported a median survival of 17.5 months in glioblastoma patients who had LAKs placed in the resection cavity compared with 13.6 months in controls. In mouse models, LAKs coated with a bispecific anti-CD3 and anti-glioma antibodies increased the LAK activity of peripheral blood lymphocytes against the xenograft gliomas.[148] The application of these coated LAKs in clinical trials showed promising results. Infusion of coated LAKs into the tumor bed in human malignant gliomas resulted in either partial or complete regression tumor radiographically in 8 of 10 patients.[149] None of the 10 patients suffered tumor recurrence during the 10- to 18-month follow-up, and 9 of the 10 control patients given untreated LAK cells developed a recurrent tumor within 1 year.[149]

Tumor-infiltrating lymphocytes (TILs) found within glioma tissue contain a higher proportion of cytotoxic (CD8+) T cells compared with the composition of the peripheral blood lymphocyte population. Presuming their recognition and activity to one or more tumor antigens, combined with the fact that they are readily expanded in culture, has made TILs potential candidates for adoptive immunotherapy. In vitro, when compared with LAKs, TILs are much more cytotoxic to glioma cells.[150]

Saris and colleagues[151] studied the antitumor activity of these TILs in a murine glioma model (GL261). TILs were incubated with enzymatically digested GL261 cells and IL-2, and then infused intraperitoneally into mice harboring gliomas in the liver or brain. The infusion reduced the number of liver metastases relative to that in animals receiving saline or IL-2 alone, but did not lengthen the survival of animals with GL261 tumors in the brain, leading the investigators to conclude that the inefficacy of TIL therapy in the brain reflects the unique challenges of the immunosuppressive tumor microenvironment, and that more efficient delivery systems need to be evaluated.[151] Subsequent studies, however, have reported success with TIL in treatment of intracranial gliomas in vitro.[152,153] Several clinical pilot studies have described the feasibility of reinfusion of IL-2 and autologous TILs expanded in vitro to patients systemically and locally, with little toxicity.[154,155] Evidence for efficacy of such technique is currently lacking. However, TILs display many dysfunctional functions that contribute to the failure to generate an effective antitumor response in vivo: altered cellular signaling, decreased proliferation, defective cytokine secretion, decreased cytotoxic capacity, and a predisposition toward apoptosis.[49,156–159] Despite their defects, the superior specificity of TILs over LAKs and early clinical success with TIL strategies warrant further investigation.

Plautz and colleagues[160] employed a novel technique using the site of tumor-rich vaccine injection. In a phase 1 clinical trial, 12 patients with astrocytoma, anaplastic glioma, or GBM were initially were given these T lymphocytes from injection site–draining lymph nodes after activation and expansion ex vivo.[161] Partial regression was observed in 4 patients, and no long-term toxicity was seen during the 2-year follow-up period.[161]

The use of MHC nonrestricted, cytotoxic T-cell lines has also been explored. TALL-104, one such clone, was established from a patient with acute T-lymphoblastic leukemia, and is able to distinguish between tumor and normal cells with MHC nonrestricted tumoricidal activity. Transfer of TALL-104 cells into tumor sites of U87 xenografts in mice significantly reduced tumor growth[162] and prolonged survival,[163] by the dual mechanisms of direct tumoricidal action and recruitment of endogenous antitumor activity.[164]

Geoerger and colleagues[165] subsequently showed evidence of significant cytotoxic activity of TALL-104 cells against several human glioblastoma and medulloblastoma cell lines in rat models, and stressed the importance of local, as opposed to systemic, administration of TALL-104 cells. Preclinical studies have characterized the cytotoxic activity, trafficking patterns, viability of TALL-104 cells under different conditions, and activity against brain tumor versus normal brain cells have concluded that TALL-104 cells are appropriate for human clinical trials.[166,167] TALL-104 implantation therapy shows killing of glioma cells, but not of normal brain cells, through a mechanism mediated by specific cytokine release, and their activity is not altered by presence of radiotherapy or corticosteroids.[166] Recent studies have further elucidated the wide array of mechanisms of cytotoxic activity against tumor cells by TALL-104 cells.[168]

Unfortunately, expression of tumor antigens, such as EGFRvIII, is not uniform among cells of a given tumor.[169] Thus, adoptive immunotherapy targeting a single tumor-specific antigen can be compounded by variants in the target, allowing evasion from immune-mediated killing. This lack of efficacy has been seen with adoptive T cell therapy directed at melanoma-specific antigens, with the result of preferential survival of tumors with antigenic variants.[170] Therefore, it is likely that the most successful adoptive cell transfer therapies will target multiple tumor antigens. Adoptive immunotherapy, like cytokine therapy, although not fully effective by itself, may become an important adjuvant to standard treatments and other immunotherapies for primary brain tumors.

## Active Immunotherapy

Active immunotherapy involves priming or augmenting patients' immunity in vivo by vaccination against tumor antigen. Tumor vaccines for malignant glioma have been the focus of great interest in recent years. Successful development of glioma vaccines, however, requires proper presentation of tumor antigens and induction of effective, durable antigen-specific T cell immune response. Early efforts in active immunotherapy used vaccines containing autologous tumor cells as a source of tumor antigens, given with various cytokines for immune stimulation.[171–174] Despite evidence of safety and feasibility of such techniques, challenges remain due to innate poor antigen-presenting capacity of tumor cells, with low levels of expressed costimulatory molecules.

To augment the process of antigen presentation, professional APCs have also been used in glioma vaccines. Recent interest has turned to dendritic cells (DCs), which have an abundant expression of costimulatory molecules and have great capacity for activating T lymphocytes. DCs are exposed to tumor antigens, then used to initiate an antitumor response in the patient's endogenous T cells.[175] More specifically, autologous DCs are obtained from peripheral blood mononuclear cells or bone marrow, primed to maturation, exposed to whole tumor cell lysate or tumor antigen ex vivo, and reintroduced to the patient. In vitro experiments have established the ability of DCs exposed to tumor antigens in inducing T cell proliferation and generating cytotoxic responses.[176,177]

In clinical trials, DCs have been exposed to tumor antigens in a variety of ways, including whole tumor cells, isolated peptides, tumor lysates, or tumor RNA. An early phase 1 trial used peptide-pulsed DCs isolated from peripheral blood and showed the generation of robust T cell infiltration into the tumor.[178] Early efforts by Kikuchi and colleagues[179] employed DCs fused to glioma cells and injected intradermally for patients with malignant gliomas. No adverse reactions, but a partial response in only 2 of 8 patients, was observed.[179] In a subsequent study by these investigators, IL-12 was added to the formulation and more robust response was seen: there was a 50% radiographic reduction of the tumor in 4 of 15 patients, with similar safety profiles.[180] A complete regression of glioma was achieved in the murine GL261 model when a regimen of intrasplenic vaccination with DC/tumor fused cells, local cranial radiotherapy, and anti-CD134 mAb 7 was given.[181] Other strategies of DC exposure to antigens have involved using tumor lysates.[182,183] Reintroduction of DCs preloaded with total tumor RNA rather than tumor antigen also produced a strong cytotoxic T cell response against autologous glioma cells.[183] These early clinical trials have yielded encouraging results regarding generating responses and improving survival in patients.[179,183–185] Liau and colleagues[185] proposed that the most promising patient subgroup for DC vaccine therapy may be patients with small, quiescent tumors with low expression of tumor TGF-β. The phase 2 randomized trial using tumor lysate pulsed DC vaccine is ongoing.

The use of unselected tumor extracts to prime DCs in such nonspecific approaches risks inducing autoimmunity against antigens of normal brain.[186] In efforts to avoid this potential hazard, focus has turned to more specific approaches using tumor-specific antigens, such as EGFRvIII

as targets for glioma vaccines. Preliminary studies using EGFRvIII peptide-pulsed DCs showed generation of cytotoxic activity against the U87 human glioma cell line.[187] When the same vaccine was given to mice that subsequently received intracerebral injections of syngeneic melanoma expressing the murine homologue of EGFRvIII, animals that were immunized survived 6 times as long as those that were not immunized.[188] Among immunized mice, 63% survived long term and 100% survived rechallenge with melanoma, indicating evidence of immunologic memory against the tumor.[188]

A peptide-based vaccine targeting the tumor-specific mutated portion of EGFRvIII is also under investigation. A phase 1 trial with enrollment of 19 patients has been completed. The therapy was shown to be well tolerated, and treated patients had progression-free survival of 12 months and median overall survival of 18 months.[189] Of note, recurrent tumors after the vaccine showed no expression of EGFRvIII.[189] The phase 2/3 randomized trial of the EGFRvIII peptide vaccine with radiation and temozolomide is currently ongoing.

Another peptide-based vaccine currently under study is based on heat-shock protein gp96 and its associated peptides isolated from the patient's autologous tumor acquired at time of surgery. Preliminary results of the ongoing phase 1/2 trial have demonstrated the vaccine to be well tolerated, with evidence of induction of tumor-specific responses.

Alternative active immunotherapeutic approaches have aimed at initiating an immune response to tumor in vivo through lymphocytes. In one such study, peripheral lymphocytes removed from patients with high-grade gliomas were cultured with irradiated tumor cells in the presence of bacillus Calmette-Guérin and IL-2, then systemically reinfused into patients, with minimal toxicity.[190] Two of 9 patients experienced increased survival with evidence of tumor regression, 1 had tumor regression but not increased survival, and the remaining 6 had neither.[190]

Infectious agents have also been used to induce an antigen-specific immune response to gliomas. These vaccines contain viral or bacterial vectors carrying tumor antigen genes, and the concept involves that an immune response to the highly immunogenic infectious agent should augment the response to the tumor antigen as well. Such an approach in animal models using Listeria monocytogenes have shown efficacy against extracranial but not intracranial tumor, suggesting potential for improved efficacy in gliomas with improved delivery systems to the CNS.[191,192] In a phase 1 trial, recombinantly modified vaccinia virus Ankara carrying the cDNA for a melanoma antigen has proven safe, and capable of eliciting a strong response against the virus but not against the antigen.[193]

## MULTIMODALITY IMMUNOTHERAPY

Cytokine and active immunotherapy strategies have been combined by introducing tumor cells or fibroblasts transfected to produce cytokines, such as IL-2, IL-4, IL-12, IL-18, IFN-$\alpha$ and granulocyte macrophage colony stimulating factor (GM-CSF) alone or in combination with DCs.[17,194–197] Several studies suggest the promise of this strategy. Intratumoral administration of IL-2–producing tumor cells along with recombinant IL-12 significantly prolonged survival in mice.[198] Tumor cells producing GM-CSF or B7-2, a costimulatory molecule, when injected locally to the tumor, also increased survival in mice.[199] In rat models, when cDNA of IFN-$\gamma$,[200] TNF-$\alpha$,[77] and IL-4[201] were delivered retrovirally to glioma cells in situ, a strong immune response was generated and complete elimination of established tumors was seen.

## SUMMARY

The continued poor prognosis of patients with gliomas, despite current treatment protocols, warrants new therapeutic approaches. Advance stage clinical trials of several promising immunotherapies are currently ongoing, and their results will determine the clinical value of these modalities. Challenges to immunotherapy remain numerous. Although immunotherapy and chemotherapy can potentially serve as coadjuvants, the current practice of administering temozolomide during and 6 months after radiation therapy is an impediment to clinical testing of immunotherapies, which may be compromised both by concurrent chemotherapy and immunosuppression that accrues with time.

Another large hurdle in developing effective immunotherapy is the immunosuppressive characteristics that are the hallmark of malignant gliomas. Effective therapeutic strategies will require overcoming these mechanisms, by augmenting tumor antigen presentation, perhaps in a setting isolated from the tumor microenvironment. The heterogeneity of potential glioma antigens warrants targeting of multiple tumor-specific antigens, and discovery and investigation of additional antigens. The optimal immunotherapy will likely employ several of the strategies reviewed here and will become a standard component of a combined multimodal approach to malignant gliomas.

## REFERENCES

1. Stupp R, Mason WP, van den Bent MJ, et al. Radiotherapy plus concomitant and adjuvant temozolomide for glioblastoma. N Engl J Med 2005; 352(10):987–96.
2. Pardoll D, Allison J. Cancer immunotherapy: breaking the barriers to harvest the crop. Nat Med 2004;10:887–92.
3. Medawar P. Immunity to homologous grafted skin; the fate of skin homografts transplanted to the brain, to subcutaneous tissue, and to the anterior chamber of the eye. Br J Exp Pathol 1948;29(1):58–69.
4. Cserr HF, Knopf PM. Cervical lymphatics, the blood-brain barrier, and the immunoreactivity of the brain. In: Keane RW, Hickey WF, editors. Immunology of the nervous system. New York: Oxford University Press; 1997. p. 134–52.
5. Lampson L, Hickey WF. Monoclonal antibody analysis of MHC expression in human brain biopsies. Tissue ranging from "histologically normal" to that showing different levels of glial tumor involvement. J Immunol 1986;136:4052–62.
6. Yang I, Kremen TJ, Giovannone AJ, et al. Modulation of major histocompatibility complex class I molecules and major histocompatibility complex-bound immunogenic peptides induced by interferon-alpha and interferon-gamma treatment of human glioblastoma multiforme. J Neurosurg 2004;100(2):310–9.
7. Levi-Strauss M, Mallat M. Primary cultures of murine astrocytes produce C3 and factor B, two components of the alternative pathway of complement activation. J Immunol 1987;139:2361–6.
8. Bernheimer H, Lassmann H, Suchanek G. Dynamics of IgG+, IgA+, and IgM+ plasma cells in the central nervous system of guinea pigs with chronic relapsing experimental allergic encephalomyelitis. Neuropathol Appl Neurobiol 1988;14: 157–67.
9. Sandberg-Wollheim M, Zweiman B, Levinson AI, et al. Humoral immune responses within the human central nervous system following systemic immunization. J Neuroimmunol 1986;11(3):205–14.
10. Aloisi F, Ria F, Columba-Cabezas S, et al. Relative efficiency of microglia, astrocytes, dendritic cells and B cells in naive CD4+ T cell priming and Th1/Th2 cell restimulation. Eur J Immunol 1999; 29(9):2705–14.
11. Aloisi F, Ria F, Penna G, et al. Microglia are more efficient than astrocytes in antigen processing and in Th1 but not Th2 cell activation. J Immunol 1998;160(10):4671–80.
12. Brannan CA, Roberts MR. Resident microglia from adult mice are refractory to nitric oxide-inducing stimuli due to impaired NOS2 gene expression. Glia 2004;48(2):120–31.

13. Hickey WF, Kimura H. Graft-vs-host disease elicits expression of class I and class II histocompatibility antigens and the presence of scattered T lymphocytes in rat central nervous system. Proc Natl Acad Sci U S A 1987;84(7):2082–6.

14. Krakowski M, Owens T. Naive T lymphocytes traffic to inflamed central nervous system, but require antigen recognition for activation. Eur J Immunol 2000;60:5731–9.

15. Hickey WF, Hsu BL, Kimura H. T-lymphocyte entry into the central nervous system. J Neurosci Res 1991;28(2):254–60.

16. Hickey WF. Basic principles of immunological surveillance of the normal central nervous system. Glia 2001;36(2):118–24.

17. Sampson J, Archer GE, Ashley DM, et al. Subcutaneous vaccination with irradiated, cytokine-producing tumor cells stimulates CD8+ cell-mediated immunity against tumors located in the "immunologically privileged" central nervous system. Proc Natl Acad Sci U S A 1996;93(19):10399–404.

18. Gordon LB, Nolan SC, Cserr HF, et al. Growth of P511 mastocytoma cells in BALB/c mouse brain elicits CTL response without tumor elimination: a new tumor model for regional central nervous system immunity. J Immunol 1997;159(5):2399–408.

19. Badie B, Schartner JM, Paul J, et al. Dexamethasone-induced abolition of the inflammatory response in an experimental glioma model: a flow cytometry study. J Neurosurg 2000;93(4):634–9.

20. Sawamura Y, Hosokawa M, Kuppner MC, et al. Antitumor activity and surface phenotypes of human glioma-infiltrating lymphocytes after in vitro expansion in the presence of interleukin 2. Cancer Res 1989;49(7):1843–9.

21. Das S, Raizer JJ, Muro K. Immunotherapeutic treatment strategies for primary brain tumors. Curr Treat Options Oncol 2008;9(1):32–40.

22. Parney I, Hao C, Petruk K. Glioma immunology and immunotherapy. Neurosurgery 2000;46(4):778–91.

23. Facoetti A, Nano R, Zelini P, et al. Human leukocyte antigen and antigen processing machinery component defects in astrocytic tumors. Clin Cancer Res 2005;11(23):8304–11.

24. Parney IF, Waldron JS, Parsa AT. Flow cytometry and in vitro analysis of human glioma-associated macrophages. Laboratory investigation. J Neurosurg 2009;110(3):572–82.

25. Flugel A, Labeur MS, Grasbon-Frodi EM, et al. Microglia only weakly present glioma antigen to cytotoxic T cells. Int J Dev Neurosci 1999;17(5–6):547–56.

26. Schartner JM, Hagar AR, Van Handel M, et al. Impaired capacity for upregulation of MHC class II in tumor-associated microglia. Glia 2005;51(4):279–85.

27. Kostianovsky AM, Maier LM, Anderson RC, et al. Astrocytic regulation of human monocytic/microglial activation. J Immunol 2008;181(8):5425–32.

28. Roszman TL, Brooks WH. Neural modulation of immune function. J Neuroimmunol 1985;10(1):59–69.

29. Roszman TL, Brooks WH, Steele C, et al. Pokeweed mitogen-induced immunoglobulin secretion by peripheral blood lymphocytes from patients with primary intracranial tumors. Characterization of T helper and B cell function. J Immunol 1985;134(3):1545–50.

30. Elliott LH, Brooks WH, Roszman TL. Cytokinetic basis for the impaired activation of lymphocytes from patients with primary intracranial tumors. J Immunol 1984;132(3):1208–15.

31. Brooks WH, Markesbery WR, Gupta GD, et al. Relationship of lymphocyte invasion and survival of brain tumor patients. Ann Neurol 1978;4(3):219–24.

32. Palma L, Di Lorenzo N, Guidetti B. Lymphocytic infiltrates in primary glioblastomas and recidivous gliomas. Incidence, fate, and relevance to prognosis in 228 operated cases. J Neurosurg 1978;49(6):854–61.

33. Dunn GP, Dunn IF, Curry WT. Focus on TILs: prognostic significance of tumor infiltrating lymphocytes in human glioma. Cancer Immun 2007;7:12.

34. Safdari H, Hochberg FH, Richardson EP Jr. Prognostic value of round cell (lymphocyte) infiltration in malignant gliomas. Surg Neurol 1985;23(3):221–6.

35. Hussain SF, Heimberger AB. Immunotherapy for human glioma: innovative approaches and recent results. Expert Rev Anticancer Ther 2005;5(5):777–90.

36. Gerosa MA, Olivi A, Rosenblum ML, et al. Impaired immunocompetence in patients with malignant gliomas: the possible role of Tg-lymphocyte subpopulations. Neurosurgery 1982;10(5):571–3.

37. El Andaloussi A, Lesniak MS. An increase in CD4+CD25+FOXP3+ regulatory T cells in tumor-infiltrating lymphocytes of human glioblastoma multiforme. Neuro Oncol 2006;8(3):234–43.

38. Fecci PE, Mitchell DA, Whitesides JF, et al. Increased regulatory T-cell fraction amidst a diminished CD4 compartment explains cellular immune defects in patients with malignant glioma. Cancer Res 2006;66(6):3294–302.

39. Thornton AM, Shevach EM. CD4+CD25+ immunoregulatory T cells suppress polyclonal T cell activation in vitro by inhibiting interleukin 2 production. J Exp Med 1998;188(2):287–96.

40. Camara NO, Sebille F, Lechler RI. Human CD4+CD25+ regulatory cells have marked and sustained effects on CD8+ T cell activation. Eur J Immunol 2003;33(12):3473–83.

41. Piccirillo CA, Shevach EM. Cutting edge: control of CD8+ T cell activation by CD4+CD25+ immuno-regulatory cells. J Immunol 2001;167(3):1137–40.

42. Dieckmann D, Bruett CH, Ploettner H, et al. Human CD4(+)CD25(+) regulatory, contact-dependent T cells induce interleukin 10-producing, contact-independent type 1-like regulatory T cells [corrected]. J Exp Med 2002;196(2):247–53.

43. Liu VC, Wong LY, Jang T, et al. Tumor evasion of the immune system by converting CD4+CD25- T cells into CD4+CD25+ T regulatory cells: role of tumor-derived TGF-beta. J Immunol 2007;178(5):2883–92.

44. Zheng Y, Manzotti CN, Liu M, et al. CD86 and CD80 differentially modulate the suppressive function of human regulatory T cells. J Immunol 2004;172(5): 2778–84.

45. Fecci PE, Sweeney AE, Grossi PM, et al. Systemic anti-CD25 monoclonal antibody administration safely enhances immunity in murine glioma without eliminating regulatory T cells. Clin Cancer Res 2006;12(14 Pt 1):4294–305.

46. El Andaloussi A, Han Y, Lesniak MS. Prolongation of survival following depletion of CD4+CD25+ regulatory T cells in mice with experimental brain tumors. J Neurosurg 2006;105(3):430–7.

47. Nitta T, Hishii M, Sato K, et al. Selective expression of interleukin-10 gene within glioblastoma multi-forme. Brain Res 1994;649(1-2):122–8.

48. Fontana A, Kristensen F, Dubs R, et al. Production of prostaglandin E and an interleukin-1 like factor by cultured astrocytes and C6 glioma cells. J Immunol 1982;129(6):2413–9.

49. Sawamura Y, Diserens AC, de Tribolet N. In vitro prostaglandin E2 production by glioblastoma cells and its effect on interleukin-2 activation of oncolytic lymphocytes. J Neurooncol 1990;9(2):125–30.

50. Couldwell WT, Yong VW, Dore-Duffy P, et al. Production of soluble autocrine inhibitory factors by human glioma cell lines. J Neurol Sci 1992; 110(1–2):178–85.

51. Dix A, Brooks WH, Roszman TL, et al. Immune defects observed in patients with primary malignant brain tumors. J Neuroimmunol 1999; 100(1–2):216–32.

52. Bodmer S, Strommer K, Frei K, et al. Immunosuppression and transforming growth factor-beta in glioblastoma. Preferential production of transforming growth factor-beta 2. J Immunol 1989;143(10): 3222–9.

53. Fontana A, Hengartner H, de Tribolet N, et al. Glioblastoma cells release interleukin 1 and factors inhibiting interleukin 2-mediated effects. J Immunol 1984;132(4):1837–44.

54. Fontana A, Frei K, Bodmer S, et al. Transforming growth factor-beta inhibits the generation of cytotoxic T cells in virus-infected mice. J Immunol 1989;143(10):3230–4.

55. Suzumura A, Sawada M, Yamamoto H, et al. Transforming growth factor-beta suppresses activation and proliferation of microglia in vitro. J Immunol 1993;151(4):2150–8.

56. Liau L, Fakhrai H, Black K. Prolonged survival of rats with intracranial C6 gliomas by treatment with TGF-beta antisense gene. Neurol Res 1998;20(8):742–7.

57. Fakhrai H, Dorigo O, Shawler DL, et al. Eradication of established intracranial rat gliomas by transforming growth factor beta antisense gene therapy. Proc Natl Acad Sci U S A 1996;93(7):2909–14.

58. Yang BC, Lin HK, Hor WS, et al. Mediation of enhanced transcription of the IL-10 gene in T cells, upon contact with human glioma cells, by Fas signaling through a protein kinase A-independent pathway. J Immunol 2003;171(8):3947–54.

59. Parsa AT, Waldron JS, Panner A, et al. Loss of tumor suppressor PTEN function increases B7-H1 expression and immunoresistance in glioma. Nat Med 2007;13(1):84–8.

60. Ichinose M, Masuoka J, Shiraishi T, et al. Fas ligand expression and depletion of T-cell infiltration in astrocytic tumors. Brain Tumor Pathol 2001;18(1): 37–42.

61. Hahn HP, Pang M, He J, et al. Galectin-1 induces nuclear translocation of endonuclease G in caspase- and cytochrome c-independent T cell death. Cell Death Differ 2004;11(12):1277–86.

62. Rorive S, Belot N, Decaestecker C, et al. Galectin-1 is highly expressed in human gliomas with relevance for modulation of invasion of tumor astrocytes into the brain parenchyma. Glia 2001;33(3): 241–55.

63. Badie B, Schartner J, Prabakaran S, et al. Expression of Fas ligand by microglia: possible role in glioma immune evasion. J Neuroimmunol 2001; 120(1-2):19–24.

64. Dong H, Strome SE, Salomao DR, et al. Tumor-associated B7-H1 promotes T-cell apoptosis: a potential mechanism of immune evasion. Nat Med 2002;8(8):793–800.

65. Magnus T, Schreiner B, Korn T, et al. Microglial expression of the B7 family member B7 homolog 1 confers strong immune inhibition: implications for immune responses and autoimmunity in the CNS. J Neurosci 2005;25(10):2537–46.

66. Barshes NR, Goodpastor SE, Goss JA. Pharmacologic immunosuppression. Front Biosci 2004;9: 411–20.

67. Lesniak MS, Gabikian P, Tyler BM, et al. Dexamethasone mediated inhibition of local IL-2 immunotherapy is dose dependent in experimental brain tumors. J Neurooncol 2004;70(1):23–8.

68. Su YB, Sohn S, Krown SE, et al. Selective CD4+ lymphopenia in melanoma patients treated with temozolomide: a toxicity with therapeutic implications. J Clin Oncol 2004;22(4):610–6.

69. Kikuchi T, Joki T, Abe T, et al. Antitumor activity of killer cells stimulated with both interleukin-2 and interleukin-12 on mouse glioma cells. J Immunother 1999;22(3):245–50.

70. Jereb B, Petric J, Lamovec J, et al. Intratumor application of human leukocyte interferon-alpha in patients with malignant brain tumors. Am J Clin Oncol 1989;12(1):1–7.

71. Farkkila M, Jaaskelainen J, Kallio M, et al. Randomised, controlled study of intratumoral recombinant gamma-interferon treatment in newly diagnosed glioblastoma. Br J Cancer 1994;70(1):138–41.

72. Merchant RE, McVicar DW, Merchant LH, et al. Treatment of recurrent malignant glioma by repeated intracerebral injections of human recombinant interleukin-2 alone or in combination with systemic interferon-alpha. Results of a phase I clinical trial. J Neurooncol 1992;12(1):75–83.

73. Buckner JC, Schomberg PJ, McGinnis WL, et al. A phase III study of radiation therapy plus carmustine with or without recombinant interferon-alpha in the treatment of patients with newly diagnosed high-grade glioma. Cancer 2001;92(2):420–33.

74. Chamberlain MC. A phase II trial of intra-cerebrospinal fluid alpha interferon in the treatment of neoplastic meningitis. Cancer 2002;94(10):2675–80.

75. Liu Y, Ehtesham M, Samoto K, et al. In situ adenoviral interleukin 12 gene transfer confers potent and long-lasting cytotoxic immunity in glioma. Cancer Gene Ther 2002;9(1):9–15.

76. Ren H, Boulikas T, Lundstrom K, et al. Immunogene therapy of recurrent glioblastoma multiforme with a liposomally encapsulated replication-incompetent Semliki forest virus vector carrying the human interleukin-12 gene—a phase I/II clinical protocol. J Neurooncol 2003;64(1-2):147–54.

77. Ehtesham M, Samoto K, Kabos P, et al. Treatment of intracranial glioma with in situ interferon-gamma and tumor necrosis factor-alpha gene transfer. Cancer Gene Ther 2002;9(11):925–34.

78. Lichtor T, Glick RP, Kim TS, et al. Prolonged survival of mice with glioma injected intracerebrally with double cytokine-secreting cells. J Neurosurg 1995;83:1038–44.

79. Lichtor T, Glick RP, Tarlock K, et al. Application of interleukin-2-secreting syngeneic/allogeneic fibroblasts in the treatment of primary and metastatic brain tumors. Cancer Gene Ther 2002;9(5):464–9.

80. Glick RP, Lichtor T, Panchal R, et al. Treatment with allogeneic interleukin-2 secreting fibroblasts protects against the development of malignant brain tumors. J Neurooncol 2003;64(1-2):139–46.

81. Kikuchi T, Joki T, Saitoh S, et al. Anti-tumor activity of interleukin-2-producing tumor cells and recombinant interleukin 12 against mouse glioma cells located in the central nervous system. Int J Cancer 1999;80(3):425–30.

82. Benedetti S, Pirola B, Pollo B, et al. Gene therapy of experimental brain tumors using neural progenitor cells. Nat Med 2000;6(4):447–50.

83. Ehtesham M, Kabos P, Kabosova A, et al. The use of interleukin 12-secreting neural stem cells for the treatment of intracranial glioma. Cancer Res 2002;62(20):5657–63.

84. Yuan X, Hu J, Belladonna ML, et al. Interleukin-23-expressing bone marrow-derived neural stem-like cells exhibit antitumor activity against intracranial glioma. Cancer Res 2006;66(5):2630–8.

85. Mizuno M, Yoshida J. Effect of human interferon beta gene transfer upon human glioma, transplanted into nude mouse brain, involves induced natural killer cells. Cancer Immunol Immunother 1998;47(4):227–32.

86. Natsume A, Mizuno M, Ryuke Y, et al. Antitumor effect and cellular immunity activation by murine interferon-beta gene transfer against intracerebral glioma in mouse. Gene Ther 1999;6(9):1626–33.

87. Natsume A, Tsujimura K, Mizuno M, et al. IFN-beta gene therapy induces systemic antitumor immunity against malignant glioma. J Neurooncol 2000;47(2):117–24.

88. Rhines LD, Sampath P, DiMeco F, et al. Local immunotherapy with interleukin-2 delivered from biodegradable polymer microspheres combined with interstitial chemotherapy: a novel treatment for experimental malignant glioma. Neurosurgery 2003;52(4):872–9 [discussion: 879–80].

89. Hanes J, Sills A, Zhao Z, et al. Controlled local delivery of interleukin-2 by biodegradable polymers protects animals from experimental brain tumors and liver tumors. Pharm Res 2001;18(7):899–906.

90. Hsu W, Lesniak MS, Tyler B, et al. Local delivery of interleukin-2 and adriamycin is synergistic in the treatment of experimental malignant glioma. J Neurooncol 2005;74(2):135–40.

91. Puri RK, Leland P, Kreitman RJ, et al. Human neurological cancer cells express interleukin-4 (IL-4) receptors which are targets for the toxic effects of IL4-Pseudomonas exotoxin chimeric protein. Int J Cancer 1994;58(4):574–81.

92. Joshi BH, Leland P, Asher A, et al. In situ expression of interleukin-4 (IL-4) receptors in human brain tumors and cytotoxicity of a recombinant IL-4 cytotoxin in primary glioblastoma cell cultures. Cancer Res 2001;61(22):8058–61.

93. Joshi BH, Leland P, Silber J, et al. IL-4 receptors on human medulloblastoma tumours serve as a sensitive target for a circular permuted IL-4-Pseudomonas exotoxin fusion protein. Br J Cancer 2002;86(2):285–91.

94. Rand RW, Kreitman RJ, Patronas N, et al. Intratumoral administration of recombinant circularly permuted interleukin-4-Pseudomonas exotoxin in

patients with high-grade glioma. Clin Cancer Res 2000;6(6):2157–65.

95. Weber FW, Floeth F, Asher A, et al. Local convection enhanced delivery of IL4-*Pseudomonas* exotoxin (NBI-3001) for treatment of patients with recurrent malignant glioma. Acta Neurochir Suppl 2003;88:93–103.

96. Weber F, Asher A, Bucholz R, et al. Safety, tolerability, and tumor response of IL4-*Pseudomonas* exotoxin (NBI-3001) in patients with recurrent malignant glioma. J Neurooncol 2003;64(1–2): 125–37.

97. Kioi M, Kawakami K, Puri RK. Analysis of antitumor activity of an interleukin-13 (IL-13) receptor-targeted cytotoxin composed of IL-13 antagonist and *Pseudomonas* exotoxin. Clin Cancer Res 2004;10(18 Pt 1):6231–8.

98. Joshi BH, Leland P, Puri RK. Identification and characterization of interleukin-13 receptor in human medulloblastoma and targeting these receptors with interleukin-13-pseudomonas exotoxin fusion protein. Croat Med J 2003;44(4): 455–62.

99. Husain SR, Joshi BH, Puri RK. Interleukin-13 receptor as a unique target for anti-glioblastoma therapy. Int J Cancer 2001;92(2):168–75.

100. Kunwar S. Convection enhanced delivery of IL13-PE38QQR for treatment of recurrent malignant glioma: presentation of interim findings from ongoing phase 1 studies. Acta Neurochir Suppl 2003;88:105–11.

101. Kunwar S, Prados MD, Chang SM, et al. Direct intracerebral delivery of cintredekin besudotox (IL13-PE38QQR) in recurrent malignant glioma: a report by the Cintredekin Besudotox Intraparenchymal Study Group. J Clin Oncol 2007;25(7): 837–44.

102. Parney IF, Kunwar S, McDermott M, et al. Neuroradiographic changes following convection-enhanced delivery of the recombinant cytotoxin interleukin 13-PE38QQR for recurrent malignant glioma. J Neurosurg 2005;102(2):267–75.

103. Kioi M, Seetharam S, Puri RK. Targeting IL-13Ralpha2-positive cancer with a novel recombinant immunotoxin composed of a single-chain antibody and mutated *Pseudomonas* exotoxin. Mol Cancer Ther 2008;7(6):1579–87.

104. Vogelbaum MA, Sampson JH, Kunwar S, et al. Convection-enhanced delivery of cintredekin besudotox (interleukin-13-PE38QQR) followed by radiation therapy with and without temozolomide in newly diagnosed malignant gliomas: phase 1 study of final safety results. Neurosurgery 2007;61(5): 1031–7 [discussion: 1037–8].

105. Heimbrook DC, Stirdivant SM, Ahern JD, et al. Transforming growth factor alpha-*Pseudomonas* exotoxin fusion protein prolongs survival of nude mice bearing tumor xenografts. Proc Natl Acad Sci U S A 1990;87(12):4697–701.

106. Phillips PC, Levow C, Catterall M, et al. Transforming growth factor-alpha-*Pseudomonas* exotoxin fusion protein (TGF-alpha-PE38) treatment of subcutaneous and intracranial human glioma and medulloblastoma xenografts in athymic mice. Cancer Res 1994;54(4):1008–15.

107. Sampson JH, Akabani G, Archer GE, et al. Progress report of a phase I study of the intracerebral microinfusion of a recombinant chimeric protein composed of transforming growth factor (TGF)-alpha and a mutated form of the *Pseudomonas* exotoxin termed PE-38 (TP-38) for the treatment of malignant brain tumors. J Neurooncol 2003; 65(1):27–35.

108. Sampath P, Hanes J, DiMeco F, et al. Paracrine immunotherapy with interleukin-2 and local chemotherapy is synergistic in the treatment of experimental brain tumors. Cancer Res 1999;59(9): 2107–14.

109. Hopkins K, Papanastassiou V, Kemshead JT. The treatment of patients with recurrent malignant gliomas with intratumoral radioimmunoconjugates. Recent Results Cancer Res 1996;141: 159–75.

110. Prasad G, Wang H, Hill DL, et al. Recent advances in experimental molecular therapeutics for malignant gliomas. Curr Med Chem Anticancer Agents 2004;4(4):347–61.

111. Bourdon MA, Wikstrand CJ, Furthmayr H, et al. Human glioma-mesenchymal extracellular matrix antigen defined by monoclonal antibody. Cancer Res 1983;43(6):2796–805.

112. Lee Y, Bullard DE, Humphrey PA, et al. Treatment of intracranial human glioma xenografts with [131]I-labeled antitenascin monoclonal antibody 81C6. Cancer Res 1988;48(10):2904–10.

113. Lee YS, Bullard DE, Zalutsky MR, et al. Therapeutic efficacy of antiglioma mesenchymal extracellular matrix [131]I-radiolabeled murine monoclonal antibody in a human glioma xenograft model. Cancer Res 1988;48(3):559–66.

114. Zalutsky MR, Moseley RP, Coakham HB, et al. Pharmacokinetics and tumor localization of [131]I-labeled anti-tenascin monoclonal antibody 81C6 in patients with gliomas and other intracranial malignancies. Cancer Res 1989;49(10):2807–13.

115. Bigner DD, Brown MT, Friedman AH, et al. Iodine-131-labeled antitenascin monoclonal antibody 81C6 treatment of patients with recurrent malignant gliomas: phase I trial results. J Clin Oncol 1998; 16(6):2202–12.

116. Brown M, Coleman RE, Friedman AH, et al. Intrathecal [131]I-labeled antitenascin monoclonal antibody 81C6 treatment of patients with leptomeningeal neoplasms or primary brain tumor

resection cavities with subarachnoid communication: phase I trial results. Clin Cancer Res 1996; 2(6):963–72.

117. Riva P, Fraceschi G, Arista A, et al. Local application of radiolabeled monoclonal antibodies in the treatment of high grade malignant gliomas: a six-year clinical experience. Cancer 1997;80(Suppl 12):2733–42.

118. Akabani G, Cokgor I, Coleman RE, et al. Dosimetry and dose-response relationships in newly diagnosed patients with malignant gliomas treated with iodine-131-labeled anti-tenascin monoclonal antibody 81C6 therapy. Int J Radiat Oncol Biol Phys 2000;46(4):947–58.

119. Reardon DA, Akabani G, Coleman RE, et al. Salvage radioimmunotherapy with murine iodine-131-labeled antitenascin monoclonal antibody 81C6 for patients with recurrent primary and metastatic malignant brain tumors: phase II study results. J Clin Oncol 2006;24(1):115–22.

120. Akabani G, Reardon DA, Coleman RE, et al. Dosimetry and radiographic analysis of $^{131}$I-labeled anti-tenascin 81C6 murine monoclonal antibody in newly diagnosed patients with malignant gliomas: a phase II study. J Nucl Med 2005; 46(6):1042–51.

121. Reardon DA, Akabani G, Coleman RE, et al. Phase II trial of murine (131)I-labeled antitenascin monoclonal antibody 81C6 administered into surgically created resection cavities of patients with newly diagnosed malignant gliomas. J Clin Oncol 2002; 20(5):1389–97.

122. Cokgor I, Akabani G, Kuan CT, et al. Phase I trial results of iodine-131-labeled antitenascin monoclonal antibody 81C6 treatment of patients with newly diagnosed malignant gliomas. J Clin Oncol 2000;18(22):3862–72.

123. Reardon DA, Quinn JA, Akabani G, et al. Novel human IgG2b/murine chimeric antitenascin monoclonal antibody construct radiolabeled with $^{131}$I and administered into the surgically created resection cavity of patients with malignant glioma: phase I trial results. J Nucl Med 2006;47(6):912–8.

124. Kalofonos HP, Pawikowska TR, Hemingway A, et al. Antibody guided diagnosis and therapy of brain gliomas using radiolabeled monoclonal antibodies against epidermal growth factor receptor and placental alkaline phosphatase. J Nucl Med 1989; 30(10):1636–45.

125. Dadparvar S, Krishna L, Miyamoto C, et al. Indium-111-labeled anti-EGFr-425 scintigraphy in the detection of malignant gliomas. Cancer 1994; 73(Suppl 3):884–9.

126. Faillot T, Magdelenat H, Mady E, et al. A phase I study of an anti-epidermal growth factor receptor monoclonal antibody for the treatment of malignant gliomas. Neurosurgery 1996;39(3):478–83.

127. Crombet T, Torres O, Neninger E, et al. Phase I clinical evaluation of a neutralizing monoclonal antibody against epidermal growth factor receptor. Cancer Biother Radiopharm 2001;16(1): 93–102.

128. Stragliotto G, Vega F, Stasiecki P, et al. Multiple infusions of anti-epidermal growth factor receptor (EGFR) monoclonal antibody (EMD 55,900) in patients with recurrent malignant gliomas. Eur J Cancer 1996;32(4):636–40.

129. Wersall P, Ohlsson I, Biberfeld P, et al. Intratumoral infusion of the monoclonal antibody, mAb 425, against the epidermal-growth-factor receptor in patients with advanced malignant glioma. Cancer Immunol Immunother 1997;44(3):157–64.

130. Ramos TC, Figueredo J, Catala M, et al. Treatment of high-grade glioma patients with the humanized anti-epidermal growth factor receptor (EGFR) antibody h-R3: report from a phase I/II trial. Cancer Biol Ther 2006;5(4):375–9.

131. Brady LW. A new treatment for high grade gliomas of the brain. Bull Mem Acad R Med Belg 1998; 153(5–6):255–61 [discussion: 261–2].

132. Brady LW, Markoe AM, Woo DV, et al. Iodine-125-labeled anti-epidermal growth factor receptor-425 in the treatment of glioblastoma multiforme. A pilot study. Front Radiat Ther Oncol 1990;24:151–60 [discussion: 161–5].

133. Brady LW, Miyamoto C, Woo DV, et al. Malignant astrocytomas treated with iodine-125 labeled monoclonal antibody 425 against epidermal growth factor receptor: a phase II trial. Int J Radiat Oncol Biol Phys 1992;22(1):225–30.

134. Snelling L, Miyamoto CT, Bender H, et al. Epidermal growth factor receptor 425 monoclonal antibodies radiolabeled with iodine-125 in the adjuvant treatment of high-grade astrocytomas. Hybridoma 1995;14(2):111–4.

135. Jungbluth AA, Stockert E, Huang JH, et al. A monoclonal antibody recognizing human cancers with amplification/overexpression of the human epidermal growth factor receptor. Proc Natl Acad Sci U S A 2003;100(2):639–44.

136. Sampson JH, Crotty LE, Lee S, et al. Unarmed, tumor-specific monoclonal antibody effectively treats brain tumors. Proc Natl Acad Sci U S A 2000;97(13):7503–8.

137. Mishima K, Johns TG, Luwor RB, et al. Growth suppression of intracranial xenografted glioblastomas overexpressing mutant epidermal growth factor receptors by systemic administration of monoclonal antibody (mAb) 806, a novel monoclonal antibody directed to the receptor. Cancer Res 2001;61(14):5349–54.

138. Mamot C, Drummond DC, Greiser U, et al. Epidermal growth factor receptor (EGFR)-targeted immunoliposomes mediate specific and efficient

drug delivery to EGFR- and EGFRvIII-overexpressing tumor cells. Cancer Res 2003;63(12):3154–61.

139. Mamot C, Drummond DC, Noble CO, et al. Epidermal growth factor receptor-targeted immunoliposomes significantly enhance the efficacy of multiple anticancer drugs in vivo. Cancer Res 2005;65(24):11631–8.

140. Hall WA. Targeted toxin therapy for malignant astrocytoma. Neurosurgery 2000;46(3):544–51 [discussion: 552].

141. Jacobs SK, Wilson SK, Kronblith PL, et al. Interleukin-2 and autologous lymphokine-activated killer cells in the treatment of malignant glioma. Preliminary report. J Neurosurg 1986;64(5):743–9.

142. Merchant RE, Grant AJ, Merchant LH, et al. Adoptive immunotherapy for recurrent glioblastoma multiforme using lymphokine activated killer cells and recombinant interleukin-2. Cancer 1988;62(4):665–71.

143. Merchant RE, Merchant LH, Cook SH, et al. Intralesional infusion of lymphokine-activated killer (LAK) cells and recombinant interleukin-2 (rIL-2) for the treatment of patients with malignant brain tumor. Neurosurgery 1988;23(6):725–32.

144. Barba D, Saris SC, Holder C, et al. Intratumoral LAK cell and interleukin-2 therapy of human gliomas. J Neurosurg 1989;70(2):175–82.

145. Lillehei KO, Mitchell DH, Johnson SD, et al. Long-term follow-up of patients with recurrent malignant gliomas treated with adjuvant adoptive immunotherapy. Neurosurgery 1991;28(1):16–23.

146. Hayes RL, Koslow M, Hiesiger EM, et al. Improved long term survival after intracavitary interleukin-2 and lymphokine-activated killer cells for adults with recurrent malignant glioma. Cancer 1995;76(5):840–52.

147. Dillman RO, Duman CM, Schiltz PM, et al. Intracavitary placement of autologous lymphokine-activated killer (LAK) cells after resection of recurrent glioblastoma. J Immunother 2004;27(5):398–404.

148. Nitta T, Sato K, Okumura K, et al. Induction of cytotoxicity in human T cells coated with anti-glioma x anti-CD3 bispecific antibody against human glioma cells. J Neurosurg 1990;72(3):476–81.

149. Nitta T, Sato K, Yagita H, et al. Preliminary trial of specific targeting therapy against malignant glioma. Lancet 1990;335(8686):368–71.

150. Tsurushima H, Lui SQ, Tsuboi K, et al. Induction of human autologous cytotoxic T lymphocytes against minced tissues of glioblastoma multiforme. J Neurosurg 1996;84(2):258–63.

151. Saris SC, Spiess P, Lieberman DM, et al. Treatment of murine primary brain tumors with systemic interleukin-2 and tumor-infiltrating lymphocytes. J Neurosurg 1992;76(3):513–9.

152. Holladay FP, Heitz T, Wood GW. Antitumor activity against established intracerebral gliomas exhibited by cytotoxic T lymphocytes, but not by lymphokine-activated killer cells. J Neurosurg 1992;77(5):757–62.

153. Holladay FP, Hetiz T, Chen YL, et al. Successful treatment of a malignant rat glioma with cytotoxic T lymphocytes. Neurosurgery 1992;31(3):528–33.

154. Holladay F, Heitz T, Wood GW, et al. Autologous tumor cell vaccination combined with adoptive cellular immunotherapy in patients with grade III/IV astrocytoma. J Neuro oncol 1996;27(2):179–89.

155. Quattrocchi KB, Miller CH, Cush S, et al. Pilot study of local autologous tumor infiltrating lymphocytes for the treatment of recurrent malignant gliomas. J Neurooncol 1999;45(2):141–57.

156. Miescher S, Stoeck M, Whiteside TL, et al. Altered activation pathways in T lymphocytes infiltrating human solid tumors. Transplant Proc 1988;20(2):344–6.

157. Miescher S, Whiteside TL, de Tribolet N, et al. In situ characterization, clonogenic potential, and antitumor cytolytic activity of T lymphocytes infiltrating human brain cancers. J Neurosurg 1988;68(3):438–48.

158. Roszman T, Elliott L, Brooks W. Modulation of T-cell function by gliomas. Immunol Today 1991;12(10):370–4.

159. Prins RM, Graf MR, Merchant RE. Cytotoxic T cells infiltrating a glioma express an aberrant phenotype that is associated with decreased function and apoptosis. Cancer Immunol Immunother 2001;50(6):285–92.

160. Plautz G, Barnett GH, Miller DW, et al. Systemic T cell adoptive immunotherapy of malignant gliomas. J Neurosurg 1998;89(1):42–51.

161. Plautz GE, Miller DW, Barnett GH, et al. T cell adoptive immunotherapy of newly diagnosed gliomas. Clin Cancer Res 2000;6(6):2209–18.

162. Cesano A, Visonneau S, Santoli D. Treatment of experimental glioblastoma with a human major histocompatibility complex nonrestricted cytotoxic T cell line. Cancer Res 1995;55(1):96–101.

163. Cesano A, Visonneau S, Santoli D. TALL-104 cell therapy of human solid tumors implanted in immunodeficient (SCID) mice. Anticancer Res 1998;18(4A):2289–95.

164. Cesano A, Visonneau S, Pasquini S, et al. Antitumor efficacy of a human major histocompatibility complex nonrestricted cytotoxic T-cell line (TALL-104) in immunocompetent mice bearing syngeneic leukemia. Cancer Res 1996;56(19):4444–52.

165. Geoerger B, Tang CB, Cesano A, et al. Antitumor activity of a human cytotoxic T-cell line (TALL-104) in brain tumor xenografts. Neuro Oncol 2000;2(2):103–13.

166. Kruse CA, Visonneau S, Kleinschmidt-DeMasters BK, et al. The human leukemic T-cell

line, TALL-104, is cytotoxic to human malignant brain tumors and traffics through brain tissue: implications for local adoptive immunotherapy. Cancer Res 2000;60(20):5731–9.

167. Gomez GG, Read SB, Gerschenson LE, et al. Interactions of the allogeneic effector leukemic T cell line, TALL-104, with human malignant brain tumors. Neuro Oncol 2004;6(2):83–95.

168. Brando C, Mukhopadhyay S, Kovacs E, et al. Receptors and lytic mediators regulating antitumor activity by the leukemic killer T cell line TALL-104. J Leukoc Biol 2005;78(2):359–71.

169. Wikstrand CJ, Bigner DD. Prognostic applications of the epidermal growth factor receptor and its ligand, transforming growth factor-alpha. J Natl Cancer Inst 1998;90(11):799–801.

170. Lozupone F, Rivoltini L, Luciani F, et al. Adoptive transfer of an anti-MART-1(27-35)-specific CD8+ T cell clone leads to immunoselection of human melanoma antigen-loss variants in SCID mice. Eur J Immunol 2003;33(2):556–66.

171. Steiner HH, Bonsanto MM, Beckhove P, et al. Antitumor vaccination of patients with glioblastoma multiforme: a pilot study to assess feasibility, safety, and clinical benefit. J Clin Oncol 2004;22(21): 4272–81.

172. Sloan AE, Dansey R, Zamorano L, et al. Adoptive immunotherapy in patients with recurrent malignant glioma: preliminary results of using autologous whole-tumor vaccine plus granulocyte-macrophage colony-stimulating factor and adoptive transfer of anti-CD3-activated lymphocytes. Neurosurg Focus 2000;9(6):e9.

173. Ishikawa E, Tsuboi K, Yamamoto T, et al. Clinical trial of autologous formalin-fixed tumor vaccine for glioblastoma multiforme patients. Cancer Sci 2007;98(8):1226–33.

174. Okada H, Lieberman FS, Walter KA, et al. Autologous glioma cell vaccine admixed with interleukin-4 gene transfected fibroblasts in the treatment of patients with malignant gliomas. J Transl Med 2007;5:67.

175. Thurner B, Roder C, Dieckmann D, et al. Generation of large numbers of fully mature and stable dendritic cells from leukapheresis products for clinical application. J Immunol Methods 1999;223(1):1–15.

176. Siesjö P, Visse E, Sjögren H. Cure of established, intracerebral rat gliomas induced by therapeutic immunizations with tumor cells and purified APC or adjuvant IFN-gamma treatment. J Immunother Emphasis Tumor Immunol 1996;19(5):334–45.

177. Liau L, Black KL, Prins RM, et al. Treatment of intracranial gliomas with bone marrow-derived dendritic cells pulsed with tumor antigens. J Neurosurg 1999;90(6):1115–24.

178. Yu JS, Wheeler CJ, Zeltzer PM, et al. Vaccination of malignant glioma patients with peptide-pulsed dendritic cells elicits systemic cytotoxicity and intracranial T-cell infiltration. Cancer Res 2001; 61(3):842–7.

179. Kikuchi T, Akasaki Y, Irie M, et al. Results of a phase I clinical trial of vaccination of glioma patients with fusions of dendritic and glioma cells. Cancer Immunol Immunother 2001;50(7):337–44.

180. Kikuchi T, Akasaki Y, Abe T, et al. Vaccination of glioma patients with fusions of dendritic and glioma cells and recombinant human interleukin 12. J Immunother 2004;27(6):452–9.

181. Kjaergaard J, Wang LX, Kuriyama H, et al. Active immunotherapy for advanced intracranial murine tumors by using dendritic cell-tumor cell fusion vaccines. J Neurosurg 2005;103(1):156–64.

182. Yu JS, Lui G, Ying H, et al. Vaccination with tumor lysate-pulsed dendritic cells elicits antigen-specific, cytotoxic T-cells in patients with malignant glioma. Cancer Res 2004;64(14):4973–9.

183. Yamanaka R, Abe T, Yajima N, et al. Vaccination of recurrent glioma patients with tumour lysate-pulsed dendritic cells elicits immune responses: results of a clinical phase I/II trial. Br J Cancer 2003;89(7):1172–9.

184. Rutkowski S, De Vleeschouwer S, Kaempgen E, et al. Surgery and adjuvant dendritic cell-based tumour vaccination for patients with relapsed malignant glioma, a feasibility study. Br J Cancer 2004;91(9):1656–62.

185. Liau LM, Prins RM, Kierscher SM, et al. Dendritic cell vaccination in glioblastoma patients induces systemic and intracranial T-cell responses modulated by the local central nervous system tumor microenvironment. Clin Cancer Res 2005;11(15): 5515–25.

186. Ludewig B, Oschesenbein AF, Odermatt B, et al. Immunotherapy with dendritic cells directed against tumor antigens shared with normal host cells results in severe autoimmune disease. J Exp Med 2000;191(5):795–804.

187. Wu AH, Xiao J, Anker L, et al. Identification of EGFRvIII-derived CTL epitopes restricted by HLA A0201 for dendritic cell based immunotherapy of gliomas. J Neurooncol 2006;76(1):23–30.

188. Heimberger AB, Archer GE, Crotty LE, et al. Dendritic cells pulsed with a tumor-specific peptide induce long-lasting immunity and are effective against murine intracerebral melanoma. Neurosurgery 2002;50(1):158–64 [discussion 164–6].

189. Heimberger AB, Crotty LE, Archer GE, et al. Epidermal growth factor receptor VIII peptide vaccination is efficacious against established intracerebral tumors. Clin Cancer Res 2003;9(11): 4247–54.

190. Wood GW, Holladay FP, Turner T, et al. A pilot study of autologous cancer cell vaccination and cellular immunotherapy using anti-CD3 stimulated

lymphocytes in patients with recurrent grade III/IV astrocytoma. J Neurooncol 2000;48(2):113–20.

191. Liau LM, Jensen ER, Kremen TJ, et al. Tumor immunity within the central nervous system stimulated by recombinant *Listeria monocytogenes* vaccination. Cancer Res 2002;62(8):2287–93.

192. Brockstedt DG, Giedlin MA, Leong ML, et al. Listeria-based cancer vaccines that segregate immunogenicity from toxicity. Proc Natl Acad Sci U S A 2004;101(38):13832–7.

193. Meyer RG, Britten CM, Siepmann U, et al. A phase I vaccination study with tyrosinase in patients with stage II melanoma using recombinant modified vaccinia virus Ankara (MVA-hTyr). Cancer Immunol Immunother 2005;54(5):453–67.

194. Yang L, Ng KY, Lillehei KO. Cell-mediated immunotherapy: a new approach to the treatment of malignant glioma. Cancer Control 2003;10(2):138–47.

195. Kuwashima N, Nishimura F, Eguchi J, et al. Delivery of dendritic cells engineered to secrete IFN-alpha into central nervous system tumors enhances the efficacy of peripheral tumor cell vaccines: dependence on apoptotic pathways. J Immunol 2005; 175(4):2730–40.

196. Okada H, Pollack IF, Lieberman F, et al. Gene therapy of malignant gliomas: a pilot study of vaccination with irradiated autologous glioma and dendritic cells admixed with IL-4 transduced fibroblasts to elicit an immune response. Hum Gene Ther 2001;12(5):575–95.

197. Yamanaka R, Honma J, Tsuchiya N, et al. Tumor lysate and IL-18 loaded dendritic cells elicits Th1 response, tumor-specific CD8+ cytotoxic T cells in patients with malignant glioma. J Neurooncol 2005;72(2):107–13.

198. Kikuchi T, et al. Antitumor activity of interleukin 12 against interleukin 2-transduced mouse glioma cells. Cancer Lett 1999;135(1):47–51.

199. Parney IF, Petruk KC, Zhang C, et al. Granulocyte-macrophage colony-stimulating factor and B7-2 combination immunogene therapy in an allogeneic Hu-PBL-SCID/beige mouse-human glioblastoma multiforme model. Hum Gene Ther 1997;8(9): 1073–85.

200. Saleh M, Jonas NK, Wiegmans A, et al. The treatment of established intracranial tumors by in situ retroviral IFN-gamma transfer. Gene Ther 2000; 7(20):1715–24.

201. Benedetti S, Bruzzone MG, Pollo B, et al. Eradication of rat malignant gliomas by retroviral-mediated, in vivo delivery of the interleukin 4 gene. Cancer Res 1999;59(3):645–52.

# Mechanisms of Local Immunoresistance in Glioma

Emilia Albesiano, PhD[a], James E. Han, BA[b], Michael Lim, MD[b],*

**KEYWORDS**

- Glioblastoma multiforme • Immunotherapy
- Oncogenic signaling pathway • Immunoresistance

Glioblastoma multiforme (GBM) is a malignant tumor of the central nervous system (CNS) comprising 40% of all primary brain tumors. Of the astrocytomas, GBM is the most malignant, high-grade type of glioma that kills 13,000 Americans every year. Without treatments, most patients face a severe prognosis, surviving fewer than 6 months. The mean duration of survival is only 14 months even after intensive therapy, combining gross total resection, radiation, and chemotherapy.[1,2] Several obstacles prevent standard therapies from effectively fighting malignant gliomas. GBMs exhibit robust proliferation, angiogenesis, genetic instability, and immunosuppression. In addition, it is a very infiltrative tumor that diffuses through white matter tracts and periventricular/perivascular areas, resulting in migration to the contralateral hemisphere.[3] As a result, the tumor cells may migrate far beyond what is visualized radiographically at the time of diagnosis. Thus, although surgical resection can remove the visible tumor mass, it cannot eradicate invasive and migratory cells. These challenges underscore the need for novel strategies to improve the outcome of patients with GBM. Immunotherapy is a strategy that would allow for surveillance and eradication of this local and distant disease.

Another factor that contributes to GBM malignancy is the high degree of genetic instability that generates cellular heterogeneity.[4] This hinders cancer cells from responding equally to radiation and chemotherapy, causing further relapses. In addition, chemotherapy has generally been unsuccessful because of poor drug delivery. The presence of active efflux transporters in the blood-brain barrier (BBB) prevents systemically administrated drugs from entering the brain,[5] thus highlighting the need for new comprehensive strategies to overcome this physical obstacle.[6]

Historically, the CNS has been viewed as immune privileged.[7,8] The CNS was considered unique relative to other organ systems by the virtues of the BBB restricting the migration of immune cells and cytokines into the brain, the absence of a lymphatic drainage system, the presence of a high concentration of immunosuppressive factors, and the lack of major histocompatibility complex (MHC) molecule expression in normal CNS cells.[9–11] However, newer data suggest that the CNS is a perfectly adequate environment for immune responses as evidenced by the presence of both humoral and cell-mediated CNS immunity.[12–14] In addition, lymphocytes have been shown to traffic to normal brain (both naive lymphocytes and activated T cells),[15] by crossing the BBB without antigen specificity.[15–17] Furthermore, many types of lymphocytes appear in the CNS during illness, such as infection or autoimmune processes.[18–20]

## THE TUMOR IMMUNE MICROENVIRONMENT

Many tumors, including GBM, create an immunosuppressive local environment to shield themselves from the body's normal immune response. The immune microenvironment created by GBM

[a] Department of Oncology, Sidney Kimmel Comprehensive Cancer Center, Johns Hopkins University School of Medicine, Baltimore, MD 21231, USA
[b] Department of Neurosurgery, Johns Hopkins University School of Medicine, Baltimore, MD 21231, USA
* Corresponding author.
E-mail address: mlim3@jhmi.edu (M. Lim).

Neurosurg Clin N Am 21 (2010) 17–29
doi:10.1016/j.nec.2009.08.008

likely plays a much larger role in immune evasion than the general BBB, which is typically compromised by the tumor. GBM evades the immune system using several strategies: (1) aberrant antigen recognition leading to insufficient immune cell activation, (2) promotion of suppressor immune cells to induce T-cell tolerance or apoptosis, (3) upregulation of co-inhibitory molecules, (4) secretion of immune inhibiting molecules, (5) recruitment of suppressor immune cells, and (6) activation of immunosuppressive pathways.

### Abnormal Antigen Recognition and Immune Cell Activation

One mechanism by which GBM evades the immune system is by preventing normal antigen recognition. This process is orchestrated by the MHC, also known in humans as human leukocyte antigen (HLA), which displays fragmented pieces of self or non-self-antigens on the host cell surface. Normally, T cells interact with MHC via the T-cell receptor molecules to determine if the antigen is self or foreign. A second signal is also required for T cells to become fully activated, the costimulatory signal. If this process occurs properly, T cells will ignore self-peptides and react appropriately to the foreign peptides (**Fig. 1A**).

### MHC

Parney and colleagues[21] found that most GBMs expressed low levels of class I MHC and no class II MHC. These data are supported by Lampson's[22] finding that class I MHC can be upregulated in gliomas after interferon γ (IFNγ) exposure in vitro.

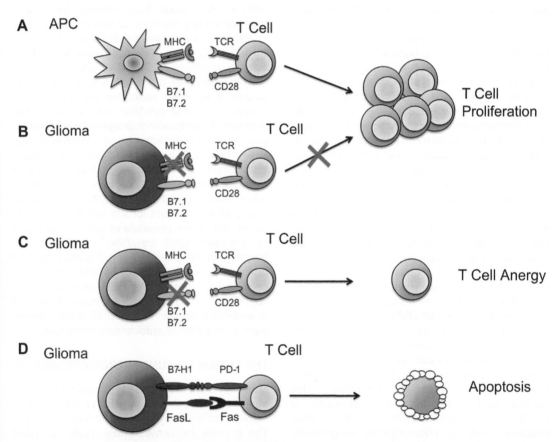

**Fig. 1.** Strategies adopted by glioma cells to inhibit T-cell proliferation and activation by interfering with the antigen presenting process. (A) Classical antigen presentation by antigen presenting cells through expression of MHC and costimulatory molecules. T cells interact with MHC via the T-cell receptors to determine if the antigen is self or foreign. When T cells identify non-self-peptides, they start to proliferate and activate to mount an immune response. Tumors disrupt this interaction by (B) downregulating the expression of MHC molecules on the cell surface. Loss of MHC molecules blocks the cross talk between tumor cells and the tumor-interacting immune cells. (C) Downregulation of the costimulatory molecules, such as B7.1 and B7.2, to induce T-cell anergy. (D) Upregulation of inhibitory B7 molecules, such as B7-H1, or death signals, such as FasL, cause T-cell apoptosis via binding with their receptors.

There are several reasons why class I and class II MHC molecules are not expressed on the glioma cell surface. First, gliomas have been reported to express immunoinhibitory factors, such as transforming growth factor β (TGF-β)[23] and prostaglandin $E_2$ (PGE$_2$),[24] that downregulate class II MHC on glioma cells. Second, most GBM lesions express mutated class I HLA molecules. HLA class I antigen loss significantly correlates with tumor grade[25] and with immunotherapy refractory tumors.[26] The antigen processing machinery (APM) components were also investigated, and tapasin expression was found to be downregulated in GBM lesions. Those aberrations seem to be linked with the mutations of HLA class I antigen expression and significantly correlates with the clinical course of the disease. These findings suggest that mutations in HLA class I antigen and in APM components may provide a mechanism for GBM to escape immune recognition and killing by cytotoxic T lymphocytes (CTLs). These findings emphasize the need to monitor HLA class I antigen and APM component expression in GBM lesions when selecting patients for T-cell–based immunotherapy treatment.[25]

### Costimulatory molecules

T-cell costimulation is necessary for T-cell proliferation, differentiation, and survival. Activation of T cells without costimulation may lead to T-cell anergy, T-cell deletion, or the development of immune tolerance. CD28, one of the best characterized costimulatory molecules expressed by T cells, interacts with CD80 (B7.1) and CD86 (B7.2) on the membrane of antigen presenting cells (APCs) (see **Fig. 1**A).

In addition to expressing low levels of MHC peptide (see **Fig. 1**B), cancer cells downregulate the costimulatory molecules that are required for activating a proper immune response (see **Fig. 1**C). Lack of T-cell costimulation is another mechanism by GBM to avoid immune surveillance. So far, B7 molecule expression is found to be absent on glioma cells.[27] In addition, peripheral blood T cells from patients with glioma typically show a high degree of anergy to GBM antigens that results from the absence of costimulatory molecules.

Studies have also shown that the receptors for the costimulatory molecules on tumor-infiltrating APCs are downregulated. Researchers have shown that the human glioma-infiltrated microglia or macrophages (GIMs) completely lack CD80/CD40 expression and show minimal CD86 expression, which could explain their inability to properly activate naive T cells.[28] Another study conducted on intracranial RG2 glioma-bearing rodents showed

that GIMs from brain tumors respond differently to general activators, such as CpG oligodeoxynucleotides (CpG ODN) and IFNγ/lipopolysaccharide (LPS), when compared with those from normal brain. CpG ODN induced the upregulation of B7 molecules but had little effect on MHC-II expression, whereas IFNγ/LPS had the opposite effect. Both upregulations were significantly lower in tumor-associated GIMs, in comparison with GIMs from normal brain. Further studies are necessary to understand if these diminished effects are a result of the local GBM immunocompromising environment, abnormal signaling, or mutated receptor expression on the tumor-infiltrating GIMs.[29]

The B7 costimulatory family includes activating and inhibiting molecules that regulate immune responses positively and negatively. Among the latter group, B7-H1, one of the newly identified B7 family member, has been shown to provide negative signals that control and suppress T-cell responses.[30] The regulation of B7-H1 seems to be pivotal in shaping the immune response to tumors because it can exert costimulatory and immune regulatory functions.[31] Although B7-H1 has been shown to mediate tumor evasion by binding to programmed death-1 (PD-1) receptor, additional counter receptors can also control the functions of B7-H1.[32]

Human and rodent cancer cells and immune cells in the cancer microenvironment have been shown to upregulate expression of inhibitory B7 molecules. Analysis of multiple glioma cell lines and human specimens have also shown high levels of B7-H1 (see **Fig. 1**D).[27,33] This high level of expression reduces glioma cell immunogenicity by suppressing T-cell cytokine production and activation. A study by Parsa and colleagues[34] demonstrates a potential relationship between B7-H1 and the phosphatase and tensin homolog-phosphatidylinositol 3-kinase (PTEN-PI3K) pathway. They show that the loss of PTEN and the activation of the PI3K-pathway lead to elevated post-transcriptional expression of B7-H1. This represents a novel mechanism of immunoresistance mediated by B7-H1, further demonstrating the importance of this molecule in tumor evasion of immune surveillance. B7-H1 has even been reported to correlate with the malignancy grade of gliomas.[35] These studies demonstrate the potential benefits of using neutralizing antibodies specific for B7-H1 and PD-1 in the treatment of patients with malignant brain tumors.

### Deregulation of Cell-mediated Immunity

During the past 3 decades, many studies of patients harboring glioma revealed that these individuals exhibit a broad suppression of cell-mediated immunity in a manner similar to those involved in autoimmunity processes. Studies have suggested that the immune cells from patients with GBM behave in a manner that is reminiscent to autoimmune diseases, such as cutaneous anergy to common bacterial antigens,[36] lymphopenia,[37] impaired antibody production,[37] and abnormal delayed-type hypersensitivity response to common recall antigens or neoantigens in vivo.[37,38] It seems that the lymphocytes in patients with GBM present intrinsic cellular abnormalities that render potentially reactive T cells unresponsive. Peripheral blood lymphocytes (PBLs) obtained from patients with GBM did not proliferate or minimally proliferated in response to mitogen stimulation in vitro. Elliott and colleagues[39] showed that PBLs obtained from patients with GBM have approximately 6 times fewer phytohemagglutinin (PHA)-reactive lymphocytes than those obtained from normal subjects. These lymphocytes fail to expand into a pool of proliferating cells in vitro. In addition, the supernatant fluids of PHA-stimulated lymphocytes obtained from patients contain a substantial reduction of interleukin-2 (IL-2) and IFN$\gamma$ compared with lymphocytes obtained from normal donors. Moreover, T cells obtained from patients with GBM are unable to offer helper activity in allogeneic pokeweed mitogen cultures in vitro.[39–41] This comprehensive depression in cellular immune function is not typical of head trauma or other tumors of the brain. Hence, it must be the complex GBM tumor microenvironment that compromises T-cell compartments and their functions.

In addition to the alterations of the intrinsic activation pathways in T cells, GBM also induces accumulation of immunosuppressive cells in the microenvironment. GBM promotes impaired immunocompetence by taking advantage of the normal immunosuppressive mechanisms by stimulating the proliferation of the regulatory T (T$_{reg}$) cells. In vivo depletion of T$_{reg}$ cells causes severe autoimmune disease, which can be reversed by reconstitution.[42] Moreover, the regression of tolerogenic tumors after depletion of T$_{reg}$ cells has been observed in vivo.[43]

Fecci and colleagues[44] reported an unbalanced ratio between CD4$^+$ T cells and T$_{reg}$ cells in GBM. Although both fractions were greatly reduced in patients with malignant glioma, T$_{reg}$ cells often represented most of the CD4 population. It is well known that T$_{reg}$ cells can inhibit T-cell activation and proliferation by downregulating IL-2 and IFN$\gamma$ production in the target cells.[25,28,29,45–48] This would also explain the shift from T$_H$1 to T$_H$2 cytokines, which propagate the regulatory phenotype.[49,50] As a demonstration of this, depletion of T$_{reg}$ cells in vitro reestablishes the normal CD4 functions in the T cells that are isolated from patients with GBM and reverses the cytokine production to the T$_H$1 type.[44] Tumor tolerance induced by T$_{reg}$ cells is also common in other solid tumors.

In addition to T$_{reg}$ cells, there are other suppressive cell types in the tumor microenvironment. Recruitment of suppressive myeloid cells, such as regulatory dendritic cells (DCs), characterized by indoleamine-pyrrole 2,3 dioxygenase (IDO) expression[51] and myeloid-derived suppressor cells (MDSCs) at the tumor site is another way to inhibit immune responses.[52]

Munn and colleagues documented IDO expression in human and murine myeloid DCs. IDO$^+$ DCs catabolize tryptophan to block local T- lymphocyte clonal expansion, causing T-cell death by apoptosis, anergy, or immune deviation.[51,53–56] Suppressive myeloid cells would directly contribute to induction of T$_{reg}$ cells in the tumor microenvironment and vice versa; T$_{reg}$ cells can induce IDO expression in DCs and effectively convert them into regulatory DCs.[57]

MDSCs also infiltrate tumors, inhibiting immune response and facilitating tumor growth and metastasis.[58] MDSCs inhibit T cell activation by anti-CD3 and superantigen, and by secretion of reactive nitrogen compounds (peroxynitrites) and immunosuppressive cytokines (TGF-$\beta$).[52] Human MDSCs were originally described in patients with head and neck cancer[59] and in the peripheral blood of patients with renal cell carcinoma.[60] Tumor-infiltrated MDSCs have been described in mouse GL261[61] and rat T9 glioma models.[62] In the latter example, the authors reported that MDSCs were recruited at the brain T9 tumor site after subcutaneous vaccination with irradiated T9 glioma cells, which inhibited T-cell function and resulted in tumor progression.

In addition to GBM-induced mechanisms, immunosuppression can also be iatrogenic. Corticosteroids may cause immunosuppression by inhibiting cytokine production and causing sequestration of CD4$^+$ T cells.[63] Newer data suggest, however, that such immunosuppression may be dose dependent; and at therapeutic levels, corticosteroids may not interfere with immunotherapy.[64] Chemotherapy can also contribute to the inhibition of the immune response to tumor. Temozolomide, for example, can cause CD4$^+$ lymphopenia,[65] which may negatively affect immunotherapeutic approaches that use a CD4$^+$ T-cell response. Newer agents, such as rapamycin, inhibit the T-cell proliferative cytokine IL-2.[63]

## Immunosuppressive Factors

The tumor microenvironment modulates various cytokines and chemokines expressed by tumor cells or lymphocytes. The glioma microenvironment contains very high levels of immunosuppressive cytokines, which contribute to impaired lymphocyte response in patients with glioma (**Fig. 2**).[66]

### TGF-β

One of the most well-characterized immunosuppressive factors is TGF-β, originally called glioblastoma cell-derived T-cell suppressor factor (see **Fig. 2**).[67] TGF-β regulates inflammation, angiogenesis, and proliferation.[68] Glioblastoma is known to produce high levels of TGF-β in the microenvironment, where it inhibits T-cell and B-cell proliferation, activation,[69,70] and maturation and function of professional APCs.[71] In particular, TGF-β directly inhibits CTL function by blocking the production of cytotoxic molecules, IFNγ, and Fas ligand (FasL).[72,73] This may also explain the inactive state of the tumor-infiltrated T cells. Furthermore, TGF-β is responsible for the downregulation of MHC class II on glioma cells,[23] which serves as another mechanism of tumor escape. TGF-β is an important growth factor for glioma cells expressing TGF-β surface receptor,[74] and it also seems to play a role in maintaining the $T_{reg}$ cell phenotype.

### IL-10

The role of IL-10, known as cytokine synthesis inhibitory factor, is similar to TGF-β.[75] IL-10 is secreted by glioma cells[76] and $T_{reg}$ cells[77]; it

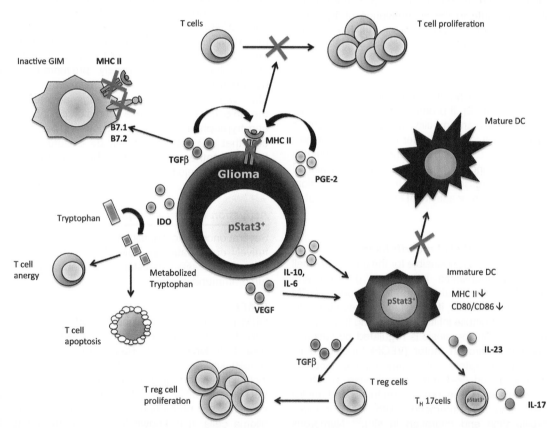

**Fig. 2.** Immunosuppressive factors secreted by glioma cells in the tumor microenvironment. (Starting from the top and proceeding clockwise) TGF-β and PGE$_2$ downregulate class II MHC molecules on glioma cells and on GIMs. As a consequence, the antigen presenting process is compromised and T cells cannot proliferate. IL-10, IL-6, and VEGF are STAT3-dependent cytokines that represent potent STAT3 activators. The tumor microenvironment has many immunosuppressive activities, and these activities are responsible for activation of STAT3 in immune cells. When DC progenitors become STAT3$^+$, they remain immature and are unable to express class II MHC and costimulatory molecules. Therefore, they cannot efficiently prime T cells, and they in turn start to secrete more inhibitory factors, including TGF-β and IL-23, which promote $T_{reg}$ cells and $T_H$17 cells accumulation, respectively. IDO$^+$ gliomas are able to actively metabolize tryptophan, and lack of tryptophan in the microenvironment blocks T-cell proliferation. In this condition, T cells can become anergic or undergo apoptosis.

inhibits production of IFNγ by lymphocytes and tumor necrosis factor α by monocytes and down-regulates class II MHC on GIMs.[76] IL-10 also induces glioma cell proliferation and motility in vitro.[78] Controversially, IL-10 has been shown to inhibit brain tumor growth in vivo.[79] New studies are necessary to clarify the conflicting roles of this cytokine in the tumor microenvironment.

Another important immunosuppressive quality of IL-10 is the ability to induce signal transducer and activator of transcription 3 (STAT3) in DC progenitors and in other immune cells, including innate immune cells and T cells (see **Fig. 2**).[80] Immunostimulatory molecule expression is reduced in immune cells that show constitutive activation of STAT3. Also, their ability to mount an antitumor immune response is defective. Moreover, they seem to produce immunosuppressive factors, such as TGF-β, IL-23, and more IL-10, that contribute to the accumulation of $T_{reg}$ cells and possibly $T_H17$ cells in the tumor microenvironment.

### PGE$_2$

PGE$_2$ has profound effects on glioma and immune cells (see **Fig. 2**). It promotes tumor cell invasion, angiogenesis, and motility. It also downregulates MHC class II.[24] On the other hand, PGE$_2$ downregulates $T_H1$ cytokine production and upregulates $T_H2$, enhancing $T_{reg}$ phenotype and proliferation.[81] It also suppresses T-cell activation, proliferation, and the antitumor activity of lymphokine-activated killer cells.[82]

### Vascular endothelial growth factor

Angiogenesis is responsible for the growth of small localized neoplasms into larger growing and potentially metastatic tumors. Although GBM rarely metastasizes, it almost always recurs locally because of diffuse infiltration resulting from angiogenesis.[83] Angiogenesis is regulated by vascular endothelial growth factor (VEGF) binding to its specific receptors, flt-1 (fms-related tyrosine kinase 1) and flk-1 (fetal liver kinase 1). These receptors are only expressed on tumor endothelial cells, and their interaction with VEGF induces proliferation and migration in situ.[84] Numerous studies have demonstrated the prevalence of VEGF expression and its isoforms in GBM.[85] In vitro and in vivo studies have confirmed a correlation between tumor grade and VEGF expression in gliomas. In addition, studies in animal models have shown that inhibiting VEGF function inhibits growth of glioma cells and causes regression of blood vessels.[83] Within GBM, cells adjacent to necrotic areas are thought to upregulate VEGF,

secondary to hypoxia. VEGF expression has been shown to strongly correlate with hypoxia.[86]

In a similar way to IL-10, VEGF has been well characterized as an inhibitor of DC maturation and activation (see **Fig. 2**).[87]

### IDO

IDO is a kynurenine pathway enzyme that catalyzes the catabolism of tryptophan,[53] an amino acid essential for T-cell proliferation and differentiation. It has been shown to play various roles within the immune system.[51,88] Uyttenhove and colleagues[89] detected positive expression of IDO in various human tumor specimens, including GBM (see **Fig. 2**). They demonstrated that IDO$^+$ tumors were successful at evading the immune response. However, they were also able to reverse these effects by using an IDO inhibitor, clearly indicating that this protein may play a possible role in tumor evasion of the immune system. Miyazaki and colleagues[90] demonstrated the same IDO mechanism at work in 4 human GBM cell lines. They demonstrated that an IDO inhibitor, 1-methyltryptophan (1MT), effectively prevented the depletion of tryptophan. In addition, combining 1MT with chemotherapeutic drugs augmented the inhibitory effect of these agents on cell growth and tryptophan degradation. These studies indicate that IDO could potentially be a useful target for immunotherapy against GBM by preserving tryptophan levels for T cells.

### Activation of Immunosuppressive Pathways

Several oncogenic signaling pathways are constitutively upregulated in GBM. They contribute to tumor progression, resistance to therapies, and tumor immune evasion.

### STAT3

GBM presents several signal transduction pathways that are overly activated, such as phosphoinositide-3 kinase, Akt, Ras, mitogen-activated protein kinases, and receptor tyrosine kinases, including epidermal growth factor receptor and VEGF receptor.[65,91] All of these pathways actively stimulate the promotion and the progression of glioma cells. It is known that they converge to specific transcription factors, including STAT3. Aberrant activation of STAT3 has been found in many cancer types,[80,92–94] including GBM.[95] STAT3 activation in tumors prevents apoptosis and promotes cellular proliferation, angiogenesis, and tissue invasion.[80] In glioma cells, STAT3 triggers the expression of antiapoptotic factors, such as Bcl-2, Bcl-XL, Mcl-1, survivin, and cFlip.[96,97] Knockdown of STAT3 expression by siRNA causes apoptosis in several glioma cell lines but not in primary human astrocytes.[97]

In addition to promoting oncogenesis, STAT3 plays an important role in immune evasion by inhibiting the expression of $T_H1$ mediators[98] and stimulating production of diverse immunosuppressive factors,[73] such as IL-10 and VEGF. This inhibits the induction of a tumor-specific T-cell response[99] and also retains DCs in their immature state, turning them into tolerogenic DCs[100] that are able to promote expansion of $T_{reg}$ cells.[101]

STAT3 has been found to be constitutively activated in tumor-infiltrating DCs and myeloid cells,[73] most probably due to the presence of IL-10 and VEGF, which are potent STAT3 activators in the tumor microenvironment (see Fig. 2).[98] STAT3 activity in DCs inhibits the expression of MHC class II molecules, B7-1, B7-2, and IL-12 secretion,[98] thus preventing their maturation and affecting their ability to activate tumor-specific T cells and natural killer (NK) cells. Hussain and colleagues[102] described a similar tolerogenic phenotype on GBM infiltrated microglia or macrophages and their inability to properly activate T cells. Blocking STAT3 with a small molecule inhibitor can reverse immune tolerance in patients with GBM. In particular, costimulatory molecules can be upregulated on GIMs and the production of IL-2, IL-4, IL-12, and IL-15 can be increased, thus inducing proliferation of T cells.[103]

New tumor-infiltrated T-cell populations have been described, and they all have the capacity of secreting IL-17.[104] IL-17 T cells have been originally described in the pathogenesis of autoimmune disease.[105,106] STAT3-induced IL-6/TGF-β costimulation is necessary to promote IL-17 differentiation, and IL-23 is necessary to maintain the IL-17 phenotype.[107–109] Because tumor-infiltrated myeloid cells are the principal source of IL-23[110] and IL-23 is responsible for tumor-associated inflammation and angiogenesis,[108] it is reasonable to speculate that IL-17 T cells might have a potential role in cancer development.

### Fas/FasL

Fas is a member of the tumor necrosis factor receptor family.[111] It is an apoptotic receptor that binds to FasL. This binding triggers an intracellular cascade resulting in cell death.[112,113] However, a study involving GBM shows that Fas receptor activation results in cell survival and proliferation rather than apoptosis.[114]

FasL expression has been detected in various tumor types.[115–118] Although FasL expression has been predominantly identified in activated immune cells, such as T cells, phagocytes, and NK cells,[112,113,119,120] its role in immune reaction suppression still remains unclear.

Cancer cell acquisition of FasL expression has been shown to deliver death signals to activated Fas-positive T lymphocytes.[121–124] This counterattack hypothesis is thought to grant the tumor an immune-privileged status. This concept originated from initial studies in transplantation, which demonstrated that the Fas-FasL interaction was fundamental to maintaining an immune-privileged status.[125,126] However, later studies contradicted these previous results, showing that FasL expression resulted in rapid rejection accompanied by inflammation.[127–130] Other contradictory studies report that FasL can also have proinflammatory and antitumoral effects.[131,132] These conflicting findings regarding Fas-FasL highlight that this system is not fully understood and that certain environmental conditions, tumor type, activated pathways, and presence or absence of immune cell populations are involved in this response.[133,134]

In GBM, the use of conventional chemotherapeutic drugs (such as camptothecin and etoposide) can sensitize the tumor cells to Fas-dependent apoptosis.[135,136] The use of decoy receptor 3, a soluble decoy for FasL, has also been shown to reduce the number of tumor-infiltrating CD4 and CD8 T cells in a 9L gliosarcoma model.[137] The administration of topotecan, a Fas-enhancing chemotherapeutic agent, before immunotherapy may also amplify apoptotic receptors, further sensitizing glioma cells for immune clearance.[138] These results demonstrate the potential benefits of combination therapy involving chemotherapy with immunotherapy in patients with glioma by focusing on Fas-FasL.

### Galectin-1

Galectin-1, a prototype member of the galectin family, is a homodimeric adhesion molecule and carbohydrate-binding protein with affinity for β-galactosides.[139] Galectin-1 plays a multifaceted role in promoting brain tumor malignancy.[140] This protein contributes to the invasive and migratory potential,[141–144] angiogenesis,[145] and chemoresistance[146] of glioma cells. Galectin-1 expression levels in glioma have even been shown to directly correlate with tumor grade.[142,147]

Galectin-1 also plays an important role in regulating immune cell homeostasis and inflammation.[148–150] Galectin-1 promotes apoptosis of activated T cells,[151–154] induces partial T-cell activation,[155] and blocks proinflammatory cytokine secretion.[156,157] Galectin-1 also contributes to tumor-induced immunosuppression in vitro and in vivo.[147] In patients with head and neck squamous cell carcinoma, Le and colleagues[158] demonstrate an inverse relationship between galectin-1 expression and the presence of T cells, suggesting that galectin-1 is a negative regulator of T-cell activation and survival. These results support the concept that galectin-1 contributes to immune privilege of tumors by negatively regulating the survival of effector T cells. Galectin-1 is also thought to play similar roles in gliomas, yet its immunosuppressive role has not been determined in these particular tumors.

## SUMMARY

Gliomas are specialized in evading the host immune system and current immunotherapies. An important component of this efficient immune escape is harbored in the complexity of the glioma microenvironment. Many immunosuppressive mechanisms are active simultaneously, and they can self-sustain themselves by creating a positive feedback loop and enhancing their effects. The glioma-derived suppressor factors generate a shift from $T_H1$ to $T_H2$ cytokines, resulting in deregulation of cell-mediated immunity, accompanied by accumulation of immunosuppressive type of cells. In addition, regulatory cell secretion of active immunosuppressive factors and activation of immunosuppressive pathways allow for tumor escape mechanisms at multiple levels. These phenomena provide difficult challenges in designing immunotherapies. However, it is clear that targeting multiple points in the immunosuppressive response and continual improvements in current vaccines will lead to improved immunotherapies. In addition, one has begun to appreciate that pathways and mechanisms affect multiple processes. For example, STAT3 affects cell proliferation and angiogenesis in addition to immunotherapy. Continuous studies of the glioma cells and their cross talk with the immune cells are paramount to overcome tumor tolerance and in the development of strategies to cure hopeless patients with GBM.

## REFERENCES

1. Buckner JC, et al. A phase III study of radiation therapy plus carmustine with or without recombinant interferon-alpha in the treatment of patients with newly diagnosed high-grade glioma. Cancer 2001;92:420–33.
2. Stupp R, et al. Radiotherapy plus concomitant and adjuvant temozolomide for glioblastoma. N Engl J Med 2005;352:987–96.
3. Hochberg FH, Pruitt A. Assumptions in the radiotherapy of glioblastoma. Neurology 1980;30: 907–11.
4. Louis DN, Gusella JF. A tiger behind many doors: multiple genetic pathways to malignant glioma. Trends Genet 1995;11:412–5.
5. Doolittle ND, Abrey LE, Bleyer WA, et al. New frontiers in translational research in neuro-oncology and the blood-brain barrier: report of the tenth annual Blood-Brain Barrier Disruption Consortium Meeting. Clin Cancer Res 2005;11:421–8.
6. Dunn GP, Bruce AT, Ikeda H, et al. Cancer immunoediting: from immunosurveillance to tumor escape. Nat Immunol 2002;3:991–8.
7. Murphy J, Sturm E. Conditions determining the transplantability of tissues in the brain. J Exp Med 1923;38:183–97.
8. Medawar P. Immunity to homologous grafted skin. III. The fate of skin homografts transplanted to the brain, to subcutaneous tissue, and to the anterior chamber of the eye. Br J Exp Pathol 1948;29: 58–69.
9. Lampson LA, Hickey WF. Monoclonal antibody analysis of MHC expression in human brain biopsies: tissue ranging from "histologically normal" to that showing different levels of glial tumor involvement. J Immunol 1986;136:4054–62.
10. Cserr HF, Knopf PM. In: Keane R, Hickey WF, editors. Immunology of the nervous system. New York: Oxford University Press; 1997.
11. Lampson L. In: Youmans J, editor. Neurological surgery. Philadelphia: WB Saunders Co; 2004.
12. Sandberg-Wollheim M, Zweiman B, Levinson AI, et al. Humoral immune responses within the human central nervous system following systemic immunization. J Neuroimmunol 1986;11:205–14.
13. Bernheimer H, Lassmann H, Suchanek G. Dynamics of IgG+, IgA+, and IgM+ plasma cells in the central nervous system of guinea pigs with chronic relapsing experimental allergic encephalomyelitis. Neuropathol Appl Neurobiol 1988;14: 157–67.
14. Levi-Strauss M, Mallat M. Primary cultures of murine astrocytes produce C3 and factor B, two components of the alternative pathway of complement activation. J Immunol 1987;139:2361–6.
15. Hickey WF, Kimura H. Graft-vs.-host disease elicits expression of class I and class II histocompatibility antigens and the presence of scattered T lymphocytes in rat central nervous system. Proc Natl Acad Sci U S A 1987;84:2082–6.
16. Hickey WF. Basic principles of immunological surveillance of the normal central nervous system. Glia 2001;36:118–24.
17. Hickey WF, Hsu BL, Kimura H. T-lymphocyte entry into the central nervous system. J Neurosci Res 1991;28:254–60.
18. Sampson JH, Archer GE, Ashley DM, et al. Subcutaneous vaccination with irradiated, cytokine-producing tumor cells stimulates CD8+ cell-mediated immunity

against tumors located in the "immunologically privi-leged" central nervous system. Proc Natl Acad Sci U S A 1996;93:10399–404.

19. Gordon LB, Nolan SC, Cserr HF, et al. Growth of P511 mastocytoma cells in BALB/c mouse brain elicits CTL response without tumor elimination: a new tumor model for regional central nervous system immunity. J Immunol 1997;159:2399–408.

20. Gordon FL, Nguyen KB, White CA, et al. Rapid entry and downregulation of T cells in the central nervous system during the reinduction of experi-mental autoimmune encephalomyelitis. J Neuroim-munol 2001;112:15–27.

21. Parney IF, Farr-Jones MA, Chang LJ, et al. Human glioma immunobiology in vitro: implications for immunogene therapy. Neurosurgery 2000;46: 1169–77 [discussion: 1177–8].

22. Lampson LA. Interpreting MHC class I expression and class I/class II reciprocity in the CNS: recon-ciling divergent findings. Microsc Res Tech 1995; 32:267–85.

23. Zuber P, Kuppner MC, De Tribolet N. Transforming growth factor-beta 2 down-regulates HLA-DR antigen expression on human malignant glioma cells. Eur J Immunol 1988;18:1623–6.

24. Wojtowicz-Praga S. Reversal of tumor-induced immunosuppression: a new approach to cancer therapy. J Immunother 1997;20:165–77.

25. Facoetti A, Nano R, Zelini P, et al. Human leukocyte antigen and antigen processing machinery compo-nent defects in astrocytic tumors. Clin Cancer Res 2005;11:8304–11.

26. Chang CC, Campoli M, Ferrone S. HLA class I defects in malignant lesions: what have we learned? Keio J Med 2003;52:220–9.

27. Wintterle S, Schreiner B, Mitsdoerffer M, et al. Expression of the B7-related molecule B7-H1 by glioma cells: a potential mechanism of immune paralysis. Cancer Res 2003;63:7462–7.

28. Hussain SF, Heimberger AB. Immunotherapy for human glioma: innovative approaches and recent results. Expert Rev Anticancer Ther 2005;5:777–90.

29. Schartner JM, Hagar AR, Van Handel M, et al. Impaired capacity for upregulation of MHC class II in tumor-associated microglia. Glia 2005;51:279–85.

30. Chen L. Co-inhibitory molecules of the B7-CD28 family in the control of T-cell immunity. Nat Rev Immunol 2004;4:336–47.

31. Sharpe AH, Freeman GJ. The B7-CD28 super-family. Nat Rev Immunol 2002;2:116–26.

32. Butte MJ, Keir ME, Phamduy TB, et al. Pro-grammed death-1 ligand 1 interacts specifically with the B7-1 costimulatory molecule to inhibit T cell responses. Immunity 2007;27:111–22.

33. Wilmotte R, Burkhardt K, Kindler V, et al. B7-homolog 1 expression by human glioma: a new mechanism of immune evasion. Neuroreport 2005;16:1081–5.

34. Parsa AT, Waldron JS, Panner A, et al. Loss of tumor suppressor PTEN function increases B7-H1 expression and immunoresistance in glioma. Nat Med 2007;13:84–8.

35. Yao Y, Tao R, Wang X, et al. B7-H1 is correlated with the malignancy grade of gliomas but it is not the privilege of tumor stem-like cells. Neuro Oncol 2009 [Epub ahead of print].

36. Brooks WH, Netsky MG, Normansell DE, et al. Depressed cell-mediated immunity in patients with primary intracranial tumors. Characterization of a humoral immunosuppressive factor. J Exp Med 1972;136:1631–47.

37. Mahaley MS Jr, Brooks WH, Roszman TL, et al. Im-munobiology of primary intracranial tumors. Part 1: studies of the cellular and humoral general immune competence of brain-tumor patients. J Neurosurg 1977;46:467–76.

38. Young HF, Sakalas R, Kaplan AM. Inhibition of cell-mediated immunity in patients with brain tumors. Surg Neurol 1976;5:19–23.

39. Elliott LH, Brooks WH, Roszman TL. Cytokinetic basis for the impaired activation of lymphocytes from patients with primary intracranial tumors. J Im-munol 1984;132:1208–15.

40. Ausiello CM, Palma C, Maleci A, et al. Cell medi-ated cytotoxicity and cytokine production in periph-eral blood mononuclear cells of glioma patients. Eur J Cancer 1991;27:646–50.

41. Roszman TL, Brooks WH, Steele C, et al. Poke-weed mitogen-induced immunoglobulin secretion by peripheral blood lymphocytes from patients with primary intracranial tumors. Characterization of T helper and B cell function. J Immunol 1985; 134:1545–50.

42. Sakaguchi S, Sakaguchi N, Asano M, et al. Immu-nologic self-tolerance maintained by activated T cells expressing IL-2 receptor alpha-chains (CD25). Breakdown of a single mechanism of self-tolerance causes various autoimmune diseases. J Immunol 1995;155:1151–64.

43. Liyanage UK, Moore TT, Joo HG, et al. Prevalence of regulatory T cells is increased in peripheral blood and tumor microenvironment of patients with pancreas or breast adenocarcinoma. J Immunol 2002;169:2756–61.

44. Fecci PE, Mitchell DA, Whitesides JF, et al. Increased regulatory T-cell fraction amidst a dimin-ished CD4 compartment explains cellular immune defects in patients with malignant glioma. Cancer Res 2006;66:3294–302.

45. Gerosa MA, Olivi A, Rosenblum ML, et al. Impaired immunocompetence in patients with malignant gliomas: the possible role of Tg-lymphocyte subpopulations. Neurosurgery 1982;10:571–3.

46. Thornton AM, Shevach EM. CD4+CD25+ immuno-regulatory T cells suppress polyclonal T cell

activation in vitro by inhibiting interleukin 2 production. J Exp Med 1998;188:287–96.

47. Camara NO, Sebille F, Lechler RI. Human CD4+CD25+ regulatory cells have marked and sustained effects on CD8+ T cell activation. Eur J Immunol 2003;33:3473–83.

48. Piccirillo CA, Shevach EM. Cutting edge: control of CD8+ T cell activation by CD4+CD25+ immunoregulatory cells. J Immunol 2001;167:1137–40.

49. Dieckmann D, Bruett CH, Ploettner H, et al. Human CD4(+)CD25(+) regulatory, contact-dependent T cells induce interleukin 10-producing, contact-independent type 1-like regulatory T cells [corrected]. J Exp Med 2002;196:247–53.

50. Zheng SG, Wang JH, Koss MN, et al. CD4+ and CD8+ regulatory T cells generated ex vivo with IL-2 and TGF-beta suppress a stimulatory graft-versus-host disease with a lupus-like syndrome. J Immunol 2004;172:1531–9.

51. Munn DH, Sharma MD, Lee JR, et al. Potential regulatory function of human dendritic cells expressing indoleamine 2,3-dioxygenase. Science 2002;297:1867–70.

52. Talmadge JE, Donkor M, Scholar E. Inflammatory cell infiltration of tumors: Jekyll or Hyde. Cancer Metastasis Rev 2007;26(3–4):373–400.

53. Munn DH, Shafizadeh E, Attwood JT, et al. Inhibition of T cell proliferation by macrophage tryptophan catabolism. J Exp Med 1999;189:1363–72.

54. Hwu P, Du MX, Lapointe R, et al. Indoleamine 2,3-dioxygenase production by human dendritic cells results in the inhibition of T cell proliferation. J Immunol 2000;164:3596–9.

55. Kudo Y, Boyd CA, Sargent IL, et al. Tryptophan degradation by human placental indoleamine 2,3-dioxygenase regulates lymphocyte proliferation. J Physiol 2001;535:207–15.

56. Frumento G, Rotondo R, Tonetti M, et al. T cell proliferation is blocked by indoleamine 2,3-dioxygenase. Transplant Proc 2001;33:428–30.

57. Grohmann U, Orabona C, Fallarino F, et al. CTLA-4-Ig regulates tryptophan catabolism in vivo. Nat Immunol 2002;3:1097–101.

58. Bronte V, Serafini P, Apolloni E, et al. Tumor-induced immune dysfunctions caused by myeloid suppressor cells. J Immunother 2001;24:431–46.

59. Kusmartsev S, Gabrilovich DI. STAT1 signaling regulates tumor-associated macrophage-mediated T cell deletion. J Immunol 2005;174:4880–91.

60. Zea AH, Rodriguez PC, Atkins MB, et al. Arginase-producing myeloid suppressor cells in renal cell carcinoma patients: a mechanism of tumor evasion. Cancer Res 2005;65:3044–8.

61. Umemura N, Saio M, Suwa T, et al. Tumor-infiltrating myeloid-derived suppressor cells are pleiotropic-inflamed monocytes/macrophages that bear M1- and M2-type characteristics. J Leukoc Biol 2008;83:1136–44.

62. Turkson J, Zhang S, Palmer J, et al. Inhibition of constitutive signal transducer and activator of transcription 3 activation by novel platinum complexes with potent antitumor activity. Mol Cancer Ther 2004;3:1533–42.

63. Barshes NR, Goodpastor SE, Goss JA. Pharmacologic immunosuppression. Front Biosci 2004;9:411–20.

64. Lesniak MS, Gabikian P, Tyler BM, et al. Dexamethasone mediated inhibition of local IL-2 immunotherapy is dose dependent in experimental brain tumors. J Neurooncol 2004;70:23–8.

65. Guha A, Mukherjee J. Advances in the biology of astrocytomas. Curr Opin Neurol 2004;17:655–62.

66. Maxwell M, Galanopoulos T, Neville-Golden J, et al. Effect of the expression of transforming growth factor-beta 2 in primary human glioblastomas on immunosuppression and loss of immune surveillance. J Neurosurg 1992;76:799–804.

67. Fontana A, Hengartner H, de Tribolet N, et al. Glioblastoma cells release interleukin 1 and factors inhibiting interleukin 2-mediated effects. J Immunol 1984;132:1837–44.

68. Govinden R, Bhoola KD. Genealogy, expression, and cellular function of transforming growth factor-beta. Pharmacol Ther 2003;98:257–65.

69. Ranges GE, Figari IS, Espevik T, et al. Inhibition of cytotoxic T cell development by transforming growth factor beta and reversal by recombinant tumor necrosis factor alpha. J Exp Med 1987;166:991–8.

70. Gorelik L, Flavell RA. Abrogation of TGFbeta signaling in T cells leads to spontaneous T cell differentiation and autoimmune disease. Immunity 2000;12:171–81.

71. Letterio JJ, Roberts AB. Regulation of immune responses by TGF-beta. Annu Rev Immunol 1998;16:137–61.

72. Smyth MJ, Strobl SL, Young HA, et al. Regulation of lymphokine-activated killer activity and pore-forming protein gene expression in human peripheral blood CD8+ T lymphocytes. Inhibition by transforming growth factor-beta. J Immunol 1991;146:3289–97.

73. Kortylewski M, Xin H, Kujawski M, et al. Inhibiting Stat3 signaling in the hematopoietic system elicits multicomponent antitumor immunity. Nat Med 2005;11:1314–21.

74. Resnicoff M, Sell C, Rubini M, et al. Rat glioblastoma cells expressing an antisense RNA to the insulin-like growth factor-1 (IGF-1) receptor are nontumorigenic and induce regression of wild-type tumors. Cancer Res 1994;54:2218–22.

75. Grutz G. New insights into the molecular mechanism of interleukin-10-mediated immunosuppression. J Leukoc Biol 2005;77:3–15.

76. Hishii M, Nitta T, Ishida H, et al. Human glioma-derived interleukin-10 inhibits antitumor immune responses in vitro. Neurosurgery 1995;37:1160–6 [discussion: 1166–7].

77. Sakaguchi S. Naturally arising Foxp3-expressing CD25+CD4+ regulatory T cells in immunological tolerance to self and non-self. Nat Immunol 2005; 6:345–52.

78. Huettner C, Czub S, Kerkau S, et al. Interleukin 10 is expressed in human gliomas in vivo and increases glioma cell proliferation and motility in vitro. Anticancer Res 1997;17:3217–24.

79. Berman RM, Suzuki T, Tahara H, et al. Systemic administration of cellular IL-10 induces an effective, specific, and long-lived immune response against established tumors in mice. J Immunol 1996;157: 231–8.

80. Yu H, Jove R. The STATs of cancer–new molecular targets come of age. Nat Rev Cancer 2004;4:97–105.

81. Wang D, Dubois RN. Prostaglandins and cancer. Gut 2006;55:115–22.

82. Baxevanis CN, Reclos GJ, Gritzapis AD, et al. Elevated prostaglandin E2 production by monocytes is responsible for the depressed levels of natural killer and lymphokine-activated killer cell function in patients with breast cancer. Cancer 1993;72:491–501.

83. Maity A, Pore N, Lee J, et al. Epidermal growth factor receptor transcriptionally up-regulates vascular endothelial growth factor expression in human glioblastoma cells via a pathway involving phosphatidylinositol 3′-kinase and distinct from that induced by hypoxia. Cancer Res 2000;60:5879–86.

84. Steiner HH, Karcher S, Mueller MM, et al. Autocrine pathways of the vascular endothelial growth factor (VEGF) in glioblastoma multiforme: clinical relevance of radiation-induced increase of VEGF levels. J Neurooncol 2004;66:129–38.

85. Cheng SY, Nagane M, Huang HS, et al. Intracerebral tumor-associated hemorrhage caused by overexpression of the vascular endothelial growth factor isoforms VEGF121 and VEGF165 but not VEGF189. Proc Natl Acad Sci U S A 1997;94: 12081–7.

86. Ziemer LS, Koch CJ, Maity A, et al. Hypoxia and VEGF mRNA expression in human tumors. Neoplasia 2001;3:500–8.

87. Gabrilovich DI, Chen HL, Girgis KR, et al. Production of vascular endothelial growth factor by human tumors inhibits the functional maturation of dendritic cells. Nat Med 1996;2:1096–103.

88. Munn DH, Mellor AL. IDO and tolerance to tumors. Trends Mol Med 2004;10:15–8.

89. Uyttenhove C, Pilotte L, Theate I, et al. Evidence for a tumoral immune resistance mechanism based on tryptophan degradation by indoleamine 2,3-dioxygenase. Nat Med 2003;9:1269–74.

90. Miyazaki T, Moritake K, Yamada K, et al. Indoleamine 2,3-dioxygenase as a new target for malignant glioma therapy. J Neurosurg 2009;111(2):230–7.

91. Rao RD, James CD. Altered molecular pathways in gliomas: an overview of clinically relevant issues. Semin Oncol 2004;31:595–604.

92. Bromberg J. Stat proteins and oncogenesis. J Clin Invest 2002;109:1139–42.

93. Bromberg J, Darnell JE Jr. The role of STATs in transcriptional control and their impact on cellular function. Oncogene 2000;19:2468–73.

94. Yu CL, Meyer DJ, Campbell GS, et al. Enhanced DNA-binding activity of a Stat3-related protein in cells transformed by the Src oncoprotein. Science 1995;269:81–3.

95. Rahaman SO, Harbor PC, Chernova O, et al. Inhibition of constitutively active Stat3 suppresses proliferation and induces apoptosis in glioblastoma multiforme cells. Oncogene 2002;21:8404–13.

96. Rahaman SO, Vogelbaum MA, Haque SJ. Aberrant Stat3 signaling by interleukin-4 in malignant glioma cells: involvement of IL-13Ralpha2. Cancer Res 2005;65:2956–63.

97. Konnikova L, Kotecki M, Kruger MM, et al. Knockdown of STAT3 expression by RNAi induces apoptosis in astrocytoma cells. BMC Cancer 2003;3:23.

98. Wang T, Niu G, Kortylewski M, et al. Regulation of the innate and adaptive immune responses by Stat-3 signaling in tumor cells. Nat Med 2004;10: 48–54.

99. Zou W. Immunosuppressive networks in the tumour environment and their therapeutic relevance. Nat Rev Cancer 2005;5:263–74.

100. Steinman RM, Hawiger D, Nussenzweig MC. Tolerogenic dendritic cells. Annu Rev Immunol 2003; 21:685–711.

101. Liu VC, Wong LY, Jang T, et al. Tumor evasion of the immune system by converting CD4+CD25- T cells into CD4+CD25+ T regulatory cells: role of tumor-derived TGF-beta. J Immunol 2007;178:2883–92.

102. Hussain SF, Yang D, Suki D, et al. The role of human glioma-infiltrating microglia/macrophages in mediating antitumor immune responses. Neuro Oncol 2006;8:261–79.

103. Hussain SF, Kong LY, Jordan J, et al. A novel small molecule inhibitor of signal transducers and activators of transcription 3 reverses immune tolerance in malignant glioma patients. Cancer Res 2007;67: 9630–6.

104. Kryczek I, Wei S, Zou L, et al. Cutting edge: Th17 and regulatory T cell dynamics and the regulation by IL-2 in the tumor microenvironment. J Immunol 2007;178:6730–3.

105. Weaver CT, Harrington LE, Mangan PR, et al. Th17: an effector CD4 T cell lineage with regulatory T cell ties. Immunity 2006;24:677–88.

106. Iwakura Y, Ishigame H. The IL-23/IL-17 axis in inflammation. J Clin Invest 2006;116:1218–22.

107. Harris TJ, Grosso JF, Yen HR, et al. Cutting edge: an in vivo requirement for STAT3 signaling in TH17 development and TH17-dependent autoimmunity. J Immunol 2007;179:4313–7.

108. Langowski JL, Zhang X, Wu L, et al. IL-23 promotes tumour incidence and growth. Nature 2006;442:461–5.

109. Cho ML, Kang JW, Moon YM, et al. STAT3 and NF-kappaB signal pathway is required for IL-23-mediated IL-17 production in spontaneous arthritis animal model IL-1 receptor antagonist-deficient mice. J Immunol 2006;176:5652–61.

110. Kortylewski M, Xin H, Kujawski M, et al. Regulation of the IL-23 and IL-12 balance by Stat3 signaling in the tumor microenvironment. Cancer Cell 2009;15:114–23.

111. Itoh N, Yonehara S, Ishii A, et al. The polypeptide encoded by the cDNA for human cell surface antigen Fas can mediate apoptosis. Cell 1991;66:233–43.

112. Krammer PH. CD95's deadly mission in the immune system. Nature 2000;407:789–95.

113. Nagata S. Apoptosis by death factor. Cell 1997;88:355–65.

114. Shinohara H, Yagita H, Ikawa Y, et al. Fas drives cell cycle progression in glioma cells via extracellular signal-regulated kinase activation. Cancer Res 2000;60:1766–72.

115. Saas P, Walker PR, Hahne M, et al. Fas ligand expression by astrocytoma in vivo: maintaining immune privilege in the brain? J Clin Invest 1997;99:1173–8.

116. Walker PR, Saas P, Dietrich PY. Role of Fas ligand (CD95L) in immune escape: the tumor cell strikes back. J Immunol 1997;158:4521–4.

117. Husain N, Chiocca EA, Rainov N, et al. Co-expression of Fas and Fas ligand in malignant glial tumors and cell lines. Acta Neuropathol 1998;95:287–90.

118. Gastman BR, Atarshi Y, Reichert TE, et al. Fas ligand is expressed on human squamous cell carcinomas of the head and neck, and it promotes apoptosis of T lymphocytes. Cancer Res 1999;59:5356–64.

119. Badie B, Schartner J, Prabakaran S, et al. Expression of Fas ligand by microglia: possible role in glioma immune evasion. J Neuroimmunol 2001;120:19–24.

120. Mabrouk I, Buart S, Hasmim M, et al. Prevention of autoimmunity and control of recall response to exogenous antigen by Fas death receptor ligand expression on T cells. Immunity 2008;29:922–33.

121. Hahne M, Rimoldi D, Schroter M, et al. Melanoma cell expression of Fas(Apo-1/CD95) ligand: implications for tumor immune escape. Science 1996;274:1363–6.

122. O'Connell J, O'Sullivan GC, Collins JK, et al. The Fas counterattack: Fas-mediated T cell killing by colon cancer cells expressing Fas ligand. J Exp Med 1996;184:1075–82.

123. Whiteside TL. Tumor-induced death of immune cells: its mechanisms and consequences. Semin Cancer Biol 2002;12:43–50.

124. Andreola G, Rivoltini L, Castelli C, et al. Induction of lymphocyte apoptosis by tumor cell secretion of FasL-bearing microvesicles. J Exp Med 2002;195:1303–16.

125. Vaux DL. Immunology. Ways around rejection. Nature 1998;394:133.

126. Lau HT, Yu M, Fontana A, et al. Prevention of islet allograft rejection with engineered myoblasts expressing FasL in mice. Science 1996;273:109–12.

127. Allison J, Georgiou HM, Strasser A, et al. Transgenic expression of CD95 ligand on islet beta cells induces a granulocytic infiltration but does not confer immune privilege upon islet allografts. Proc Natl Acad Sci U S A 1997;94:3943–7.

128. Kang SM, Schneider DB, Lin Z, et al. Fas ligand expression in islets of Langerhans does not confer immune privilege and instead targets them for rapid destruction. Nat Med 1997;3:738–43.

129. Kang SM, Lin Z, Ascher NL, et al. Fas ligand expression on islets as well as multiple cell lines results in accelerated neutrophilic rejection. Transplant Proc 1998;30:538.

130. Kang SM, Hoffmann A, Le D, et al. Immune response and myoblasts that express Fas ligand. Science 1997;278:1322–4.

131. Restifo NP. Countering the 'counterattack' hypothesis. Nat Med 2001;7:259.

132. Simon AK, Gallimore A, Jones E, et al. Fas ligand breaks tolerance to self-antigens and induces tumor immunity mediated by antibodies. Cancer Cell 2002;2:315–22.

133. Green DR, Ferguson TA. The role of Fas ligand in immune privilege. Nat Rev Mol Cell Biol 2001;2:917–24.

134. O'Connell J, Houston A, Bennett MW, et al. Immune privilege or inflammation? Insights into the Fas ligand enigma. Nat Med 2001;7:271–4.

135. Xia S, Rosen EM, Laterra J. Sensitization of glioma cells to Fas-dependent apoptosis by chemotherapy-induced oxidative stress. Cancer Res 2005;65:5248–55.

136. Giraud S, Bessette B, Boda C, et al. In vitro apoptotic induction of human glioblastoma cells by Fas ligand plus etoposide and in vivo antitumour activity of combined drugs in xenografted nude rats. Int J Oncol 2007;30:273–81.

137. Roth W, Isenmann S, Nakamura M, et al. Soluble decoy receptor 3 is expressed by malignant gliomas and suppresses CD95 ligand-induced

apoptosis and chemotaxis. Cancer Res 2001;61: 2759–65.

138. Wei J, DeAngulo G, Sun W, et al. Topotecan enhances immune clearance of gliomas. Cancer Immunol Immunother 2009;58:259–70.

139. Fortin S, Le Mercier M, Camby I, et al. Galectin-1 is implicated in the protein kinase C epsilon/Vimentin-controlled trafficking of integrin-beta1 in glioblastoma cells. Brain Pathol 2008 [Epub ahead of print].

140. Camby I, Le Mercier M, Lefranc F, et al. Galectin-1: a small protein with major functions. Glycobiology 2006;16:137R–57R.

141. Camby I, Belot N, Rorive S, et al. Galectins are differentially expressed in supratentorial pilocytic astrocytomas, astrocytomas, anaplastic astrocytomas and glioblastomas, and significantly modulate tumor astrocyte migration. Brain Pathol 2001; 11:12–26.

142. Camby I, Belot N, Lefranc F, et al. Galectin-1 modulates human glioblastoma cell migration into the brain through modifications to the actin cytoskeleton and levels of expression of small GTPases. J Neuropathol Exp Neurol 2002;61:585–96.

143. Jung TY, Jung S, Ryu HH, et al. Role of galectin-1 in migration and invasion of human glioblastoma multiforme cell lines. J Neurosurg 2008;109:273–84.

144. Rorive S, Belot N, Decaestecker C, et al. Galectin-1 is highly expressed in human gliomas with relevance for modulation of invasion of tumor astrocytes into the brain parenchyma. Glia 2001;33:241–55.

145. Le Mercier M, Lefranc F, Mijatovic T, et al. Evidence of galectin-1 involvement in glioma chemoresistance. Toxicol Appl Pharmacol 2008;229:172–83.

146. Le Mercier M, Mathieu V, Haibe-Kains B, et al. Knocking down galectin 1 in human hs683 glioblastoma cells impairs both angiogenesis and endoplasmic reticulum stress responses. J Neuropathol Exp Neurol 2008;67:456–69.

147. Rubinstein N, Alvarez M, Zwirner NW, et al. Targeted inhibition of galectin-1 gene expression in tumor cells results in heightened T cell-mediated rejection; a potential mechanism of tumor-immune privilege. Cancer Cell 2004;5:241–51.

148. Toscano MA, Ilarregui JM, Bianco GA, et al. Dissecting the pathophysiologic role of endogenous lectins: glycan-binding proteins with cytokine-like activity? Cytokine Growth Factor Rev 2007;18: 57–71.

149. Rabinovich GA, Baum LG, Tinari N, et al. Galectins and their ligands: amplifiers, silencers or tuners of the inflammatory response? Trends Immunol 2002;23:313–20.

150. Liu FT. Galectins: a new family of regulators of inflammation. Clin Immunol 2000;97:79–88.

151. Perillo NL, Pace KE, Seilhamer JJ, et al. Apoptosis of T cells mediated by galectin-1. Nature 1995;378: 736–9.

152. Rabinovich GA, Ramhorst RE, Rubinstein N, et al. Induction of allogenic T-cell hyporesponsiveness by galectin-1-mediated apoptotic and non-apoptotic mechanisms. Cell Death Differ 2002;9: 661–70.

153. Rabinovich GA, Iglesias MM, Modesti NM, et al. Activated rat macrophages produce a galectin-1-like protein that induces apoptosis of T cells: biochemical and functional characterization. J Immunol 1998;160:4831–40.

154. Blaser C, Kaufmann M, Muller C, et al. Beta-galactoside-binding protein secreted by activated T cells inhibits antigen-induced proliferation of T cells. Eur J Immunol 1998;28:2311–9.

155. Chung CD, Patel VP, Moran M, et al. Galectin-1 induces partial TCR zeta-chain phosphorylation and antagonizes processive TCR signal transduction. J Immunol 2000;165:3722–9.

156. Rabinovich GA, Daly G, Dreja H, et al. Recombinant galectin-1 and its genetic delivery suppress collagen-induced arthritis via T cell apoptosis. J Exp Med 1999;190:385–98.

157. Rabinovich GA, Ariel A, Hershkoviz R, et al. Specific inhibition of T-cell adhesion to extracellular matrix and proinflammatory cytokine secretion by human recombinant galectin-1. Immunology 1999;97:100–6.

158. Le QT, Shi G, Cao H, et al. Galectin-1: a link between tumor hypoxia and tumor immune privilege. J Clin Oncol 2005;23:8932–41.

# Glioblastoma-Derived Mechanisms of Systemic Immunosuppression

Allen Waziri, MD

**KEYWORDS**

- Glioma • Immunity • Immunosuppression
- Immunoregulation • T cell • Monocyte

Nearly 40 years have passed since initial studies documented abnormalities of the cellular immune response in patients with malignant brain tumors.[1,2] Early observations regarding defects in circulating T-cell populations, blunted responses to mitogenic stimulation in vitro, and aberrant delayed type hypersensitivity reactions were confirmed by numerous subsequent experiments.[3] However, despite this long history of study, there is poor understanding of the underlying factors responsible for suppressing effective antitumor immunity in affected individuals.

Throughout the 1970s and 1980s, dedicated efforts were made to outline characteristic changes of the circulating T-cell compartment in patients with malignant glioma and to define the generators of the observed immunosuppressive effect. This initial experimentation was limited by a primitive understanding of the various components and functional characteristics of the cellular immune response. Associated with this lack of basic knowledge was a paucity of experimental tools for detailed study of cells involved with cellular immunity. Thus, further detailed experimentation into the source of suppression of cellular immunity associated with glioblastoma (GBM) was restricted. During the 1990s, the literature documented a shifting of research interests towards tumor-specific vaccines and other immunologically based therapies, driven by continued failures of conventional adjuvant therapies. As with many immunotherapeutic strategies, these research efforts have been largely unsubstantiated in the clinical realm. Although recent work with dendritic cell-based vaccines has shown some potentially promising results,[4] there is no effective option for a vaccine-based therapeutic approach in patients with GBM. A full discussion of these strategies is outside the scope of this article; however, the consideration of prior immunotherapeutic failures is relevant to a discussion of glioma-derived immunosuppression. More specifically, tumor-associated factors involved with suppression of cellular immune responses in patients with GBM are likely to similarly affect any antitumor immunity generated via immunotherapeutic strategies. Therefore, it is important to renew efforts towards elucidating the biologic basis of the observed suppressive effect.

During the late 1980s, the growing acquired immune deficiency syndrome (AIDS) epidemic resulted in a significant dedication of research money and effort to increasing understanding of cellular immunity, most particularly in T-cell biology. The usefulness of specific T-cell markers for phenotypic and functional characterization, and the development of powerful experimental techniques such as flow cytometry and enzyme-linked immunosorbent assay (ELISA)-based cytokine detection, allowed for more detailed study of newly described populations of immunologically relevant cells with widely divergent functional activities. More recently, increasing understanding of the complex interactions involved with regulation of the immune response, including the influence of various cell-surface proteins and

Relevant funding: AW is supported in part by an American Cancer Society-Institutional Research Grant.
Department of Neurosurgery, University of Colorado Health Sciences Center, 12631 E. 17th Avenue, Aurora, CO 80045, USA
*E-mail address:* allen.waziri@uchsc.edu

secreted factors, has provided new opportunities to revisit concepts proposed by pioneering researchers in brain-tumor immunology from prior decades.

This article summarizes critical data that contribute to current theories of the immunosuppressive effects of malignant glioma, focusing on experimentally relevant conditions that either support or preclude the likelihood that an individual factor may play in glioma-associated immunosuppression. Most early research in the field focused on proteins proposed to be expressed on the cell surface or secreted by glioma cells; this article focuses on several key proteins in each group that have been most closely studied. More recently, work has outlined abnormalities inherent to the various monocytic populations in patients with GBM, and the presence and potential functional relevance of regulatory lymphocytes in these patients. In most cases, these factors have been investigated as potential suppressors of activated T cells, putatively responsible for the functionally relevant component of antitumor immunity. This article provides a systems-based framework for understanding potential sources of the glioma-specific immunosuppressive phenomenon, based on a review of prior experimental results and viewed in the light of current immunologic knowledge of the endogenous regulators of cellular immunity.

## CAVEATS IMPORTANT TO CONSIDER WHEN EVALUATING PRIOR WORK

Several caveats should be kept in mind when reviewing the results of prior experimentation in glioma immunology. Recent insight into the endogenous suppressors of cellular immunity, increasing awareness of the complexity of regulatory circuits in immunologic systems, and more common acceptance of the limitations of glioma cell lines and animal models require more critical retrospection of prior experimentation implicating a wide spectrum of glioma-associated factors in the suppression of antitumor immunity.

Cellular heterogeneity is a sine qua non of GBM, with histologic analysis demonstrating an amalgam of presumed tumor cells, reactive astrocytes, tumor-associated microglia, trapped neurons, and various cells infiltrating from the peripheral circulation (including lymphocytes and macrophages).[5] Study of bulk (ie, "unsorted") tumor specimens does not take into consideration potentially significant differences in expression patterns amongst these varied cell types, rendering RNA and protein analysis of limited usefulness. These differences are of critical importance when attempting to categorize phenotypic and functional characteristics of cells involved with the cellular immune response. Although immunohistochemistry (IHC) can provide some specificity of cellular expression and subtumoral anatomic localization, this technique is not particularly conducive to the concurrent detection and quantitation of multiple markers necessary for identification and subclassification of relevant regulatory cells.

The use of glioma cell lines has been a mainstay of research evaluating expression patterns of immunologically relevant markers from malignant brain tumors. However, recent comparative analyses have suggested that there are in fact dissimilarities between commonly used glioma cell lines and direct ex vivo tumor specimens. A seminal series of experiments, recently reported by Howard Fine's group,[6] used comparative chromosomal analysis and microarray expression profiling between a large number of primary GBM specimens and a range of commonly used glioma cell lines (including U87, U251, and T98G). They found that the overall spectrum of genomic alterations differed substantially between primary tumors and the tested cell lines. Their analysis demonstrated that observed expression patterns and genomic abnormalities within tested glioma cell lines were more congruent to abnormalities observed in other nonglioma cell lines, suggesting that selection pressure of in vitro culture resulted in activation or alteration of common "transformation" pathways. Similar analysis of immunologically relevant markers in short passage cultures of fresh human GBM specimens has demonstrated a rapid shift in the expression of immunologically relevant markers, including downregulation of major histocompatibility complex (MHC)-I and increased expression of TGF-β.[7] Recent data supporting the role of "cancer stem cells" found at high frequencies in human GBM and proven to harbor a tumorigenic phenotypic in xenograft models mandate that future in vitro study includes these cell populations.[8,9] Cells with stemlike characteristics are notoriously sensitive to culture conditions for maintenance of a limited-differentiation phenotype, a consideration which sets in vitro experimentation with these populations apart from standardized culture cocktails used in most prior in vitro glioma experimentation. Although such observations do not obviate the results of prior studies investigating the expression of immunologically relevant factors through in vitro culture, these studies mandate that the results of in vitro testing are further confirmed in more biologically relevant systems.

Investigators have used many animal models for comparative analysis in the study of immune responses to malignant brain tumors. These models have been primarily developed in rodents, using stereotactic injection of glioma cell lines into the brains of test animals, allowing for consistent and predictable tumor growth. However, these models often bear little pathologic and immunologic similarity to human GBM. Many of the commonly used rat glioma lines grow as "pushing masses" rather than infiltrating neoplasms, and formed tumors often do not demonstrate the pathologic hallmarks of human malignant glioma.[10] From an immunologic standpoint, these models are often more representative of a transplant system, in some cases even demonstrating genetic mismatch between transferred cell lines and the host animal (rendering the immunologic relevance of these models limited at best).[11] In addition, it is possible that the procedure involved with stereotactic injection of tumor cells may alter the immunologic microenvironment of the brain, providing an increased "danger" signal and promotion of a proinflammatory environment. More recently, xenograft systems using the injection of dissociated human GBM specimens or human glioma cell lines into immunoincompetent rodents has become a commonly accepted method for studying glioma biology.[12] Deficiencies in immunity that allow for engrafting of tumor in these models concurrently prevent any meaningful study into tumor-specific immune responses. In addition, the evaluation of expression patterns of tumors initially derived from human glioma cell lines subsequently xenografted into immunodeficient animals confirms a closer correlation of derived tumors with other long-term cultured cell lines, rather than ex vivo human glioma specimens.[6] More recently, tumor models driven by retroviral targeting of white-matter progenitor cells in rodents have been developed that closely recapitulate the pathologic hallmarks of human GBM (including pseudopallisading necrosis, microvascular proliferation, and infiltrative growth).[13,14] Preliminary studies have suggested that the frequency and phenotype of tumor-infiltrating lymphocytes (TIL) within these lesions more closely resemble profiles of TIL within human GBM than do other rodent models[15–17] (B. Killory and D. Fusco, unpublished data, 2009). Although preliminary, such models may be instrumental in the further study of relevant immune responses to malignant brain tumors.

Although in vitro and animal data are important components of ongoing immunologic research in glioma, increased emphasis must be placed on the further development of more immunologically relevant models and renewed study of fresh human tissues. This article focuses on immunoregulatory factors explored or confirmed to be present within human tissue.

## OBSERVATIONS OF CELLULAR IMMUNITY IN PATIENTS WITH MALIGNANT GLIOMA

What is known about cellular immunity and the antitumor immune response in patients with malignant glioma? T cells can be found within human GBM specimens, although these cells are present at low frequencies and are primarily restricted to the perivascular spaces.[15,18] These intratumoral populations also demonstrate a skew from the expected CD8+ ("effector") phenotype towards a more dominant CD4+ representation.[15,19] Studies have also demonstrated the presence of a limited repertoire of T-cell receptor expression on TIL within GBM specimens, and the presence of a predominantly CD45RA-negative (or "memory") phenotype, suggesting that there may be an antigen-specific expansion of T-cell subsets within these lesions.[15,20,21] In addition, tumor antigen-specific T cells can be generated from bulk peripheral blood mononuclear cell (PBMC) samples from affected patients, providing evidence for potential tumor-specific cellular immunity.[18] However, these potentially tumor-specific T cells are ultimately ineffective at providing any benefit in regards to tumor control. Certain T-cell abnormalities can be temporarily reversed following tumor resection, and subsequently return with tumor recurrence, potentially confirming an association between tumor and the suppressive phenotype rather than a global defect in cellular immunity.[22]

Circulating T cells in patients with glioma-associated immunosuppression seem to be globally abnormal through in vitro analysis. Although not systemically immunocompromised, these patients generally exhibit a loss of CD4+ cells, resulting in a CD4/CD8 ratio closer to 1 (rather than the usual 2:1) and a total mild lymphopenia. CD4+ and CD8+ T cells are handicapped in their response to in vitro mitogenic stimulation, a phenomenon that has been partially attributed to decreased production of and hyporesponsiveness to interleukin 2 (IL-2).[3] Aside from widely reported anomalies of T-cell number and function in patients with GBM, further detailed analyses of various signaling pathways involved with T-cell activation have demonstrated significant abnormalities in expression levels and poststimulation phosphorylation patterns of proteins downstream from the T-cell receptor, including PLC$\gamma$1, pp100 and p56lck.[23]

The aforementioned findings offer critical insights into the nature of GBM-associated immunosuppression. First, T cells can enter the tumor microenvironment and potentially respond specifically to antigen, but these cells are somehow blocked in their ability to expand into effector populations and provide tumor clearance. Second, considering that most peripheral/circulating T cells are never physically exposed to tumor cells, and assuming that affected patients are not globally immunocompromised, the presumed tumor-specific immunosuppressive factor must extend far beyond the tumor microenvironment. Third, considering that relative immunosuppression can be transiently reversed following tumor extirpation, and returns with tumor recurrence, the tumor itself provides a driving force behind the generation of the immunosuppressive effect.

## SUPPRESSIVE SURFACE MARKERS EXPRESSED ON GLIOMA CELLS

Several studies have explored the expression of surface markers on GBM cells with putative suppressive effects on cellular immunity. The most widely explored of these factors is likely Fas ligand (FasL or CD95L). Fas (CD95) is constitutively expressed on activated T cells in CD4 and CD8 compartments, and the Fas/FasL system is known to be an important regulator of activated T-cell populations. Binding of Fas and FasL is believed to be critical in mediating activation-induced cell death (AICD). AICD is essential for downregulating activated T-cell populations at the termination of immune responses, for maintaining T-cell homeostasis, and in the prevention of autoimmunity.[24] Although FasL is primarily expressed on the surface of activated T cells, several groups have documented the expression of FasL on the surface of glioma cells.[25-28] The resulting hypothesis focuses on the potential killing of activated tumor-specific T cells through cell-cell contact with FasL-expressing glioma cells, thereby resulting in effective escape from the cellular immune response. To provide potential functional relevance for this hypothesis, Ichinose and colleagues[26] correlated the expression of FasL in 9 of 14 GBM specimens with decreased numbers of TILs in relevant samples. Yu and colleagues[19] performed double-staining IHC for FasL and endothelial cell markers, finding that approximately 30% of tested GBM samples demonstrated positive FasL staining on tumor vasculature. In contrast to the findings of Ichinose and colleagues,[26] these investigators did not find any correlation between FasL expression and extent of lymphocytic infiltration, although they did identify a shift in CD4/CD8 ratios in positive samples. Frankel and colleagues[29] identified increased levels of soluble FasL in fluid aspirated from cystic malignant gliomas. Surface-bound FasL can be cleaved by metalloproteinases, resulting in a soluble yet functional form of the protein.[24] Soluble FasL within cystic aspirates from astrocytoma was effective at inducing cell death in cultured Jurkat cells.[29] These investigators suggested that elevated FasL in cyst fluid is representative of concentrations in the tumor extracellular microenvironment and therefore potentially effective at killing infiltrating tumor-specific T cells.

The expression of nonclassic human leukocyte antigen (HLA) molecules by glioma cells has also been explored as a potential source of immunosuppression. In contrast to classically described MHC-Ia molecules, which are expressed on cells of virtually all tissue types and primarily responsible for peptide presentation to CD8+ T cells, MHC-Ib molecules bind a restricted set of peptides and have been primarily associated with natural killer (NK) cell-mediated immunity through the binding of the CD94/NKG2 class of receptors.[30] The expression of these markers, previously associated with suppression of cellular immunity, has been explored in GBM. The first of these is HLA-G, which has been identified on the surface of several glioma cell lines and a limited subset of fresh glioma samples.[31] A potential functional role for HLA-G in glioma was demonstrated through gene transfer experiments, which suggested that forced expression of HLA-G by U87 glioma cells rendered the transfected cells resistant to killing by alloreactive PBMCs.[31] Additional studies demonstrated that increased levels of soluble HLA-G can be detected in sera from patients with multiple malignancies, including glioma, although a functional role for this finding has not been defined.[32] HLA-E, a second member of the MHC-Ib family, has been similarly associated with glioma. Advanced tumor grade is paralleled by increasing levels of tumor-specific HLA-E expression, although no functional relevance has been provided for this finding.[33] A potentially contradictory association between expression of HLA-E in GBM specimens with increasing numbers of infiltrating CD8+ T cells has been reported,[34] resulting in an unclear impact of these nonclassic HLA proteins on glioma-specific cellular immunity.

More recent data have explored the potential functional relevance of glioma-specific expression of B7-homolog 1 (B7-H1, also known as programmed death ligand 1, or PD-L1). The CD28-B7 family of costimulatory molecules has been expanded to include several receptor-ligand pairs that have potent regulatory effects on antigen-specific T cells. The classic role for the canonical members of this family, CD28 (expressed on T cells) and B7-1 (expressed on antigen-presenting cells), is to provide necessary costimulation in the process of antigen-specific activation through the T-cell receptor. Newer members of this family, including B7-H1, have been suggested to be critical regulators and suppressors of activated T-cell function.[35] Involvement of B7-H1 in glioma-associated immunosuppression has been hypothesized and explored by several groups. Studies have demonstrated low-level expression of this marker on multiple glioma cell lines.[36,37] In addition, single-color IHC has provided evidence for B7-H1 positivity in the small number of GBM samples tested.[36] Further experimentation demonstrated that coculture of alloreactive T cells with B7-H1+ cell lines, in the presence of blocking antibodies, can drive increased expression of proinflammatory cytokines and T-cell activation markers. However, no evidence for increased T-cell death was identified in the absence of blocking antibodies, which argues against a baseline functional role in this system.[36] A series of experiments recently reported by Parsa and colleagues[38] identified a link between the commonly identified mutation in phosphatase and tensin homolog (PTEN) and increased expression of B7-H1. Expression levels of B7-H1 were directly correlated with loss of PTEN function, shown to be secondary to increased Akt activity and posttranscriptional upregulation of B7-H1 on the cell surface. PTEN-deleted cells were rendered less susceptible to cytotoxic T lymphocyte-mediated targeting, providing evidence for a potential functional connection between a commonly identified mutation in GBM and the immunosuppressive effect.[38]

Although the expression of immunosuppressive factors on the surface of glioma cells may provide some explanation for local effects on activated T cells, this hypothesis does not adequately define a comprehensive solution to the systemic immunosuppression problem. Again, considering that most circulating T cells do not come into direct contact with tumor cells, additional far-reaching factors are necessary to explain the characteristically global defects in affected individuals.

## GLIOMA-SECRETED FACTORS WITH POTENTIAL IMMUNOSUPPRESSIVE EFFECTS

In 1984, Fontana and colleagues[39] presented the first report providing evidence for a factor secreted from cultured glioma cells that inhibited IL-2-induced T-cell proliferation and blocked allogeneic T-cell responses in mixed lymphoid reactions. Over the next several years, continued study from this group, and others, confirmed the immunosuppressive effects of this factor.[40–42] Purification and sequencing of the responsible protein, initially named GBM-derived T-cell suppressor factor (G-TsF), demonstrated significant homology with human transforming growth factor beta (TGF-$\beta$). Subsequent study found G-TsF to be identical to TGF-$\beta$2.[43,44] Expression of all 3 isoforms of TGF-$\beta$ by GBM was ultimately documented.[45,46] This family of proteins has been shown to significantly impair activation of T cells and monocytes, and more recently TGF-$\beta$ has been associated with the generation of CD4+ T regulatory cells (Treg, discussed later). Although most data have focused on the expression of TGF-$\beta$ by glioma cells in culture, potential in vivo relevance has been provided through IHC analysis of GBM specimens, indicating that areas of high extracellular TGF-$\beta$ concentration within tumor samples have fewer numbers of infiltrating lymphocytes than do regions with lower levels of TGF-$\beta$.[47] Although the secretion of TGF-$\beta$ provides a compelling explanation for glioma-associated immunosuppression, the potential for systemic effects is unclear. Several studies using comparative analysis of TGF-$\beta$ levels in serum from GBM patients and controls identified no difference between the 2 groups, suggesting that systemic levels were not significantly altered by the presence of tumor.[48,49]

Tumor-specific production of immunosuppressive prostanoids, most notably prostaglandin E2 (PGE-2), has also been associated with suppression of antitumor immunity. Studies have demonstrated high levels of expression of cyclooxygenase type 2 (COX-2) and arachadonic acid (the substrate for prostanoid production) in malignant glioma. Elevated intratumoral levels of these factors have been correlated with increasing pathologic grade and proliferative behavior. These findings have resulted in some interest in the use of selective COX-2 inhibitors for treatment of GBM.[50] Production of PGE-2 has also been suggested to play a role in GBM-associated immunosuppression, although attempts to demonstrate PGE-2-specific immunosuppressive effects, using coculture experiments with mitogen-driven proliferation of PBMC in the presence of glioma supernatant, have provided mixed results.[51,52] A more recent study suggested that COX-2 expression by GBM, with secondary induction of IL-10 production from intermediary dendritic cells, resulted in the generation of CD4+ Treg cells.[53] This effect could be blocked by selective COX-2 inhibitors and subsequently rescued via addition of exogenous PGE-2, although in vivo correlates of these findings have yet to be provided.

Multiple studies have attempted to link expression of the immunosuppressive cytokine IL-10 with glioma-associated immune inhibition. Early reports used real-time polymerase chain reaction to demonstrate increased levels of IL-10 mRNA within bulk GBM specimens.[54,55] However, subsequent studies using in-situ hybridization confirmed that IL-10 was not expressed by putative glioma cells. Rather, IL-10 expression could be specifically localized to circulating monocytes and tumor-associated microglia/infiltrating macrophages within these tumors.[56–58] The role of immunosuppressive mononuclear cells is discussed in more detail later.

It remains difficult to conceptualize a mechanism by which factors secreted locally by glioma cells could reach serum concentrations sufficient to repress T-cell function globally. In addition, it seems unlikely that such a factor could be subsequently transferred into in vitro, tumor-free studies at a sufficient concentration to exert continued suppressive effects in experimental systems. However, GBM-secreted factors may play an important role in recruiting or driving the development of a secondary immunosuppressive agent.

## ABNORMALITIES OF MONOCYTIC POPULATIONS IN PATIENTS WITH GBM

Several studies in the early 1980s suggested that glass-adherent cell populations (notably monocytes) were involved with suppression of T-cell proliferation in response to mitogenic stimulation, secondary to observations that exclusion of these cells from PBMC cultures partially restored proliferative defects.[59,60] Since that time, few studies have focused on the potential immunosuppressive effect of this population, despite the central role that monocytes and their progeny, including the potent antigen-presenting dendritic cells, play in shaping cellular immune responses in various systems. It has been shown that a soluble factor (or factors) secreted by GBM cells in vitro can induce functionally relevant changes in monocyte cultures, including downregulation of IL-12, MHC-II, and the costimulatory molecules CD80 and CD86.[61] These changes are associated with a concomitant increase in IL-10 production,[61] consistent with prior observations identifying monocytic cells as the predominant source of IL-10 within GBM specimens. A recent study by Kostianovsky and colleagues[62] further explored the potential influence exerted by glioma cells on microglia/macrophages, demonstrating that monocytes cultured with glioma cells are rendered tolerogenic for CD4+ T cells and cocultured monocytes.

More recently, a subset of monocytic cells, which have been consolidated under the rubric of the myeloid-derived suppressor cell (MDSC), have been studied as potent inactivators of CD4+ and CD8+ T cells and have been increasingly identified in several human cancers.[63] In addition to their expression of CD11b and variable expression of CD14, MDSC have been characterized to express CD33, CD34, and decreased levels of HLA-DR.[63] Patients with GBM harbor a relative peripheral monocytosis.[60,64,65] In addition, several studies have indicated that a high percentage of circulating monocytes in patients with GBM harbor a subset of functional abnormalities previously described as characteristic of MDSC. Flow cytometry-based analysis of the expression of relevant surface markers on peripheral blood monocytes from patients with GBM demonstrates decreased numbers of HLA-DR+ cells.[49,64] Ogden and colleagues[64] also noted that peripheral monocytes from these patients harbor significant deficits in the in vitro generation of mature dendritic cells compared with circulating monocytes from patients with other intracranial tumors. Further functional characterization of these abnormal monocytic populations in GBM patients is ongoing in the authors' laboratory and others.

From a systemic standpoint, monocytes have the potential to traffic into and out of areas of immunologic activity within the central nervous system, thereby providing a hypothetical bridge between the tumor microenvironment and circulating lymphocyte populations.[66] It is therefore possible that monocytes accessing the local tumor environment are encouraged by tumor-specific factors to adopt functional characteristics of MDSC, which subsequently spill back into the circulation to exert suppressive effects on peripherally located T cells. Although these data provide intriguing preliminary evidence, confirmation of the MDSC phenotype in GBM patients has yet to be completed. In addition, a potential mechanistic link between GBM and the development of cells with possible MDSC characteristics remains to be identified.

## IDENTIFICATION AND CHARACTERIZATION OF T CELLS WITH REGULATORY CHARACTERISTICS IN GBM

Over the past decade, several newly described populations of T cells with potent regulatory properties have been studied in various immunologic systems, including malignant brain tumors. The presence of lymphocytes with suppressive effects on activated T cells in patients with GBM was initially suggested decades ago.[59,67] However, recent experimentation in other immunologic systems, focusing on the identification and characterization of regulatory cells, has provided significant insight into new mechanisms for endogenous regulation of cellular immunity.

The most well-characterized class of relevant lymphocytes is the "T regulatory cell," or "Treg." Progressive analysis of these cells has provided detailed knowledge regarding their phenotype and functional activity. Tregs are a subset of CD4+ T cells, generally found at low numbers within circulating T-cell populations of normal individuals, which have been most definitively identified by their expression of the transcription factor FoxP3.[68] In addition to their expression of CD4 and FoxP3, Tregs are typified by increased expression of the high-affinity IL-2 receptor (also known as CD25). Although all T cells upregulate CD25 in response to activation, levels of CD25 on Tregs are distinctly higher than levels expressed by other activated T cells.[68] In addition to being CD25hi, Tregs have been shown to express CTLA-4, glucocorticoid-induced tumor necrosis factor receptor (GITR), and various other markers.[69] The powerful functional activity of Tregs in the suppression and regulation of activated T cells has been described in many immunologic systems. Studies involving depletion of Tregs in animal models have confirmed their central role in preventing autoimmunity.[70] In addition, depletion of Tregs provides improved immune responses to nonself antigens (ie, bacterial infection) and tumors in several animal models.[71,72] The mechanism by which Tregs are generated or recruited remains unclear; however, studies of T-cell receptor expression on Treg populations suggest that these cells may have increased affinity for self-antigen/MHC complexes.[70] As Tregs are believed to emerge from the thymus in a previously mature state, it is possible that T cells with significant self-reactivity during early selection may be shunted into the Treg population within the thymus itself.[70] Tregs are proposed to exert their suppressive effects through secretion of cytokines (TGF-β, IL-10), perforin/granzyme-mediated killing of responder T cells, or by modulation of antigen presenting cell (APC) function.[70] Tregs have also been shown to express the endonucleosidases CD39 and CD73, responsible for extracellular generation of adenosine, which has immunosuppressive properties.[73]

Several groups have explored a potential role for Tregs in the suppression of cellular immunity in patients with GBM. Fecci and colleagues[74] identified an increased percentage of cells expressing high levels of CD25 and CD45RO within the circulating compartment of CD4+ T cells compared with normal volunteers. Further experiments using sorted populations of CD4+ T cells that were depleted of CD25+ cells demonstrated that observed deficiencies in mitogen-induced proliferation could be recovered with this strategy. Finally, using a murine intracranial glioma model, these investigators demonstrated that depletion of Treg populations using an anti-CD25 antibody resulted in improved survival. Parallel analysis of the frequency of putative Tregs within PBMC and TIL from patients with GBM was performed by El Andaloussi and colleagues,[75] who suggested that nearly 25% of all CD4+ cells within TIL were Tregs. However, it is unclear whether these cells were all truly Tregs as the gating strategy identified all CD25+ cells, a fraction which is known to contain not only Tregs but also traditional activated T cells. A series of correlative experiments were performed by Heimberger and colleagues,[76] who used single-color IHC to quantify the number of FoxP3+ cells within gliomas of varying grade and histologic subtype. They found an association between increased numbers of FoxP3+ cells with advanced tumor grade, and noted that the presence of FoxP3+ cells within GBM was associated with poorer prognosis. A caveat inherent to their analysis was a lack of phenotypic or functional confirmation of a true Treg phenotype, caused by the use of single-color IHC. This finding is particularly relevant in light of data recently presented by Ebert and colleagues,[77] who used 2-color IHC to demonstrate that FoxP3 can be expressed by ex vivo melanoma cells and a wide range of cancer cell lines, including GBM. The authors have used direct ex vivo multicolor flow cytometric analysis to quantify the frequency of Tregs within PBMC and TIL from patients with a range of intracranial tumors. Frequencies of CD4+CD25hi Tregs were similar within PBMC from patients with GBM, metastatic tumors, and meningioma. Although there was an increase in the proportion of Tregs within the CD4+ compartment of TIL from GBM, there was a nearly 10-fold increase in the number of similar cells in patients with metastatic lesions.[15] Recent data suggest that Tregs may play a role in glioma-associated immunosuppression. However, factors involved with the recruitment of these cells, and the contribution they may provide in blunting tumor-specific immune responses, remain to be determined.

A second class of lymphocytes with immunoregulatory properties is the natural killer T (NKT) cell, a diverse population that expresses an array of traditional NK cell markers (such as CD56) in addition to the T-cell receptor and the coactivation receptor CD3. In contrast to canonical T lymphocytes, NKT cells are believed to be restricted to interaction with the nonclassic HLA-like CD1d molecule, suggesting a role as a regulatory bridge between the innate and adaptive immune systems.[78] NKT cells have attracted interest because of their capacity for rapid expression of high levels of Th1 or Th2 cytokines following stimulation, supporting their role as key early regulators in the cellular immune response. The traditional, or "type I," NKT cell expresses an invariant T-cell receptor and has known responsiveness to the glycolipid α-galactosylceramide (aGalCer). In experimental stimulation paradigms, type I NKT cells have been shown to produce Th1 and Th2 cytokines, and their ability to confer potent tumor killing in animal models has encouraged the study of this subset as a possible avenue for tumor immunotherapy. More recently, a second subset of NKT cells has been described. These "type II" NKT cells remain restricted to CD1d interaction but express a variable T-cell receptor. Recent studies have implicated type II NKT cells, and more specifically the CD4 single-positive population, in the suppression of antitumor immunity and the prevention of autoimmunity.[79–81] Terabe and colleagues[82] recently elucidated the mechanism of type II NKT cell suppression of the antitumor immune response using a mouse fibrosarcoma model, in which they demonstrated that IL-13 expression by CD4+ NKT cells specifically induced the activity of CD11b+Gr-1+ myeloid suppressor cells (MDSC, discussed earlier), which were in turn directly responsible for suppression of tumor-specific cytotoxic T cells.

The authors have recently published data documenting the presence of a novel population of CD4+ NKT cells found within TIL from direct ex vivo GBM specimens. Using comparative flow cytometric analysis of fresh intracranial tumor samples, the authors demonstrated that a significant percentage of TIL from GBM were CD4+CD56+ NKT cells. Although the percentage of peripheral NKT cells was similar between patients with GBM, metastatic tumors, and meningiomas, the increased proportion of NKT cells within TIL was unique to GBM (**Fig. 1**). NKT cells within GBM demonstrated evidence for antigenic activation and intratumoral proliferation, and direct ex vivo comparative analysis of cytokine expression patterns in matched peripheral T cells and TIL from GBM, using intracellular cytokine detection, demonstrated a significant increase in the percentage of T cells expressing IL-13 within GBM specimens.[15] Studies are ongoing to provide further functional relevance for NKT cells in

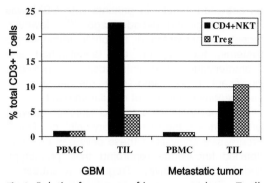

**Fig. 1.** Relative frequency of immunoregulatory T cells within PBMC and TIL from patients with GBM and metastatic lung tumors. Plots represent percentage of the total CD3+ fraction, determined by flow cytometry, that are either CD4+CD56+ NKT cells or CD4+CD25hi Treg cells.

patients with GBM and to identify potential sources of recruitment or intratumoral stimulation of these cells. Although preliminary, these studies suggest intriguing parallels between the NKT cells found within GBM and those described in animal models associated with the NKT-MSC immunosuppressive circuit.

The role that immunoregulatory lymphocytes play in glioma-associated suppression of cellular immunity, and potential tumor-specific pathways responsible for their generation or recruitment, is unclear. However, the regulatory T-cell hypothesis is attractive for several reasons. First, these cells have been increasingly identified as the primary regulators of the cellular immune response in many immunologic systems. The likelihood that these cells play a similar role in GBM offers an explanation. Second, the presence of these cells within the peripheral circulation allows for an explanation of system-wide aberrations in cellular immunity, which is otherwise difficult to explain through the action of a locally expressed factor. Finally, potential biologic relevance of these cells can be studied in animal models in a detailed and mechanistic fashion, allowing for the development of potential therapeutic strategies aimed at exclusion or functional disruption of the suppressive element.

## SUMMARY

Although glioma-associated suppression of cellular immunity has been discussed for several decades, little clinically relevant progress in the understanding of this phenomenon has occurred. The continued failure of immunotherapeutic strategies, in conjunction with exciting new insights into the endogenous regulators of cellular immunity, warrants renewed effort towards eluci- dation of factors involved with immunosuppres- sion in GBM and the pathways associated with their generation.

A continuing theoretic conundrum in the study of glioma-related immunosuppression is that locally induced factors exert powerful effects on a more systemic level. It is possible that genetic mutation or otherwise altered expression of regulatory factors by tumor cells, driven by selective immu- nologic pressure, may derive the eventual escape from antitumor immunity. However, in contrast to the more sinister hypotheses focusing on de- novo, glioma-specific expression of immunosup- pressive factors, observed defects in affected patients may simply represent tumor cooptation of endogenous, naturally regulated systems that function to shape cellular immunity. As under- standing of the significant complexity of endoge- nous immunoregulatory networks grows, it becomes increasingly unlikely that a single factor, whether cell-associated or secreted, is respon- sible for the wide-ranging immunosuppressive effects seen in patients with GBM. More likely, identification of a series of cognate regulatory events, best elucidated at the systems level, will provide a binding hypothesis for the failure of anti- tumor cellular immunity.

Further studies using glioma cell lines, nonphy- siologic culture systems, or poorly congruent animal models are not likely to provide meaningful insights into the nature of glioma-associated immunosuppression. Use of ex vivo human-tissue samples and newly developed animal models, in conjunction with correlative analysis from other immunologic systems, are more likely to provide relevant data for ongoing research. The continued participation and collaborative role of neurosur- geons in providing and studying fresh human tissues will continue to be an essential element of these research efforts, and of extending results into the clinical realm.

Suppression of cellular immune responses in patients with GBM remains poorly understood. Tumor-associated factors that function to suppress endogenous cellular immunity are likely to affect the efficacy of immunotherapeutic strate- gies similarly, therefore mandating the application of renewed effort towards the elucidation and ther- apeutic targeting of these factors. Recent obser- vations regarding endogenous systems of immune control, and initial insights into mecha- nisms by which these systems are activated and regulated, allow for potential advances in improving antitumor immunity and the develop- ment of new therapeutic options for patients with GBM.

## REFERENCES

1. Brooks WH, Netsky MG, Normansell DE, et al. Depressed cell-mediated immunity in patients with primary intracranial tumors. Characterization of a humoral immunosuppressive factor. J Exp Med 1972;136(6):1631–47.

2. Brooks WH, Caldwell HD, Mortara RH. Immune responses in patients with gliomas. Surg Neurol 1974;2(6):419–23.

3. Dix AR, Brooks WH, Roszman TL, et al. Immune defects observed in patients with primary malignant brain tumors. J Neuroimmunol 1999;100(1-2): 216–32.

4. Wheeler CJ, Black KL, Liu G, et al. Vaccination elicits correlated immune and clinical responses in glio- blastoma multiforme patients. Cancer Res 2008; 68(14):5955–64.

5. McComb RD, Bigner DD. The biology of malignant gliomas–a comprehensive survey. Clin Neuropathol 1984;3(3):93–106.

6. Li A, Walling J, Kotliarov Y, et al. Genomic changes and gene expression profiles reveal that established glioma cell lines are poorly representative of primary human gliomas. Mol Cancer Res 2008;6(1):21–30.

7. Anderson RC, Elder JB, Brown MD, et al. Changes in the immunologic phenotype of human malignant glioma cells after passaging in vitro. Clin Immunol 2002;102(1):84–95.

8. Ogden AT, Waziri AE, Lochhead RA, et al. Identifica- tion of A2B5+CD133− tumor-initiating cells in adult human gliomas. Neurosurgery 2008;62(2):505–14 [discussion: 514–5].

9. Singh SK, Hawkins C, Clarke ID, et al. Identification of human brain tumour initiating cells. Nature 2004; 432(7015):396–401.

10. Barth RF. Rat brain tumor models in experimental neuro-oncology: the 9L, C6, T9, F98, RG2 (D74), RT-2 and CNS-1 gliomas. J Neurooncol 1998;36(1): 91–102.

11. Parsa AT, Chakrabarti I, Hurley PT, et al. Limitations of the C6/Wistar rat intracerebral glioma model: implications for evaluating immunotherapy. Neuro- surgery 2000;47(4):993–9 [discussion: 999–1000].

12. Goldbrunner RH, Wagner S, Roosen K, et al. Models for assessment of angiogenesis in gliomas. J Neuro- oncol 2000;50(1-2):53–62.

13. Assanah M, Lochhead R, Ogden A, et al. Glial progenitors in adult white matter are driven to form malignant gliomas by platelet-derived growth factor-expressing retroviruses. J Neurosci 2006; 26(25):6781–90.

14. Shih AH, Dai C, Hu X, et al. Dose-dependent effects of platelet-derived growth factor-B on glial tumori- genesis. Cancer Res 2004;64(14):4783–9.

15. Waziri A, Killory B, Ogden AT 3rd, et al. Preferential in situ CD4+CD56+ T cell activation and expansion

within human glioblastoma. J Immunol 2008; 180(11):7673–80.

16. Kennedy BC, Maier LM, D'Amico R, et al. Dynamics of central and peripheral immunomodulation in a murine glioma model. BMC Immunol 2009;10:11.

17. Candolfi M, Curtin JF, Nichols WS, et al. Intracranial glioblastoma models in preclinical neuro-oncology: neuropathological characterization and tumor progression. J Neurooncol 2007;85(2):133–48.

18. Dunn GP, Dunn IF, Curry WT. Focus on TILs: prognostic significance of tumor infiltrating lymphocytes in human glioma. Cancer Immun 2007;7:12.

19. Yu JS, Lee PK, Ehtesham M, et al. Intratumoral T cell subset ratios and Fas ligand expression on brain tumor endothelium. J Neurooncol 2003;64(1-2): 55–61.

20. Perrin G, Schnuriger V, Quiquerez AL, et al. Astrocytoma infiltrating lymphocytes include major T cell clonal expansions confined to the CD8 subset. Int Immunol 1999;11(8):1337–50.

21. Ebato M, Nitta T, Yagita H, et al. Skewed distribution of TCR V alpha 7-bearing T cells within tumor-infiltrating lymphocytes of HLA-A24(9)-positive patients with malignant glioma. Immunol Lett 1993;39(1):53–64.

22. Kempuraj D, Devi RS, Madhappan B, et al. T lymphocyte subsets and immunoglobulins in intracranial tumor patients before and after treatment, and based on histological type of tumors. Int J Immunopathol Pharmacol 2004;17(1):57–64.

23. Morford LA, Elliott LH, Carlson SL, et al. T cell receptor-mediated signaling is defective in T cells obtained from patients with primary intracranial tumors. J Immunol 1997;159(9):4415–25.

24. Strasser A, Jost PJ, Nagata S. The many roles of FAS receptor signaling in the immune system. Immunity 2009;30(2):180–92.

25. Didenko VV, Ngo HN, Minchew C, et al. Apoptosis of T lymphocytes invading glioblastomas multiforme: a possible tumor defense mechanism. J Neurosurg 2002;96(3):580–4.

26. Ichinose M, Masuoka J, Shiraishi T, et al. Fas ligand expression and depletion of T-cell infiltration in astrocytic tumors. Brain Tumor Pathol 2001;18(1):37–42.

27. Husain N, Chiocca EA, Rainov N, et al. Co-expression of Fas and Fas ligand in malignant glial tumors and cell lines. Acta Neuropathol 1998;95(3):287–90.

28. Saas P, Walker PR, Hahne M, et al. Fas ligand expression by astrocytoma in vivo: maintaining immune privilege in the brain? J Clin Invest 1997; 99(6):1173–8.

29. Frankel B, Longo SL, Canute GW. Soluble Fas-ligand (sFasL) in human astrocytoma cyst fluid is cytotoxic to T-cells: another potential means of immune evasion. J Neurooncol 2000;48(1):21–6.

30. O'Callaghan CA, Bell JI. Structure and function of the human MHC class Ib molecules HLA-E, HLA-F and HLA-G. Immunol Rev 1998;163:129–38.

31. Wiendl H, Mitsdoerffer M, Hofmeister V, et al. A functional role of HLA-G expression in human gliomas: an alternative strategy of immune escape. J Immunol 2002;168(9):4772–80.

32. Rebmann V, Regel J, Stolke D, et al. Secretion of sHLA-G molecules in malignancies. Semin Cancer Biol 2003;13(5):371–7.

33. Wischhusen J, Friese MA, Mittelbronn M, et al. HLA-E protects glioma cells from NKG2D-mediated immune responses in vitro: implications for immune escape in vivo. J Neuropathol Exp Neurol 2005; 64(6):523–8.

34. Mittelbronn M, Simon P, Loffler C, et al. Elevated HLA-E levels in human glioblastomas but not in grade I to III astrocytomas correlate with infiltrating CD8+ cells. J Neuroimmunol 2007;189(1-2):50–8.

35. Greenwald RJ, Freeman GJ, Sharpe AH. The B7 family revisited. Annu Rev Immunol 2005;23:515–48.

36. Wintterle S, Schreiner B, Mitsdoerffer M, et al. Expression of the B7-related molecule B7-H1 by glioma cells: a potential mechanism of immune paralysis. Cancer Res 2003;63(21):7462–7.

37. Wilmotte R, Burkhardt K, Kindler V, et al. B7-homolog 1 expression by human glioma: a new mechanism of immune evasion. Neuroreport 2005;16(10):1081–5.

38. Parsa AT, Waldron JS, Panner A, et al. Loss of tumor suppressor PTEN function increases B7-H1 expression and immunoresistance in glioma. Nat Med 2007;13(1):84–8.

39. Fontana A, Hengartner H, de Tribolet N, et al. Glioblastoma cells release interleukin 1 and factors inhibiting interleukin 2-mediated effects. J Immunol 1984;132(4):1837–44.

40. Schwyzer M, Fontana A. Partial purification and biochemical characterization of a T cell suppressor factor produced by human glioblastoma cells. J Immunol 1985;134(2):1003–9.

41. Wrann M, Bodmer S, de Martin R, et al. T cell suppressor factor from human glioblastoma cells is a 12.5-kd protein closely related to transforming growth factor-beta. EMBO J 1987;6(6):1633–6.

42. Roszman TL, Brooks WH, Elliott LH. Inhibition of lymphocyte responsiveness by a glial tumor cell-derived suppressive factor. J Neurosurg 1987; 67(6):874–9.

43. Kuppner MC, Hamou MF, Bodmer S, et al. The glioblastoma-derived T-cell suppressor factor/transforming growth factor beta 2 inhibits the generation of lymphokine-activated killer (LAK) cells. Int J Cancer 1988;42(4):562–7.

44. Bodmer S, Strommer K, Frei K, et al. Immunosuppression and transforming growth factor-beta in glioblastoma. Preferential production of transforming growth factor-beta 2. J Immunol 1989;143(10): 3222–9.

45. Yamada N, Kato M, Yamashita H, et al. Enhanced expression of transforming growth factor-beta and

its type-I and type-II receptors in human glioblastoma. Int J Cancer 1995;62(4):386–92.

46. Constam DB, Philipp J, Malipiero UV, et al. Differential expression of transforming growth factor-beta 1, -beta 2, and -beta 3 by glioblastoma cells, astrocytes, and microglia. J Immunol 1992;148(5):1404–10.

47. Horst HA, Scheithauer BW, Kelly PJ, et al. Distribution of transforming growth factor-beta 1 in human astrocytomas. Hum Pathol 1992;23(11):1284–8.

48. Krzyszkowski T, Dziedzic T, Czepko R, et al. Decreased levels of interleukin-10 and transforming growth factor-beta 2 in cerebrospinal fluid of patients with high grade astrocytoma. Neurol Res 2008;30(3):294–6.

49. Woiciechowsky C, Asadullah K, Nestler D, et al. Diminished monocytic HLA-DR expression and ex vivo cytokine secretion capacity in patients with glioblastoma: effect of tumor extirpation. J Neuroimmunol 1998;84(2):164–71.

50. Nathoo N, Barnett GH, Golubic M. The eicosanoid cascade: possible role in gliomas and meningiomas. J Clin Pathol 2004;57(1):6–13.

51. Lauro GM, Di Lorenzo N, Grossi M, et al. Prostaglandin E2 as an immunomodulating factor released in vitro by human glioma cells. Acta Neuropathol 1986;69(3-4):278–82.

52. Couldwell WT, Dore-Duffy P, Apuzzo ML, et al. Malignant glioma modulation of immune function: relative contribution of different soluble factors. J Neuroimmunol 1991;33(2):89–96.

53. Akasaki Y, Liu G, Chung NH, et al. Induction of a CD4+ T regulatory type 1 response by cyclooxygenase-2-overexpressing glioma. J Immunol 2004; 173(7):4352–9.

54. Nitta T, Hishii M, Sato K, et al. Selective expression of interleukin-10 gene within glioblastoma multiforme. Brain Res 1994;649(1–2):122–8.

55. Huettner C, Paulus W, Roggendorf W. Messenger RNA expression of the immunosuppressive cytokine IL-10 in human gliomas. Am J Pathol 1995;146(2):317–22.

56. Huettner C, Czub S, Kerkau S, et al. Interleukin 10 is expressed in human gliomas in vivo and increases glioma cell proliferation and motility in vitro. Anticancer Res 1997;17(5A):3217–24.

57. Wagner S, Czub S, Greif M, et al. Microglial/macrophage expression of interleukin 10 in human glioblastomas. Int J Cancer 1999;82(1):12–6.

58. Samaras V, Piperi C, Korkolopoulou P, et al. Application of the ELISPOT method for comparative analysis of interleukin (IL)-6 and IL-10 secretion in peripheral blood of patients with astroglial tumors. Mol Cell Biochem 2007;304(1-2):343–51.

59. Braun DP, Penn RD, Flannery AM, et al. Immunoregulatory cell function in peripheral blood leukocytes of patients with intracranial gliomas. Neurosurgery 1982;10(2):203–9.

60. Wood GW, Morantz RA. Depressed T lymphocyte function in brain tumor patients: monocytes as suppressor cells. J Neurooncol 1983;1(2):87–94.

61. Zou JP, Morford LA, Chougnet C, et al. Human glioma-induced immunosuppression involves soluble factor(s) that alters monocyte cytokine profile and surface markers. J Immunol 1999; 162(8):4882–92.

62. Kostianovsky AM, Maier LM, Anderson RC, et al. Astrocytic regulation of human monocytic/microglial activation. J Immunol 2008;181(8):5425–32.

63. Ostrand-Rosenberg S, Sinha P. Myeloid-derived suppressor cells: linking inflammation and cancer. J Immunol 2009;182(8):4499–506.

64. Ogden AT, Horgan D, Waziri A, et al. Defective receptor expression and dendritic cell differentiation of monocytes in glioblastomas. Neurosurgery 2006; 59(4):902–9 [discussion: 909–10].

65. Rapp M, Ozcan Z, Steiger HJ, et al. Cellular immunity of patients with malignant glioma: prerequisites for dendritic cell vaccination immunotherapy. J Neurosurg 2006;105(1):41–50.

66. Hickey WF. Leukocyte traffic in the central nervous system: the participants and their roles. Semin Immunol 1999;11(2):125–37.

67. Elliott LH, Brooks WH, Roszman TL. Activation of immunoregulatory lymphocytes obtained from patients with malignant gliomas. J Neurosurg 1987; 67(2):231–6.

68. Baecher-Allan C, Anderson DE. Regulatory cells and human cancer. Semin Cancer Biol 2006;16(2): 98–105.

69. Brusko TM, Putnam AL, Bluestone JA. Human regulatory T cells: role in autoimmune disease and therapeutic opportunities. Immunol Rev 2008;223:371–90.

70. Sakaguchi S, Yamaguchi T, Nomura T, et al. Regulatory T cells and immune tolerance. Cell 2008;133(5): 775–87.

71. Shimizu J, Yamazaki S, Sakaguchi S. Induction of tumor immunity by removing CD25+CD4+ T cells: a common basis between tumor immunity and autoimmunity. J Immunol 1999;163(10):5211–8.

72. Belkaid Y, Rouse BT. Natural regulatory T cells in infectious disease. Nat Immunol 2005;6(4):353–60.

73. Dwyer KM, Deaglio S, Gao W, et al. CD39 and control of cellular immune responses. Purinergic Signal 2007;3(1-2):171–80.

74. Fecci PE, Mitchell DA, Whitesides JF, et al. Increased regulatory T-cell fraction amidst a diminished CD4 compartment explains cellular immune defects in patients with malignant glioma. Cancer Res 2006;66(6):3294–302.

75. El Andaloussi A, Lesniak MS. An increase in CD4+CD25+FOXP3+ regulatory T cells in tumor-infiltrating lymphocytes of human glioblastoma multiforme. Neuro Oncol 2006;8(3):234–43.

76. Heimberger AB, Abou-Ghazal M, Reina-Ortiz C, et al. Incidence and prognostic impact of FoxP3+ regulatory T cells in human gliomas. Clin Cancer Res 2008;14(16):5166–72.

77. Ebert LM, Tan BS, Browning J, et al. The regulatory T cell-associated transcription factor FoxP3 is expressed by tumor cells. Cancer Res 2008;68(8): 3001–9.

78. Berzofsky JA, Terabe M. NKT cells in tumor immunity: opposing subsets define a new immunoregulatory axis. J Immunol 2008;180(6):3627–35.

79. Moodycliffe AM, Nghiem D, Clydesdale G, et al. Immune suppression and skin cancer development: regulation by NKT cells. Nat Immunol 2000;1(6):521–5.

80. Park JM, Terabe M, van den Broeke LT, et al. Unmasking immunosurveillance against a syngeneic colon cancer by elimination of CD4+ NKT regulatory cells and IL-13. Int J Cancer 2005;114(1):80–7.

81. Terabe M, Berzofsky JA. The role of NKT cells in tumor immunity. Adv Cancer Res 2008;101: 277–348.

82. Terabe M, Matsui S, Park JM, et al. Transforming growth factor-beta production and myeloid cells are an effector mechanism through which CD1d-restricted T cells block cytotoxic T lymphocyte-mediated tumor immunosurveillance: abrogation prevents tumor recurrence. J Exp Med 2003; 198(11):1741–52.

# Microglia and Central Nervous System Immunity

Gurvinder Kaur, BS, Seunggu J. Han, BS,
Isaac Yang, MD*, Courtney Crane, PhD

**KEYWORDS**

- Microglia • Central nervous system
- Immunity • Glioma immunology

The central nervous system (CNS) has evolved as an immune-privileged site to protect its vital functions from damaging immune-mediated inflammation. With the protective shield of the blood-brain barrier and lack of lymphatic system, the CNS strictly regulates the entry of most peripheral immune cells, soluble factors, and plasma proteins in homeostasis.[1] However, during a CNS injury or disease such as multiple sclerosis (MS),[2] T-cell and peripheral antigen-presenting–cell (APC) infiltration are involved in the observed pathogenesis. Thus, there must be a CNS-adapted system of surveillance that continuously evaluates local changes in the nervous system and communicates to the peripheral immune system during an injury or a disease. Recent advances leading to a better understanding of the CNS disease processes has placed microglia, the CNS-based resident macrophages, at center stage in this system of active surveillance. Microglia are tightly regulated by their local environment, including neuron-microglia interactions during homeostasis, and they remain quiescent.[3] In the steady-state CNS, microglia cells express the macrophage marker CD11b and exhibit a resting phenotype characterized by a low-level expression of major histocompatibility complex (MHC) class I and II and co-stimulatory molecules like CD86 and CD40.[4–6] Conversely, in the event of an insult or injury, microglia cells increase mobility,[7] phagocytosis,[8,9] and proliferation,[10] and they contribute to resulting immune responses and inflammation by releasing various reactive oxygen intermediates, cytokines, and chemokines.[11] In comparison to macrophage responses in the peripheral tissues, microglia responses on activation are restricted, spatially and temporally, to preserve an immunologically silent CNS environment.[12] Microglia as APCs also contribute to activating T-cell responses by upregulating MHC and co-stimulatory molecules, generating specific CD4 and CD8 memory responses.[13–15] Therefore, microglia are essential components of the innate and adaptive aspects of immune responses in the CNS, similar to macrophages in the peripheral tissues.

Considering these broad immune functions, it is not surprising to see microglia accumulation in almost every CNS disease process; examples include CNS tumors, particularly malignant gliomas, which account for nearly half of primary CNS neoplasm and are known to accumulate a large number of microglia and a small population of lymphocytes. Initial observation of this high percentage of microglia in gliomas led many to deduce their role in antitumor activity and in cell death (necrosis) associated with many gliomas like glioblastoma multiforme (GBM). However, in recent years, the accumulating evidence strongly suggests that microglia cells contribute to the immunosuppressive environment of gliomas and can actually promote tumor growth.[16,17] This article discusses the role of microglia in CNS immunity and highlights key advances made in glioma immunology.

Department of Neurological Surgery, University of California at San Francisco, 505 Parnassus Avenue, One Shrader Street, Suite 650, San Francisco, CA 94117, USA
* Corresponding author.
*E-mail address:* yangi@neurosurg.ucsf.edu (I. Yang)

Neurosurg Clin N Am 21 (2010) 43–51
doi:10.1016/j.nec.2009.08.009

## ORIGIN OF MICROGLIA

Microglia constitute 5% to 20% of total glial cell population in the CNS, making them as abundant as neurons.[18–20] They were first recognized by Nissl, who named them "Staebchenzellen" or rod cells for their rod-shaped nuclei and considered them to be reactive neuroglia suggesting a capacity for migration and phagocytosis. In 1913, Santiago Ramon y Cajal described microglia as part of 3 elements of the CNS. It was del Rio Hortega, after his studies on young animals, who established microglia as distinct from other non-neuronal cell types, astrocytes and oligodendrocytes. Hortega described microglia's origin from mononuclear cells of the circulating blood and believed that these cells have the ability to transform from resting ramified form into amoeboid phagocytic macrophages.[21] These conclusions were based on Hortega's observations from stab wounds made in the mature brains of various animal species. In 1925, Wilder Penfield further usedthe special silver-staining method utilized by Hortega to provide the first detailed descriptions of microglia in glioma tissue. After a long debate over the role and origin of microglia in the CNS, they have been established as a phenotypically, developmentally, and functionally distinct population of glial cells that are of myelomonocytic origin. The microglia precursor cells of monocyte-macrophage lineage are derived from mesodermal hematopoietic cells, which in mammals originate from the yolk sac.[22] These circulating precursor cells invade the developing brain during perinatal stages and transform into microglia cells that express several macrophage-specific markers, including Toll-like receptors (TLRs),[23,24] the integrin CD11b,[25] and the glycoprotein of unknown function, F4/80, but they have lower levels of the leukocyte common antigen, CD45, when compared with macrophages.[26,27] These findings together with the phagocytic activity of microglia strongly suggest that microglia are closely related to peripheral monocytes.

Recent studies have classified microglia into 3 types according to their morphologic appearance: resting ramified microglia, activated reactive microglia, and amoeboid phagocytic microglia.[22] Furthermore, consistent with the immunologically silent nature of the CNS, the invading amoeboid microglia in perinatal life transform into ramified resting microglia during postnatal life, which represent a fairly permanent population with slower turnover when compared with macrophages of other tissues.[28,29] According to studies done by Lawson and colleagues,[19,20] the resting ramified microglia are less numerous in white matter than in gray matter, and they adapt the morphology of their cell bodies, processes, and expression of cell surface markers to their microenvironment. The microglia remain in the resting state until a stimulus from an injury, infection, or other neurodegenerative process activates them to transform back into activated amoeboid phagocytic cells.[8,9]

## MICROGLIA AS A SYSTEM OF ACTIVE SURVEILLANCE

In the steady state, the fairly quiescent-looking microglia cells undergo continuous pinocytosis to sample the surrounding microenvironment, as a way of conducting routine surveillance of the CNS.[30] Neuron-to-microglia communication also plays a key role in the surveillance, and it shapes the quiescent and reactive states of microglia. In vitro studies have provided evidence that electrically active neurons inhibit $T_H1$ cytokine interferon (IFN)-$\gamma$-induced expression of major histocompatibility complex (MHC) class II molecules on astrocytes and microglia,[31] whereas some neurotransmitter molecules like substance P[32] enhance the pro-inflammatory phenotype of microglia. These opposing actions of various neurotransmitters suggest the existence of a complex set of interactions between local inhibitory and stimulatory signals in shaping microglia responses. In vivo studies conducted by Hoek and colleagues[33,34] have led to the characterization of a previously identified membrane-bound glycoprotein termed OX2 or CD200 expressed on neurons as a key regulator of microglia. In OX2-deficient mice, microglia exhibit an activated phenotype with enhanced CD45 and complement type-3 receptor (CR3) along with less ramified morphology. In addition, OX2- deficient mice show an accelerated reactive response to an injury. Thus, neurons deliver inhibitory signals to microglia through OX2 receptor signaling pathway. These findings in combination strongly support the idea of microenvironment regulation of microglia function.

Moreover, the plasticity of microglia in function and morphology directly correlates with its interactions with the microenvironment. Granulocyte-macrophage colony-stimulating factor (GM-CSF) and M-CSF are known to play a crucial role in the terminal differentiation of tissue macrophages.[35,36] In Alzheimer disease and MS, it has been shown that levels of GM-CSF are elevated in addition to upregulation in M-CSF receptor.[37,38] With in vitro studies, Fischer and Reichmann have demonstrated that the incubation of purified microglia with GM-CSF increases microglia cell size, and it generates a heterogeneous population that contains cells resembling other tissue macrophages and microglia cells expressing CD11c and MHC class II molecules.[39] These studies indicate that microglia cells are poised to use their range of plasticity in response to their microenvironment changes.

## MICROGLIA AS MEDIATORS OF INFLAMMATION

One key similarity of microglia and peripheral macrophages is the ability to contribute significantly to innate and adaptive immune responses. The resting microglia cells are activated by various stimuli, such as lipopolysaccharide (LPS), β amyloid, IFN-γ, thrombin, and some proinflammatory cytokines, involved in infection, neurodegenerative diseases, and CNS injury.[40] Upon stimulation, the resting ramified microglia undergo a series of morphologic and functional changes to mobilize the cellular and molecular defense of the CNS. For example, it has been demonstrated that microglia express TLRs[23] that interact with bacterial cell wall components to initiate innate response such as production of cytokines, chemokines, and nitric oxide.[41,42] The molecules released by microglia in response to stimuli include (1) proinflammatory cytokines interleukin (IL)-1,[43] IL-6,[44] and tumor necrosis factor (TNF)-α[45]; and (2) monocyte chemoattractant protein-1 (MCP-1),[46] macrophage inflammatory protein 1 (MIP-1),[47,48] and regulated on activation normal T cell expressed and secreted (RANTES)[49]; and (3) chemokines involved in lymphocyte recruitment. This implicates microglia as a critical first line of defense because the adaptive immune cells typically take longer to respond to pathogens present in the CNS. Once the microenvironment of the CNS has become activated, the local cells produce proinflammatory cytokines and chemokines and upregulate immunomodulatory surface markers to contribute to local inflammatory response in addition to decreasing the stringency of the blood brain barrier. This allows the entry of soluble factors and immune effector cells from the periphery,[50] such as macrophages, natural killer cells, and lymphocytes.[51,52] Early activation of microglia before peripheral cell infiltration is supported by bone marrow chimera studies demonstrating that microglia activation precedes the entry of peripheral macrophages.[35] Microglia also exhibit phagocytic and cytotoxic functions during CNS infection and injury. On microglia activation, there is upregulation of opsonic receptors, including complement receptors (CR1, CR3, CR4) and FcγR (I,II,III), which enhances phagocytosis by binding to complement components and immunoglobulin fragments respectively.[53,54] Microglia are known to function as transitory phagocytes during CNS ontogeny to clear apoptotic neuronal cell bodies,[55] and in experimental autoimmune encephalitis (EAE), the animal model of MS, T-cell debris is phagocytosed by microglia.[56] Phagocytosis by microglia directly induces the production of reactive radicals to degrade cellular debris. Moreover, microglia secrete superoxide radicals and nitric oxide into their microenvironment in response to pathogens and cytokine stimulation.[57]

Antigen presentation is a critical event involved in the generation of T-cell responses against the pathogen, as part of pathogen-specific adaptive immune response. The antigen presentation requires interaction between the T-cell receptor and the processed antigen peptide presented on MHC molecules on the surface of APCs. MHC class I and MHC class II molecules stimulate CD8 cytotoxic cells and CD4 T-helper cells, respectively. Additional key interactions between co-stimulatory molecules, such as B7-1 (CD80), B7-2 (CD86), and CD40, expressed on the surface of APC and specific counter-receptors on T cells are required for optimal T-cell–APC adhesion and activation.[58,59] Within the CNS parenchyma under steady-state conditions, MHC class I and II expression is generally minimal or absent, and when present, it is restricted to microglia in low levels.[6,60,61] According to the studies done by Ford and colleagues[62] in normal rodent brains, microglia behave as poor APCs under resting conditions. However, in inflammatory and neurodegenerative conditions, microglia readily upregulate MHC expression[63] along with co-stimulatory molecules.[64] In particular, the interaction of CD80 and CD86 molecules on microglia with CD28 expressed on T cells is required for inducing T-cell cytokine secretion, growth, and survival.[58] Additionally, microglia CD40 interaction with CD40L on T cells enhances expression of MHC class II, nitric synthase and CD80/CD86 molecules on microglia, which in turn further promote T-cell activation.[59] In EAE, the animal model of MS, both microglia and blood-derived macrophages have been shown to express MHC class II and co-stimulatory molecules.[65] Additionally, in vivo and in vitro studies have demonstrated that IFN-γ, a cytokine secreted by pre-activated CD4 T cells and NK cells, induces and maintains MHC class II and adhesion/co-stimulatory molecule expression on microglia to maintain stimulation of T cells.[66]

In addition to initiating innate and adaptive immune responses, microglia contribute to downregulating inflammatory responses. In the absence of sufficient co-stimulatory molecules, the interaction of Fas ligand (FasL) on APCs with the Fas receptor on the T cell will lead to activation-induced T cell apoptosis.[67] In vitro[68,69] and in vivo studies of EAE[70] have detected FasL expression on microglia. Cytotoxic molecules like nitric oxide produced by microglia can also contribute to the death of immune effector response. Additionally, microglia can express Fas molecules on their surface that can interact with FasL-expressing cells, leading to their own apoptosis.[70] These studies indicate that microglia activity in a neuropathology can be self-limiting in addition to regulating other immune effector cells.

## MICROGLIA IN CNS GLIOMAS
### Microglia Chemoattraction and Proliferation in Glioma

Histopathologic studies of glioma tissue have consistently identified a high infiltrating population of microglia within gliomas.[71–75] Badie and colleagues[75] using flow cytometry showed one-third of glioma cells to be expressing resident microglia markers, and this exceeds the number of other immune cells in gliomas. It has been proposed that microglia accumulation at the site of a CNS tumor is due to the local production of chemoattractants and growth factors. For example, MCP-1 is produced by glioma cells, and microglia have been found to express the MCP-1 receptor, CCR2, on their surface.[76,77] Thus, local production of MCP-1 may help recruit microglia to the site of glioma. Furthermore, growth factors such as colony stimulating factor-1 (CSF-1), granulocyte colony-stimulating factor (G-CSF) and hepatocyte growth factor/scatter factor (HGF/SF) have been known to be secreted by various gliomas,[78–80] and these growth factors along with serving chemokine signals also promote proliferation of microglia. Therefore, gliomas are actively promoting microglia trafficking and proliferation by secreting chemokines and growth factors.

### Microglia's Role in Tumor Progression

The recruitment of microglia in brain tumors was postulated as an attempt by the CNS to destroy invading neoplastic cells.[81] However, in recent years, it has become increasingly evident that the immune defense functions of microglia against glioma are compromised because there is no strong evidence of tumor rejection, and tumors grow despite increased microglia invasion over time. Also, the microglia, instead of being localized to the area of necrosis, are found diffusely throughout tumor parenchyma and do not appear to be phagocytosing tumor cells or debris.[2] Growing evidence suggests that glioma infiltrating microglia/macrophages may actually be promoting tumor growth.[82] For instance, though MHC molecule expression has been detected on microglia cells in gliomas,[83,84] they appear to be deficient in proper antigen presentation[85] for cytotoxic and helper T-cell activation. The number of microglia cells expressing MHC class II antigen is further reduced in high-grade gliomas, despite the abundance of microglia in these CNS neoplasms. Schartner and colleagues[16] demonstrated that microglia isolated from tumor-expressing mice do not show MHC class II upregulation following in vivo stimulation, thereby preventing the induction of an efficient antitumor immune response. Additionally, the expression of MHC class II and co-stimulatory B7 molecules was significantly increased when freshly isolated microglia were cultured in the absence of glioma cells.[86] Alternatively, the interaction of microglia with T cells can inhibit T-cell function by increased expression of inhibitory molecules. In particular, increased expression of co-stimulatory molecule B7-H1 on APCs induces T cell apoptosis. Microglia express B7-H1 in homeostasis, but the expression is upregulated in pathologic conditions including gliomas.[87,88] Thus, it is likely that upregulation of inhibitory molecules like B7-H1 may contribute to inhibition of T-cell activation, and even apoptosis, regardless of the presence of MHC molecules.[89]

FasL is another inhibitory molecule expressed on tumor-associated microglia that may play a key role in limiting the ability of T cells to recognize and respond to tumor cells. FasL-expressing cells induce apoptosis of CD8 T cells and thus, the upregulation of FasL on tumor-associated microglia may serve as another mechanism to limit tumor recognition by cytotoxic cells. Microglia in intracranial tumors express FasL and the inhibition of FasL activity has been demonstrated to dramatically increase the number of peripheral immune effector cells in tumors.[90] In a study by Parney and colleagues,[91] coculturing human peripheral blood mononuclear cells with human glioma lines caused glioma-conditioned monocytes to reduce phagocytosis and induce apoptosis of activated lymphocytes when added to the glioma-monocyte culture. Kostianovsky and colleagues[92] studied microglia/monocyte activation in GBM. They found that the presence of GBM tumor cells downregulated the production of the proinflammatory cytokine TNF-$\alpha$ by microglia after LPS stimulation and instead, anti-inflammatory cytokine IL-10 was induced. The immunosuppression by microglia was maintained with different stimulus signals such as $\beta$ amyloid, suggesting that GBM tumor cells affect microglia/monocyte activation regardless of the nature of stimuli. Moreover, glioma cells produce anti-inflammatory cytokines, such as IL-6, transforming growth factor (TGF)-β2, and prostaglandin E2, and tumor-growth–promoting cytokines, such as IL-1 and bFGF.[2,93] TGF-β2 in particular inhibits proliferation and secretion of pro-inflammatory cytokines by microglia and lymphocytes.[94] These studies together suggest that the phagocytosis, pro-inflammatory cytokine secretion, and antigen presentation functions of microglia are strongly suppressed by glioma cells.

Microglia, under the influence of an immunosuppressive environment, also secrete anti-inflammatory cytokines such as IL-10 that enable rapid proliferation of tumor cells by inhibiting cytotoxic T cell.[95] Additionally in vitro studies have demonstrated that IL-10 suppresses microglia antigen presentation function by inhibiting IFN-γ–induced MHC class II expression.[96] Thus, microglia IL-10 secretion further contributes to the maintenance of an immunosuppressive environment. Microglia are known to be the cellular source of matrix metalloproteinase-2 (MMP-2), extracellular matrix-degrading enzymes, and their release into the tumor environment can help increase the spread of tumors because in the absence of extracellular matrix, tumor cells are free to proliferate.[97] Microglia also secret tumor proliferation promoting factors including epidermal growth factor (EGF) and vascular endothelial growth factor (VEGF),[38,98] which are well known to be involved in glial cell proliferation and tumor angiogenesis. These studies in combination suggest that microglia play an integrative role in the tumor progression by supporting migration (MMP-9), angiogenesis (VEGF), and proliferation (EGF) of glioma cells.

## Therapeutic Potential of Microglia in Glioma

Microglia are potent immune effector cells that display a broad range of functionality, mediating both innate and adaptive responses during CNS injury and disease while remaining quiescent in the steady state. In addition to their significant numbers in gliomas, their versatility in bridging the gap between the immune-privileged CNS and the peripheral immune system makes them a potential candidate in immunotherapy treatment. Microglia associated with CNS tumors do not seem to be active in inducing antitumor T-cell response; there is potential for overcoming glioma-induced immunosuppression, so that activated microglia can enhance CNS immunity against tumors. For instance, signal transducer and activator of transcription (Stat) 3 protein

inhibitors have been found to activate microglia and T cell immune responses in malignant glioma.[92,99–101] Signal transducers and activators of transcription proteins are a family of transcription factors activated by tyrosine kinases such as epidermal growth factor receptor (EGFR) in response to tumor-secreted factors including VEGF, IL-6, and IL-10.[102,103] On activation, the Stat proteins translocate to the nucleus and bind to specific elements within target promoters to regulate gene expression.[104] Malignant gliomas are well known for their dysregulation of the EGFR pathway via amplification, mutation of EGFR, and upregulation of Stat3 activation.[105–108] Stat signaling, in particular Stat3, regulates immune activation and tolerance by altering transcription of several genes that control tumor cell survival, resistance to apoptosis, cell cycle progression, and angiogenesis in glioma cells.[109] These findings suggest that Stat3 is abnormally activated through EGFR dysregulation and contributes to glioma proliferation and immunosuppression.

In vitro studies, Iwamaru and colleagues[100] demonstrated that a novel small molecule, WP1066—a pharmacologic derivative of the natural compound caffeic acid—inhibits Stat3 activation. Stat3 signaling inhibition downregulates gene expression of Bcl-XL, Mcl-1, and c-myc and induces apoptosis resulting in significant inhibition of tumor cell growth in human malignant glioma cell lines U87-MG and U373-MG. Studies by Hussain and colleagues[99] demonstrated that Stat3 inhibition by WP1066 reversed immune tolerance in GBM by upregulating co-stimulatory molecules CD80 and CD86 in glioma-infiltrating microglia and peripheral blood monocytes and inducing effector T cell–stimulating cytokines, such as IL-2, IL-4, IL-12, and IL-15. Collectively, these studies indicate that the inhibition of Stat3 activity could be a promising therapeutic strategy for the treatment of patients with malignant gliomas due to its potent immune adjuvant responses.

Additionally, studies by Carpentier and colleagues[110,111] demonstrated long-term survival in animals with established CNS glioma using single intratumoral injection of CpG oligodeoxynucleotide, an immunostimulatory sequence that signals through TLR9 to induce production of IFN-α, IFN-β, IL-12, and TNF-α. However, animals with macrophage/microglia depletion were unable to reject tumor after CpG treatment, showing that microglia/macrophages are a critical component of antitumor response.[112] Though CpG is fairly safe in humans, an improved understanding of microglia function in gliomas can provide better methods of manipulating the glioma microenvironment to allow effective antigen presentation to T cells.

## REFERENCES

1. Pachter JS, de Vries HE, Fabry Z. The blood-brain barrier and its role in immune privilege in the central nervous system. J Neuropathol Exp Neurol 2003;62(6):593–604.

2. Hao C, Parney IF, Rao WH, et al. Cytokine and cytokine receptor mRNA expression in human glioblastomas: evidence of Th1, Th2 and Th3 cytokine dysregulation. Acta Neuropathol (Berl) 2002; 103(2):171–8.

3. Ayoub AE, Salm AK. Increased morphological diversity of microglia in the activated hypothalamic supraoptic nucleus. J Neurosci 2003;23(21):7759–66.

4. Sedgwick JD, Schwender S, Imrich H, et al. Isolation and direct characterization of resident microglial cells from the normal and inflamed central nervous system. Proc Natl Acad Sci U S A 1991; 88(16):7438–42.

5. Aloisi F, De Simone R, Columba-Cabezas S, et al. Functional maturation of adult mouse resting microglia into an APC is promoted by granulocyte-macrophage colony-stimulating factor and interaction with Th1 cells. J Immunol 2000;164(4): 1705–12.

6. Hoftberger R, Aboul-Enein F, Brueck W, et al. Expression of major histocompatibility complex class I molecules on the different cell types in multiple sclerosis lesions. Brain Pathol 2004;14(1): 43–50.

7. Carbonell WS, Murase SI, Horwitz AF, et al. Infiltrative microgliosis: activation and long-distance migration of subependymal microglia following periventricular insults. J Neuroinflammation 2005; 2(1):5.

8. Schroeter M, Jander S, Huitinga I, et al. Phagocytic response in photochemically induced infarction of rat cerebral cortex. The role of resident microglia. Stroke 1997;28(2):382–6.

9. Zhang SC, Goetz BD, Carre JL, et al. Reactive microglia in dysmyelination and demyelination. Glia 2001;34(2):101–9.

10. Eliason DA, Cohen SA, Baratta J, et al. Local proliferation of microglia cells in response to neocortical injury in vitro. Brain Res Dev Brain Res 2002;137(1): 75–9.

11. Liu L, Persson JK, Svensson M, et al. Glial cell responses, complement, and clusterin in the central nervous system following dorsal root transection. Glia 1998;23(3):221–38.

12. Aloisi F. Immune function of microglia. Glia 2001; 36(2):165–79.

13. Brannan CA, Roberts MR. Resident microglia from adult mice are refractory to nitric oxide-inducing stimuli due to impaired NOS2 gene expression. Glia 2004;48(2):120–31.

14. Aloisi F, Ria F, Penna G, et al. Microglia are more efficient than astrocytes in antigen processing and in Th1 but not Th2 cell activation. J Immunol 1998;160(10):4671–80.

15. Aloisi F, Ria F, Columba-Cabezas S, et al. Relative efficiency of microglia, astrocytes, dendritic cells and B cells in naive CD4+ T cell priming and Th1/Th2 cell restimulation. Eur J Immunol 1999; 29(9):2705–14.

16. Schartner JM, Hagar AR, Van Handel M, et al. Impaired capacity for upregulation of MHC class II in tumor-associated microglia. Glia 2005;51(4):279–85.

17. Bettinger I, Thanos S, Paulus W. Microglia promote glioma migration. Acta Neuropathol 2002;103(4): 351–5.

18. Benveniste EN. Role of macrophages/microglia in multiple sclerosis and experimental allergic encephalomyelitis. J Mol Med 1997;75(3):165–73.

19. Lawson LJ, Perry VH, Dri P, et al. Heterogeneity in the distribution and morphology of microglia in the normal adult mouse brain. Neuroscience 1990;39(1):151–70.

20. Lawson LJ, Perry VH, Gordon S. Turnover of resident microglia in the normal adult mouse brain. Neuroscience 1992;48(2):405–15.

21. Del Rio-Hortega P. Microglia. In: Penfield W, editor. Cytology and cellular pathology of the nervous system, vol. 11. New York: Paul B Hoeber; 1932. p. 481–534.

22. Ling EA, Wong WC. The origin and nature of ramified and amoeboid microglia: a historical review and current concepts. Glia 1993;7(1):9–18.

23. Bsibsi M, Ravid R, Gveric D, et al. Broad expression of Toll-like receptors in the human central nervous system. J Neuropathol Exp Neurol 2002; 61(11):1013–21.

24. Olson JK, Miller SD. Microglia initiate central nervous system innate and adaptive immune responses through multiple TLRs. J Immunol 2004;173(6):3916–24.

25. Akiyama H, McGeer PL. Brain microglia constitutively express beta-2 integrins. J Neuroimmunol 1990;30(1):81–93.

26. Dick AD, Ford AL, Forrester JV, et al. Flow cytometric identification of a minority population of MHC class II positive cells in the normal rat retina distinct from CD45lowCD11b/c+CD4low parenchymal microglia. Br J Ophthalmol 1995;79(9): 834–40.

27. Becher B, Antel JP. Comparison of phenotypic and functional properties of immediately ex vivo and cultured human adult microglia. Glia 1996;18(1):1–10.

28. Hess DC, Abe T, Hill WD, et al. Hematopoietic origin of microglial and perivascular cells in brain. Exp Neurol 2004;186(2):134–44.

29. Kennedy DW, Abkowitz JL. Kinetics of central nervous system microglial and macrophage engraftment: analysis using a transgenic bone marrow transplantation model. Blood 1997;90(3):986–93.

30. Nimmerjahn A, Kirchhoff F, Helmchen F. Resting microglial cells are highly dynamic surveillants of brain parenchyma in vivo. Science 2005; 308(5726):1314–8.

31. Neumann H, Boucraut J, Hahnel C, et al. Neuronal control of MHC class II inducibility in rat astrocytes and microglia. Eur J Neurosci 1996;8(12):2582–90.

32. McCluskey LP, Lampson LA. Local neurochemicals and site-specific immune regulation in the CNS. J Neuropathol Exp Neurol 2000;59(3):177–87.

33. Hoek RM, Ruuls SR, Murphy CA, et al. Down-regulation of the macrophage lineage through interaction with OX2 (CD200). Science 2000;290(5497): 1768–71.

34. Wright GJ, Puklavec MJ, Willis AC, et al. Lymphoid/neuronal cell surface OX2 glycoprotein recognizes a novel receptor on macrophages implicated in the control of their function. Immunity 2000;13(2): 233–42.

35. Schilling M, Besselmann M, Leonhard C, et al. Microglial activation precedes and predominates over macrophage infiltration in transient focal cerebral ischemia: a study in green fluorescent protein transgenic bone marrow chimeric mice. Exp Neurol 2003;183(1):25–33.

36. De Simone R, Ajmone-Cat MA, Tirassa P, et al. Apoptotic PC12 cells exposing phosphatidylserine promote the production of anti-inflammatory and neuroprotective molecules by microglial cells. J Neuropathol Exp Neurol 2003;62(2):208–16.

37. Kreuzfelder E, Menne S, Ferencik S, et al. Assessment of peripheral blood mononuclear cell proliferation by [2-3H]adenine uptake in the woodchuck model. Clin Immunol Immunopathol 1996;78(3): 223–7.

38. Tsai JC, Goldman CK, Gillespie GY. Vascular endothelial growth factor in human glioma cell lines: induced secretion by EGF, PDGF-BB, and bFGF. J Neurosurg 1995;82(5):864–73.

39. Fischer HG, Reichmann G. Brain dendritic cells and macrophages/microglia in central nervous system inflammation. J Immunol 2001;166(4): 2717–26.

40. Dheen ST, Kaur C, Ling EA. Microglial activation and its implications in the brain diseases. Curr Med Chem 2007;14(11):1189–97.

41. Banati RB, Gehrmann J, Schubert P, et al. Cytotoxicity of microglia. Glia 1993;7(1):111–8.

42. Nakamichi K, Saiki M, Sawada M, et al. Double-stranded RNA stimulates chemokine expression in microglia through vacuolar pH-dependent activation of intracellular signaling pathways. J Neurochem 2005;95(1):273–83.

43. Hartlage-Rubsamen M, Lemke R, Schliebs R. Interleukin-1beta, inducible nitric oxide synthase, and nuclear factor-kappaB are induced in morphologically distinct microglia after rat hippocampal lipopolysaccharide/interferon-gamma injection. J Neurosci Res 1999;57(3):388–98.

44. Suzumura A, Sawada M, Marunouchi T. Selective induction of interleukin-6 in mouse microglia by granulocyte-macrophage colony-stimulating factor. Brain Res 1996;713(1–2):192–8.

45. Floden AM, Li S, Combs CK. Beta-amyloid-stimulated microglia induce neuron death via synergistic stimulation of tumor necrosis factor alpha and NMDA receptors. J Neurosci 2005;25(10):2566–75.

46. Babcock AA, Kuziel WA, Rivest S, et al. Chemokine expression by glial cells directs leukocytes to sites of axonal injury in the CNS. J Neurosci 2003;23(21): 7922–30.

47. Si Q, Cosenza M, Zhao ML, et al. GM-CSF and M-CSF modulate beta-chemokine and HIV-1 expression in microglia. Glia 2002;39(2):174–83.

48. Takami S, Nishikawa H, Minami M, et al. Induction of macrophage inflammatory protein MIP-1alpha mRNA on glial cells after focal cerebral ischemia in the rat. Neurosci Lett 1997;227(3):173–6.

49. Chen CJ, Chen JH, Chen SY, et al. Upregulation of RANTES gene expression in neuroglia by Japanese encephalitis virus infection. J Virol 2004; 78(22):12107–19.

50. Lu J, Moochhala S, Kaur C, et al. Cellular inflammatory response associated with breakdown of the blood-brain barrier after closed head injury in rats. J Neurotrauma 2001;18(4):399–408.

51. Tonra JR, Reiseter BS, Kolbeck R, et al. Comparison of the timing of acute blood-brain barrier breakdown to rabbit immunoglobulin G in the cerebellum and spinal cord of mice with experimental autoimmune encephalomyelitis. J Comp Neurol 2001;430(1):131–44.

52. Baldwin AC, Kielian T. Persistent immune activation associated with a mouse model of Staphylococcus aureus-induced experimental brain abscess. J Neuroimmunol 2004;151(1–2):24–32.

53. Peress NS, Fleit HB, Perillo E, et al. Identification of Fc gamma RI, II and III on normal human brain ramified microglia and on microglia in senile plaques in Alzheimer's disease. J Neuroimmunol 1993;48(1):71–9.

54. Barnum SR. Inhibition of complement as a therapeutic approach in inflammatory central nervous system (CNS) disease. Mol Med 1999;5(9):569–82.

55. Ferrer I, Bernet E, Soriano E, et al. Naturally occurring cell death in the cerebral cortex of the rat and removal of dead cells by transitory phagocytes. Neuroscience 1990;39(2):451–8.

56. Nguyen KB, Pender MP. Phagocytosis of apoptotic lymphocytes by oligodendrocytes in experimental

autoimmune encephalomyelitis. Acta Neuropathol 1998;95(1):40–6.

57. Chao CC, Hu S, Peterson PK. Modulation of human microglial cell superoxide production by cytokines. J Leukoc Biol 1995;58(1):65–70.

58. Slavik JM, Hutchcroft JE, Bierer BE. CD28/CTLA-4 and CD80/CD86 families: signaling and function. Immunol Res 1999;19(1):1–24.

59. van Kooten C, Banchereau J. CD40-CD40 ligand. J Leukoc Biol 2000;67(1):2–17.

60. Stoll M, Capper D, Dietz K, et al. Differential microglial regulation in the human spinal cord under normal and pathological conditions. Neuropathol Appl Neurobiol 2006;32(6):650–61.

61. Gehrmann J, Matsumoto Y, Kreutzberg GW. Microglia: intrinsic immuneffector cell of the brain. Brain Res Brain Res Rev 1995;20(3):269–87.

62. Ford AL, Foulcher E, Lemckert FA, et al. Microglia induce CD4 T lymphocyte final effector function and death. J Exp Med 1996;184(5):1737–45.

63. Kreutzberg GW. Microglia: a sensor for pathological events in the CNS. Trends Neurosci 1996; 19(8):312–8.

64. De Simone R, Giampaolo A, Giometto B, et al. The costimulatory molecule B7 is expressed on human microglia in culture and in multiple sclerosis acute lesions. J Neuropathol Exp Neurol 1995;54(2): 175–87.

65. Li H, Cuzner ML, Newcombe J. Microglia-derived macrophages in early multiple sclerosis plaques. Neuropathol Appl Neurobiol 1996;22(3):207–15.

66. Shrikant P, Benveniste EN. The central nervous system as an immunocompetent organ: role of glial cells in antigen presentation. J Immunol 1996; 157(5):1819–22.

67. Pender MP, Rist MJ. Apoptosis of inflammatory cells in immune control of the nervous system: role of glia. Glia 2001;36(2):137–44.

68. Spanaus KS, Schlapbach R, Fontana A. TNF-alpha and IFN-gamma render microglia sensitive to Fas ligand-induced apoptosis by induction of Fas expression and down-regulation of Bcl-2 and Bcl-xL. Eur J Immunol 1998;28(12):4398–408.

69. Frigerio S, et al. Modulation of fas-ligand (Fas-L) on human microglial cells: an in vitro study. J Neuroimmunol 2000;105(2):109–14.

70. Kohji T, Matsumoto Y. Coexpression of Fas/FasL and Bax on brain and infiltrating T cells in the central nervous system is closely associated with apoptotic cell death during autoimmune encephalomyelitis. J Neuroimmunol 2000;106(1–2):165–71.

71. Rossi ML, Jones NR, Candy E, et al. The mononuclear cell infiltrate compared with survival in high-grade astrocytomas. Acta Neuropathol 1989; 78(2):189–93.

72. Roggendorf W, Strupp S, Paulus W. Distribution and characterization of microglia/macrophages in human brain tumors. Acta Neuropathol 1996; 92(3):288–93.

73. Streit WJ. Cellular immune response in brain tumors. Neuropathol Appl Neurobiol 1994;20(2): 205–6.

74. Wierzba-Bobrowicz T, Kuchna I, Matyja E. Reaction of microglial cells in human astrocytomas (preliminary report). Folia Neuropathol 1994;32(4):251–2.

75. Badie B, Schartner JM, Paul J, et al. Dexamethasone-induced abolition of the inflammatory response in an experimental glioma model: a flow cytometry study. J Neurosurg 2000;93(4):634–9.

76. Prat E, Baron P, Meda L, et al. The human astrocytoma cell line U373MG produces monocyte chemotactic protein (MCP)-1 upon stimulation with beta-amyloid protein. Neurosci Lett 2000; 283(3):177–80.

77. Galasso JM, Stegman LD, Blaivas M, et al. Experimental gliosarcoma induces chemokine receptor expression in rat brain. Exp Neurol 2000;161(1): 85–95.

78. Suzuki Y, Funakoshi H, Machide M, et al. Regulation of cell migration and cytokine production by HGF-like protein (HLP)/macrophage stimulating protein (MSP) in primary microglia. Biomed Res 2008;29(2):77–84.

79. Alterman RL, Stanley ER. Colony stimulating factor-1 expression in human glioma. Mol Chem Neuropathol 1994;21(2-3):177–88.

80. Badie B, Schartner J, Klaver J, et al. In vitro modulation of microglia motility by glioma cells is mediated by hepatocyte growth factor/scatter factor. Neurosurgery 1999;44(5):1077–82 [discussion: 1082–3].

81. Morantz RA, Wood GW, Foster M, et al. Macrophages in experimental and human brain tumors. Part 2: studies of the macrophage content of human brain tumors. J Neurosurg 1979;50(3): 305–11.

82. Badie B, Schartner J. Role of microglia in glioma biology. Microsc Res Tech 2001;54(2):106–13.

83. Proescholdt MA, Merrill MJ, Ikejiri B, et al. Site-specific immune response to implanted gliomas. J Neurosurg 2001;95(6):1012–9.

84. Tran CT, Wolz P, Egensperger R, et al. Differential expression of MHC class II molecules by microglia and neoplastic astroglia: relevance for the escape of astrocytoma cells from immune surveillance. Neuropathol Appl Neurobiol 1998;24(4):293–301.

85. Flugel A, Labeur MS, Grasbon-Frodl EM, et al. Microglia only weakly present glioma antigen to cytotoxic T cells. Int J Dev Neurosci 1999;17(5–6): 547–56.

86. Badie B, Bartley B, Schartner J. Differential expression of MHC class II and B7 costimulatory molecules by microglia in rodent gliomas. J Neuroimmunol 2002;133(1–2):39–45.

87. Magnus T, Schreiner B, Korn T, et al. Microglial expression of the B7 family member B7 homolog 1 confers strong immune inhibition: implications for immune responses and autoimmunity in the CNS. J Neurosci 2005;25(10):2537–46.

88. Parsa AT, Waldron JS, Panner A, et al. Loss of tumor suppressor PTEN function increases B7-H1 expression and immunoresistance in glioma. Nat Med 2007;13(1):84–8.

89. Dong H, Strome SE, Salomao DR, et al. Tumor-associated B7-H1 promotes T-cell apoptosis: a potential mechanism of immune evasion. Nat Med 2002;8(8):793–800.

90. Badie B, Schartner J, Prabakaran S, et al. Expression of Fas ligand by microglia: possible role in glioma immune evasion. J Neuroimmunol 2001; 120(1–2):19–24.

91. Parney IF, Waldron JS, Parsa AT. Flow cytometry and in vitro analysis of human glioma-associated macrophages. J Neurosurg 2009;110(3):572–82.

92. Kostianovsky AM, Maier LM, Anderson RC, et al. Astrocytic regulation of human monocytic/microglial activation. J Immunol 2008;181(8):5425–32.

93. Parney IF, Hao C, Petruk KC. Glioma immunology and immunotherapy. Neurosurgery 2000;46(4): 778–91 [discussion: 791–2].

94. Suzumura A, Sawada M, Yamamoto H, et al. Transforming growth factor-beta suppresses activation and proliferation of microglia in vitro. J Immunol 1993;151(4):2150–8.

95. Hishii M, Nitta T, Ishida H, et al. Human glioma-derived interleukin-10 inhibits antitumor immune responses in vitro. Neurosurgery 1995;37(6):1160–6 [discussion: 1166–7].

96. O'Keefe GM, Nguyen VT, Benveniste EN. Class II transactivator and class II MHC gene expression in microglia: modulation by the cytokines TGF-beta, IL-4, IL-13 and IL-10. Eur J Immunol 1999;29(4): 1275–85.

97. Rao JS. Molecular mechanisms of glioma invasiveness: the role of proteases. Nat Rev Cancer 2003; 3(7):489–501.

98. Lafuente JV, Adan B, Alkiza K, et al. Expression of vascular endothelial growth factor (VEGF) and platelet-derived growth factor receptor-beta (PDGFR-beta) in human gliomas. J Mol Neurosci 1999;13(1–2):177–85.

99. Hussain SF, Kong LY, Jordan J, et al. A novel small molecule inhibitor of signal transducers and activators of transcription 3 reverses immune tolerance in malignant glioma patients. Cancer Res 2007; 67(20):9630–6.

100. Iwamaru A, Szymanski S, Iwado E, et al. A novel inhibitor of the STAT3 pathway induces apoptosis in malignant glioma cells both in vitro and in vivo. Oncogene 2007;26(17):2435–44.

101. Zhang L, Alizadeh D, Van Handel M, et al. Stat3 inhibition activates tumor macrophages and abrogates glioma growth in mice. Glia 2009;57(13): 1458–67.

102. Gabrilovich DI, Chen HL, Girgis KR, et al. Production of vascular endothelial growth factor by human tumors inhibits the functional maturation of dendritic cells. Nat Med 1996;2(10):1096–103.

103. Kortylewski M, Kujawski M, Wang T, et al. Inhibiting Stat3 signaling in the hematopoietic system elicits multicomponent antitumor immunity. Nat Med 2005;11(12):1314–21.

104. Darnell JE Jr. STATs and gene regulation. Science 1997;277(5332):1630–5.

105. Raizer JJ. HER1/EGFR tyrosine kinase inhibitors for the treatment of glioblastoma multiforme. J Neuro-oncol 2005;74(1):77–86.

106. Salomon DS, Brandt R, Ciardiello F, et al. Epidermal growth factor-related peptides and their receptors in human malignancies. Crit Rev Oncol Hematol 1995;19(3):183–232.

107. Tang P, Steck PA, Yung WK. The autocrine loop of TGF-alpha/EGFR and brain tumors. J Neurooncol 1997;35(3):303–14.

108. Schaefer LK, Ren Z, Fuller GN, et al. Constitutive activation of Stat3alpha in brain tumors: localization to tumor endothelial cells and activation by the endothelial tyrosine kinase receptor (VEGFR-2). Oncogene 2002;21(13):2058–65.

109. Yu H, Jove R. The STATs of cancer–new molecular targets come of age. Nat Rev Cancer 2004;4(2): 97–105.

110. Carpentier AF, Xie J, Mokhtari K, et al. Successful treatment of intracranial gliomas in rat by oligodeoxynucleotides containing CpG motifs. Clin Cancer Res 2000;6(6):2469–73.

111. Carpentier AF, Auf G, Delattre JY. CpG-oligonucleotides for cancer immunotherapy: review of the literature and potential applications in malignant glioma. Front Biosci 2003;8:e115–27.

112. Auf G, Carpentier AF, Chen L, et al. Implication of macrophages in tumor rejection induced by CpG-oligodeoxynucleotides without antigen. Clin Cancer Res 2001;7(11):3540–3.

# Immunostimulants for Malignant Gliomas

Nicholas Butowski, MD

**KEYWORDS**

- Glioblastoma multiforme • Novel therapy
- Immunostimulant • Immunotherapy • Cytokine

Despite advances in surgical-, radiation-, and chemotherapy-based strategies, malignant gliomas continue to be associated with a poor prognosis. Immunostimulants offer a novel treatment approach. This article reviews immunostimulant treatment approaches and understanding for malignant glioma and relevant clinical trials. Early attempts at glioma therapy based on immunostimulants failed to demonstrate effectiveness. Current immunostimulant therapies have shifted to a more multifaceted approach combining two or more different immunotherapeutic strategies. As understanding of the immune system's role in brain cancer increases, continued efforts will move toward potentially more effective therapies.

Glioblastoma mutiforme (GBM) is challenging to treat and associated with a high degree of morbidity and mortality. Standard treatment consists of cytoreductive surgery followed by radiation therapy in combination with temozolomide chemotherapy followed by adjuvant temozolomide, which leads to a median survival of 14.6 months.[1] Based on several meta-analyses, other types of adjuvant chemotherapy, mainly nitrosoureas, seem to add some survival benefit, but the gain is modest.[2,3] Continuous efforts are ongoing to develop more novel, effective agents or combinations of agents that may improve overall survival or prolong time to progression.

Immunotherapy, and in particular immunostimulants (also known as biologic modifiers), are an example of an area of research into novel therapy for use in high- and low-grade gliomas. Immunotherapy, or treatment that uses the body's immune system to combat tumors is attractive for cancer therapy for several reasons, including the conviction that it would be less toxic than the traditional cytotoxic therapies and may lead to sustained responses through immunologic memory. Nevertheless, various advances and promising preclinical results seen in both in vitro and animal models have not yet translated into positive human clinical trials for glioma, although these studies provide more insight and guidance for future studies. Consequently, a considerable interest in immunotherapy persists, and combined with accumulating evidence of the immune system's role (or suppression) in the genesis of cancer, immunotherapy studies in glioma are ongoing and are increasingly frequent.[4] This article highlights the use of immunostimulants in glioma. Other articles in this issue provide a further review of other forms of active immunotherapy and passive immunotherapy.

## THE IMMUNE SYSTEM'S ROLE IN CANCER GENESIS

The genesis of cancer and the genesis of immunosuppression are related.[5,6] It is thought that under ideal circumstances, immune surveillance identifies neoplastic cells and subsequently destroys them. Tumor cells, however, manage to avoid detection by the immune system, and the cancer cells that avoid surveillance are able to proliferate and acquire additional immunoevasive mechanisms. As such, by the time the tumor is clinically apparent, it is adept at avoiding the immune system in various ways.[7] For example, glioma patients have been found to have decreased T-cell responsiveness, T-cell receptor-mediated signaling, and antibody production. These immunosuppressive effects are mediated by tumor cells in numerous ways, including cytokine

Department of Neurological Surgery, University of California San Francisco, 400 Parnassus Avenue, A808, San Francisco, CA 94143, USA
*E-mail address:* butowski@neurosurg.ucsf.edu

neurosurgery.theclinics.com

dysregulation. For instance, tumor-expressed cytokines like transforming growth factor beta (TGF-β), prostaglandin E2 (PGE2), and interleukin (IL)-10 suppress immune responses, and these cytokines are often overexpressed in glioma. Other immunosuppressive measures consist of down-regulating major histocompatability complex (MHC) molecules, thereby decreasing the body's ability to see or recognize and destroy tumor. Immunostimulants as a cancer treatment are appealing, because boosting impaired tumor responses can in theory eradicate tumor by over-coming tumor-associated immunosuppression. The complexity of this process continues to be worked out, and a broader understanding of the immunosuppressive environment of the tumor, the low avidity of T-cells for tumor antigen ex-pressed on tumor, and the poor immune response will lead to more effective therapies.

## IMMUNOSTIMULANTS

Immunostimulants are generally cytokines or che-mokines. Not all immunostimulants or biologic modifiers, however, fall into this class of mole-cules. In fact, the first immunotherapy studies in glioma involved active immunization with agents such as bacilli Calmette-Guerin (BCG) and Imu-vert, which is derived from *Serratia marcescens* bacterium.[8,9] These studies did not yield positive clinical results for patients with gliomas, but they did serve as the foundation for future studies both in glioma and other cancers. Cytokines have been used in most further immunostimulant studies. Different T-helper cells (Th) secrete cyto-kines, the characteristics of which vary with the nature of immune response.[10] Cytokines tradition-ally are divided into three classes:

> The Th1 cytokine class, such as interferon (IFN)-γ, interleukin (IL)-2), and IL-12, promotes cell-mediated immune responses and are capable of exerting antitumor responses.
> Th2 class cytokines such as IL-4 stimulate humeral responses or may be immunosup-pressive like IL-10.
> Cytokines in the Th3 class including the trans-forming growth factor (TGF) family are by and large immunosuppressive.[11,12]

Immunostimulants may be delivered to patients intravenously or intratumorally to potentiate immune surveillance and cell-mediated antitumor responses. These responses can be divided into one of three categories of response:

1. Exert direct toxic effects on the tumor

2. Enhance tumor immunogenicity alone or in the setting of other therapies, immune-based or not
3. Support depressed antitumor cell-mediated immune responses

Initial studies attempted systemic, intratumoral, or intrathecal delivery, but resulted in significant toxicity. Endeavors to reduce toxicity led to engi-neering cells, using gene transfer techniques, to secrete cytokines directly. These cells then can be transplanted into central nervous system (CNS) tumors and achieve production of cytokine without the need for systemic administration.[7] More recent strategies use intratumoral delivery of engineered cytokine gene-bearing attenuated viral vectors, which have the advantage of deliv-ering high viral titers into tumor with subsequent infection and cytokine secretion by tumor cells; this manner of viral vector delivery also obviates the concern of immune rejection of transplanted cytokine secreting cells. More recent attention has focused on cell-based cytokine delivery via neural stem cells (NSCs). NSCs are capable of intracranial migration and are tropic for migrating glioma, which invades brain parenchyma beyond the main tumor mass. Cytokine-secreting NSCs are therefore capable of tracking and delivering cytokines to areas of tumor beyond the surgical resection cavity, the radiation field, and perhaps beyond the distance that traditional chemotherapy can penetrate. This neural stem cell system is particularly attractive for glioma, which is a highly invasive and disseminated tumor, a characteristic that has limited treatment success to date.

## CYTOKINES

Cytokine therapy for cancer has received consid-erable attention. The initial use of cytokines used systemic recombinant therapy with the intent of delivering a high, potent dose to stimulate tumor-icidal responses. This strategy worked in mouse models but was limited in people because of toxicity and short half-lives.[13,14] In regard to primary brain tumors, the use of cytokine therapy must afford for the blood–brain barrier and the privileged state of the CNS. Given these chal-lenges, some studies have focused on local delivery or intratumoral delivery of cytokines, but these studies also often resulted in significant toxicity.

Particular to glioma, attention has focused on the promotion of T-cell activity by using IL-2, IL-4, IL-12, IFN-α, and IFN-γ.[15–23] IFN-γ also may inhibit tumor induced neovascularization.[24] Cytokines like tumor necrosis factor (TNF)-α have been used to induce up-regulation of cell surface

MHC, thereby increasing visibility of tumor to the immune system. TNF-$\alpha$ associated chemokine, TRAIL (TNF-related apoptosis inducing ligand) also has been used to induce tumor cell death by triggering apoptotic cascades within cancer cells only.[25–27] Further discussion of the most common cytokines used in glioma studies to date follows.

## IL-2

IL-2 was among the first cytokines to be studied in glioma. IL-2 is an important T-cell growth factor involved in the proliferation of CD8+ T-cells and blockade of the immunosuppressive effects of transforming growth factor (TGF)-$\beta$.[28–30] High systemic doses are required to achieve effective levels in the brain for therapy against brain tumors.[31] Early, small clinical trials using IL-2 for patients with glioma, generally in combination with lymphokine-activated killer cells (LAK), did not have positive results.[32,33] These trials involved systemic, intrathecal, and intratumoral administration of IL-2 but resulted in significant toxicity, including cerebral edema, which was caused by IL-2 increasing vascular permeability. Other trials used IL-2 with IFN-$\alpha$ but had similar negative results and toxicity.[34]

Further preclinical studies concentrated on different delivery methods. For example, in one study, allogeneic fibroblasts were engineered to secrete interleukin IL-2 and subsequently administered either subcutaneously or intracerebrally to mice with intracranial glioma.[16] This treatment led to a significant prolongation of survival in mice with intracranial glioma treated intracerebrally relative to the survival of mice with treated subcutaneously. Other similar studies have shown a cytotoxic antitumor response that leads to significant prolongation of survival in mice challenged with melanoma.[35] More recent studies demonstrated that local IL-2 therapy in the brain not only generates an immediate local antitumor immune response, but also establishes long-term immunologic memory capable of eliminating subsequent tumor challenges within and outside of the CNS.[36] IL-2 also has been combined with traditional cytotoxic chemotherapy in a study that showed that the combination of paracrine immunotherapy, with nonreplicating genetically engineered tumor cells that produce IL-2, and local delivery of chemotherapy by biodegradable polymers prolonged survival in a synergistic manner in mice challenged intracranially with murine brain tumor.[37] Finally, an injectable polymeric system for the long-term localized delivery of IL-2 has been studied in the rat brain; antitumor efficacy studies performed in brain tumor models

in rats appeared promising and indicative of long-lasting immunity.[38]

More recent studies in human patients used IL-2 as a transgene and in combination with HSV-tk transgene; the genes were carried by a retroviral virus on vector-producing cells. Twelve patients with recurrent GBM were treated with an intratumoral injection of the construct followed by systemic administration of acyclovir.[39] The treatment was tolerated well, and several patients had radiographic responses. Another clinical trial in 40 patients with recurrent GBM performed by Dillman and colleagues[40] used IL-2 to generate autologous LAKs. After generating LAK, these cells were injected intratumorally. This approach was tolerated well, and a clinical benefit was seen, with a median survival of 9 months, and a 1-year survival rate of 34%. Further studies for both the aforementioned clinical trials are being considered.

## IL-4

IL-4 overexpression may impair tumorigenicity of glioma, and several studies have determined that IL-4 may have a role in tumor treatment. For example, the ability of IL-4 to mediate an antitumor response to human gliomas was studied in nude mice using a transfected tumor cell line expressing IL-4.[21] This study showed a significant inhibition of growth of U87 human glioma cells, with a prolongation of survival when compared with control nude mice. Histologic analysis revealed the presence of an eosinophil infiltrate and tumor necrosis.

Other evidence of the antitumor effect of IL-4 was provided after in vivo gene transfer into malignant gliomas.[15] In this study, GBM cells and retroviral producer cells, secreting 20 ng and 50 ng of IL-4 were implanted into rats.[15] Several rats were cured of their tumors and developed an immunologic memory and thus rejected a rechallenge with tumor cells. Immunohistology showed inflammatory infiltrates in IL-4-treated tumors in which CD8+ T-lymphocytes were more abundant, although CD4+ T-lymphocytes, B-lymphocytes, and macrophages were also present. Another study found that implantation of gliosarcoma cells expressing IL-4 into rats induced a specific, protective, immune response against rechallenge with tumors and suggested that tumor-specific reactivity among CD4+ T-cells was critical for developing tumor resistance.[41] Other findings support the use of tumor cell vaccines expressing IL-4.[42] Benedetti and colleagues[43] have described the use of IL-4 secreting neural stem cells for treating mice with intracranial gliomas, and results are indicative of promise, although more work needs to be done. Overall, these findings suggest that IL-4 gene transfer is a new, promising approach for treating malignant gliomas. Interestingly, it also has been shown that dexamethasone significantly reduced the antitumor effect of IL-4.[44] This result is relevant to patients with brain tumors who often take steroids for cerebral edema.

## IL-12

IL-12 is a cytokine that promotes an antitumor Th1-type pattern of differentiation in naïve T-cells. Recent studies also have found that IL-12 is needed to overcome the immunosuppressive effects of TGF-β. A recent, extensive review of immunotherapy by IL-12 based cytokine combinations also describes several other potential effects of IL-12 on the immune system.[45]

Despite its therapeutic success in multiple animal cancer models, the utility of systemically administered recombinant IL-12 has been limited by its toxicity. This has encouraged the development of local IL-12 delivery systems through gene transfer. Using such techniques and direct intratumoral administration of IL-12 into mice with gliomas, researchers demonstrated that survival was prolonged significantly, and immunohistochemistry demonstrated robust CD4+ and CD8+ T-cell infiltration in these mice compared with the two control groups.[23] Another study demonstrated that local delivery of IL-12 into the rat brain by genetically engineered gliosarcoma cells significantly prolonged survival time in animals challenged intracranially with a malignant glioma. Survivors appeared to develop an antitumor immunologic memory, as surviving rats were immune to rechallenging with a second injection of tumor cells.[46] Other studies have shown the potent antitumor effects observed for paracrine gene-delivered administration of IL-12 in multiple tumor cell types and in multiple murine strains.[47] Interestingly, IL-12 secreting neural stem cells also have been studied preclinically, and it has been shown that these cells exhibit tropism for tumor and result in long-term survival.[22]

Kikuchi and colleagues conducted a study with IL-12 that included 15 people varying gliomas. Treatment consisted of subcutaneous administration of recombinant IL-12 in combination with a fusion of autologous dendritic and glioma cells.[48] Augmentation of CD8+ cytolytic activity on glioma cells was documented after treatment, and there was a modest radiographic response.

## GRANULOCYTE–MACROPHAGE COLONY-STIMULATING FACTOR

Granulocyte-macrophage colony-stimulating factor (GM-CSF) is secreted by macrophages, cells, mast cells, endothelial cells, and fibroblasts. GM-CSF stimulates stem cells to produce granulocytes (neutrophils, eosinophils, and basophils) and monocytes. Monocytes exit the circulation and migrate into tissue, whereupon they mature into macrophages. It is thus part of the immune/inflammatory cascade, by which activation of a small number of macrophages can rapidly lead to an increase in their numbers, a process crucial for fighting infection.

GM-CSF exerts its antineoplastic effects by producing a cytotoxic T-cell response. GM-CSF also induces the recruitment of antigen-presenting cells and may activate antigen presentation pathways for MHC class 1-mediated processes. Most studies relevant to glioma have used GM-CSF to derive dendritic cells by exposing monocytes to GM-CSF.[49] GM-CSF also has been shown to stimulate intracranial responses to irradiated tumor cell vaccines.[50,51] Clinical studies with GM-CSF as an immunotherapy for gliomas are limited, but GM-CSF may serve as a useful vaccine adjuvant with limited toxicity in human clinical trials of antiglioma vaccine therapy.[52] In fact, it is being used currently as an adjuvant in a phase 2 study of CDX-110 in patients with newly diagnosed GBM. Objectives of the study are to investigate the anticancer activity, impact on survival, and safety of CDX-110 plus GM-CSF when administered concurrently with temozolomide and continuing until disease progression. Of note, CDX-110 is a vaccine-based therapy that targets the tumor-specific molecule called EGFRvIII, a functional variant of the epidermal growth factor receptor (EGFR), a protein that has been validated as a target for cancer therapy. Unlike EGFR, EGFRvIII is not present in normal tissues, suggesting this target will enable the development of a tumor-specific therapy for cancer patients. More information is available at: http://www.celldextherapeutics.com/wt/page/cdx_110.

### TNF-α

TNF-α, also known as cachexin or cachectin, is a cytokine involved in systemic inflammation, and it is a member of a group of cytokines that stimulate the acute phase reaction. The primary role of TNF-α is in the regulation of immune cells. TNF-α is also able to induce apoptotic cell death, to induce inflammation, and to inhibit tumorigenesis and viral replication. Dysregulation and, in particular, overproduction of TNF, has been implicated in various human diseases, including cancer. Built on proof of concept from prior studies, a 2009 study of retroviral vector-mediated TNF-$\alpha$ given with IFNs (see section on IFN) increased tumor antigen expression through the up-regulation of MHC class 1 and 2 molecules.[53] Tumor regression was seen in animal models, but the benefit to people remains uncertain. It is worth mentioning that glioma-bearing mice deficient in TNF-$\alpha$ developed larger tumors and had reduced survival compared with their wild-type controls.[54]

## MISCELLANEOUS CYTOKINES

Several other cytokines have been used in glioma studies. For example, recent studies have incorporated the Flt3L ligand, which can expand dendritic cells and enhance immunogenicity and can promote tumor death when given with other immunotherapies.[55] Further studies on this novel cytokine demonstrate that Flt3L has distinct effects on dendritic cell development, suggesting an important role for Flt3L in generating dendritic cells that have tolerogenic effects on T-cells.[56]

IL-21 also has received relatively recent interest. IL-21 has potent regulatory effects on cells of the immune system, including natural killer cells and cytotoxic T-cells that can destroy virally infected or cancerous cells. Preclinical studies have focused on gene-modified cell delivery and generally in tandem with other cytokines.[57] Interestingly, researchers discovered that IL-21 is produced by Hodgkin's lymphoma (HL) cells (which was surprising, because IL-21 was thought until then to be produced only by T-cells).[58] This discovery may explain a great deal of the behavior of classical HL, including clusters of other immune cells gathered around HL cells in cultures. Targeting IL-21 may be a potential treatment or possibly a test for the disease.

## IFN

INFs are glycoproteins, which are cell-signaling molecules produced by the cells of the immune system in response to challenges such as viruses and tumor cells. IFNs assist the immune response by inhibiting viral replication within host cells, activating natural killer cells and macrophages, increasing antigen presentation to lymphocytes, and inducing the resistance of host cells to viral infection.[4] Early preclinical studies with IFN-$\alpha$ and IFN-$\beta$ showed promise, but these clinical studies suffered from poor design and lack of strict patient eligibility and selection.[18,59–62] Imaging analysis

and tumor grading also made it difficult to appropriately assess efficacy.

### IFN-$\alpha$

IFN-$\alpha$ is associated with accumulation of CD4+, CD8+, and dendritic cells within the established tumor, demonstrating induction of antitumor immune responses.[63] Preclinical testing has led to various clinical trials. For example, IFN-$\alpha$ was tested in a phase 3 clinical trial for patients with recurrent high-grade gliomas.[64] The study included 214 patients with anaplastic astrocytoma, anaplastic oligiodendroglioma, GBM, and gliosarcoma. The patients initially were treated with radiation and BCNU (carmustine). Following radiotherapy, patients without disease progression were stratified and randomized into two groups: BCNU and BCNU plus IFN-$\alpha$. Unfortunately, there was no difference in response rates between the two treatment arms in the final evaluation. A recent phase 1 clinical trial combined IFN-$\alpha$ with BCNU wafers in patients with recurrent GBM.[65] Patients were treated with surgical resection and implantation of BCNU wafers; then a week later, IFN was initiated three times a week at a dose of 3 mU/m(2), which was escalated in increments of 3 mU/m(2). Dose-limiting toxicity in the form of fatigue occurred at 9 mU/m(2). There were nine evaluable patients, and two had complete imaging responses. Further studies are in the planning stages.

### IFN-$\beta$

IFN-$\beta$ exerts its antitumor effect by inhibiting glioma in the S phase, enhancing natural killer cell and cytotoxic T-cell activity, and perhaps synergizing with cytotoxic chemotherapies.[10] IFN-$\beta$ has been delivered successfully to the brains of mice using bone marrow cells.[66] A small phase 1 study of seven patients in 1989 used recombinant IFN-$\beta$ in escalating dosages intravenously three times weekly.[67] There was no evidence of response in any patient, either on clinical examination or by computerized tomography (CT), and four patients had immediate progression of disease. Another phase 1 study administered IFN-$\beta$ intrathecally three times weekly to 20 patients with recurrent malignant gliomas. Adverse effects occurred in only one patient and consisted of nausea, vomiting, fever, and chills. Problems with the Ommaya reservoir (obstruction in two patients and infection in four patients) led to six patients being terminated from the study. Although this was primarily a study of toxicity, of 12 evaluable patients, 3 had stable disease for 148,

192, and 539 days, respectively; 9 had progressive disease. Other similar clinical studies have yielded mixed results.[68,69] A Japanese cooperative group has just opened a multicenter phase 1 clinical trial, the Integrated Japanese Multicenter Clinical Trial: A phase I study of interferon-beta and temozolomide for glioma in combination with radiotherapy (INTEGRA Study).[70] This study is being conducted for patients with high-grade glioma to evaluate the safety, feasibility, and preliminary clinical effectiveness of the combination of IFN-β and temozolomide. The primary endpoint is toxicity, and secondary endpoints are progression-free survival time and overall survival time. In addition, objective tumor response will be evaluated in a subpopulation of patients with the measurable disease. Planned enrollment is 10 newly diagnosed and 10 recurrent patients.

## IFN-γ

IFN-γ causes increased major histocompatability complex expression on brain cells, class 1 antigen on local endothelial and ependymal cells, and class 2 antigen on microglial, ependymal, and perivascular cells.[71] It also recruits lymphocytes and other inflammatory cells.

IFN-γ has demonstrated tumoricidal effects in various cancers. Preclinical studies show that IFN-γ produces an antiglioma response mediated predominantly by natural killer/lymphokine-activated killer cells.[72] Studies have made use of in situ adenoviral-mediated IFN-γ gene transfer in glioma-bearing rodents and have found that survival was prolonged.[73] These effects were accompanied by significant up-regulation of tumor MHC-1 and MHC-2 expression. In addition, therapy down-regulated the expression of endothelial Fas ligand, a cell membrane protein implicated as a contributor to immune privilege in cancer. Other studies using IFN-γ secreting allogeneic cells showed that the survival of mice with glioma injected with the cells was prolonged significantly relative to the survival of mice receiving equivalent numbers of glioma cells alone.[74] A clinical trial in pediatric high-grade glioma patients treated with IFN-γ and low-dose cyclophosphamide after radiation has been performed. Forty patients were enrolled (median age: 8.5 years). The median overall survival of 1 year was not significantly different from a historical control group.[75]

## PATHOGEN-ASSOCIATED MOLECULAR PATTERN AS ADJUVANTS

Early efforts focused on the use of nonspecific immune stimulators to expand antitumor immune response. More recently, the focus has been on immunostimulatory agents that act directly on antigen-presenting cells and effector cells of the immune system via pattern recognition receptors such as toll-like receptor (TLR) agonists.[7] Another term for these immunostimulatory agents is pathogen-associated molecular patterns, or PAMPs, which are small molecular motifs conserved within a class of microbes.[76] PAMPs are recognized by pattern recognition receptors, which after identifying nonself molecules, elicit an innate immune response and thus protect the host from infection.[77] Pattern recognition receptor agonists include lipopolysaccharide (LPS), heat shock protein, imiquimod, and CpG oligonucleotides.[78] Other PAMPs include bacterial flagellin, lipoteichoic acid from gram-positive bacteria, peptidoglycan, and nucleic acid variants normally associated with viruses, such as double-stranded RNA (dsRNA) or unmethylated CpG motifs.[76,77,79,80]

TLRs are among the best-described pattern recognition receptors, and their activation results in the up-regulation of costimulatory molecules and cytokine production. Additionally, the anticancer effects of several microbial components, used as adjuvants for the immunotherapy of cancers, are thought to be mediated through TLR signaling. Studies have demonstrated that TLR stimulation triggers several proteins and kinases, leading to the induction of proinflammatory mediators but also anti-inflammatory and antitumor cytokines and enhanced antigen presentation.[79] Other studies show another effect of TLR stimulation on malignant cells; they can be proapoptotic or promote survival under different conditions.[80] In essence, data indicate that activation of innate immune responses via TLR in the brain and elsewhere in the body is not homogeneous but rather tailored according to cell type and environmental signal.[81] It is therefore crucial to design further studies in glioma and cancer in general assessing the biology of these receptors in normal and transformed cells. Additionally, although the agonists listed alone can enhance physiologic antitumor response, most studies with demonstrated antitumor efficacy use the agonists in combination with some other form of immunotherapy. Studies also have used cocktails of PAMPs like LPS and muramyl dipeptide in combination with TNF-α; while others used heat shock protein gene therapy.[82–85] In way of further example, recent studies have shown that IL-12 and TLR activation by a cocktail of polyinosinic-polycytidilic acid stabilized with polylysine and carbox (poly-ICLC), IL-1, and INF-γ is needed to overcome glioma-induced immunosuppression by TGF-β.[86]

## OLIGODEOXYNUCLEOTIDES

Oligodeoxynucleotides containing CpG motifs (CpG ODNs) display a strong immunostimulating activity and drive the immune response toward the Th1 phenotype.[87] A preclinical study investigated whether radiotherapy could be used advantageously with intratumoral injections of CpG-ODN.[88] In this study, rats with glioma were treated with various combinations of radiotherapy (RT) and CpG-28. When both treatments were combined, complete tumor remission was achieved in two thirds of the animals; this response was better than with either treatment alone. A possible trial in people is in the planning stage. Other preclinical studies using CpG ODNs in animal models have yielded similar results.[89,90]

A phase 1 trial in people administered CpG-ODN intratumorally by convection-enhanced delivery in patients with recurrent GBM.[91] Twenty-four patients entered the trial, and CpG-ODN was tolerated well at doses up to 20 mg per injection. Adverse effects possibly or probably related to the study drug consisted of worsening of neurologic conditions, fever above 38°C that disappeared within a few days, and reversible grade 3 lymphopenia. Only one patient experienced a dose-limiting toxicity. Preliminary evidence of activity was suggested by a minor response observed in two patients and an overall median survival of 7.2 months.

## POLY-ICLC/HILTONOL

Poly-ICLC, also known as Hiltinol, is a double-stranded RNA (dsRNA) molecule previously used as an IFN inducer and immune-modulating agent at high doses in various clinical trials. These trials were based on studies that demonstrated that dsRNA possessed antineoplastic activity, including in glioma cell lines, that was thought to be caused by induction of IFN and an IFN-independent immune-enhancing effect that involved an increased antibody response to antigen and activation of natural killer cells, T-cells, macrophages, and cytokines.[92–98] These original trials showed various results with significant toxicity; thus the use of poly-ICLC was discarded when IFNs became available via recombinant DNA technology.[99–104] As it became apparent that lower doses of poly-ICLC may elicit different results, ensuing studies were performed with these lower doses, resulting in less toxicity and a broader host defense stimulation, including activation of T-cells, natural killer cells, and myeloid dendritic cells via TLR3, as well as induction of a mix of IFNs and cytokines. The host defense stimulation

also resulted in a antiviral and antiproliferative effect mediated by activation of IFN-inducible dsRNA-dependent enzyme systems that regulate such cell functions as protein synthesis, proliferation, and apoptosis.[92,105–111]

An early glioma clinical trial of various histologies (newly diagnosed or recurrent GBM or anaplastic astrocytoma) performed by Salazar and colleagues[112] had patients treated with low-dose poly-ICLC intramuscularly. Twenty of 38 patients also received concurrent lomustine (CCNU) at 120 mg/m$^2$ once every 6 weeks, while others received no chemotherapy. Sixty-six percent of patients receiving poly-ICLC showed regression or stabilization of enhancing tumor volume on magnetic resonance imaging (MRI) for at least 6 months from study entry. Median survival was 19 months for 18 newly diagnosed GBM patients receiving poly-ICLC. In effect, this pilot study demonstrated the safety of long-term, low-dose intramuscularly administered poly-ICLC in patients with malignant glioma, but it was too small and the patients too heterogeneous to provide reliable evidence of efficacy.

Salazar's pilot study led to a phase 2 trial with the objective of determining whether poly-ICLC with concurrent radiation followed by adjuvant poly-ICLC could improve the median survival time of patients with newly diagnosed GBM. This clinical trial was initiated before temozolomide became incorporated into the standard of care for patients with newly diagnosed GBM.[1] Accrual to this study was discontinued after the results of the phase 3 study defined the standard of care for newly diagnosed patients as radiotherapy plus concomitant and adjuvant temozolomide. The study demonstrated that poly-ICLC and RT were tolerated well, and no patients went off-study because of toxicity. The median survival for this study was 65 weeks. Compared with a matched historical group, this appeared to be better than radiation therapy alone; however, there was no statistical difference in survival compared with a historical group treated with adjuvant chemotherapy (not including temozolomide). The toxicity experienced by patients in this trial, however, was less than that of chemotherapy agents such as nitrosoureas.[3] Comparing the results of this trial with those trials involving temozolomide use in newly diagnosed GBM patients, overall survival of 65 weeks or 15 months is not different from that found in the original 2002 Stupp and colleagues[1,113] study of RT and concurrent temozolomide (TMZ) followed by adjuvant TMZ (16 months). Overall survival is also similar to that in the landmark European Organization for Research and Treatment of Cancer (EORTC) trial (2005) that established temozolomide as part of the standard of care for newly diagnosed GBM (14.6 months).[1] Based on these results, combining temozolomide and poly-ICLC represents an interesting possibility. The NABTT (New Approaches to Brain Tumor Therapy) Consortium has an ongoing Phase 2 trial of RT plus temozolomide followed by adjuvant temozolomide and poly-ICLC in patients with newly diagnosed GBM (see http://www.nabtt.org/protocols/poly.htm), with initial data indicative of increased efficacy compared with chemoradiation with adjuvant temozolomide only (ASCO 2009 abstract).

The question arises whether poly-ICLC (or other PAMPs) and temozolomide would augment or interfere with each other's efficacy. It traditionally has been thought that chemotherapy may counteract the cellular processes needed to produce an immune response; yet, recent data suggest that chemotherapy may augment immune effects through preferential elimination of regulatory components or amplification of antigen exposure following cytotoxic cell damage. It appears that the immune system recovering from a cytotoxic insult may be activated acutely and particularly responsive because of stimulatory cytokines and reduced regulatory elements.[114–116] Research on this issue is ongoing but mostly devoted to the combined use of cytotoxic agents and vaccine therapy rather than to agents such as poly-ICLC. On the other hand, it does appear that poly-ICLC or other PAMPs may improve the efficacy of anti-CNS tumor peptide-based vaccinations by augmenting the overall immune response to the vaccine.[117]

There are nearly a dozen ongoing clinical trials using Hiltonol as the adjuvant for various vaccine platforms in patients with gliomas and prostate, breast, ovarian, cervical, colon, liver and pancreatic cancers, melanomas, and lymphomas. Another recently completed phase 2 trial in glioma patients examined whether poly-ICLC could improve the 6-month progression-free survival in patients with multiply recurrent anaplastic glioma. The 6-month progression free survival (PFS) for the study was 24%, similar to the 6-month PFS of 31% from a study performed by Wong and colleagues,[118] which pooled the results of eight consecutive, negative phase 2 trials in patients with recurrent grade 3 astrocytomas. The authors raised the point that the use of poly-ICLC at initial diagnosis or first recurrence for patients with anaplastic glioma may produce improved results that more closely resemble the results of the pilot study of poly-ICLC, in which patients with newly diagnosed anaplastic astrocytoma (AA) had a PFS of 77 months. An equally important point to consider is that the pilot study also allowed the use of combination CCNU chemotherapy in 10 of 11 newly diagnosed patients with AA.

## SUMMARY

Many immunologic approaches have been studied for treating gliomas. The advent of recombinant DNA technology led to a nonspecific immune strategy via administration of cytokines or immune biologic modifiers. These agents were administered systemically with the hope that they would boost the immune response in patients with brain tumors. Most systemic treatments have been met with only modest results and a high degree of toxicity. Local injection of cytokines also has led to mixed results and adverse effects. In trying to more closely mimic their natural activity, cytokines recently have been delivered either by implanting genetically transduced cells or by using in vivo gene transfer techniques. Although effective in animal models, these strategies either have not moved into human clinical trials or have failed to eradicate gliomas. Combining more than one mode of immunotherapy may provide better results. For example, peptide vaccinations may be used in conjunction with a cytokine adjuvant to produce more widespread immune responses. Pursuits continue to tease out the optimal mix of IFNs, cytokines, chemokines, and PAMPs for responding to particular pathogens, such that one can begin to harness these systems. Advances also must be made in understanding how to overcome the immunologic privilege of the CNS and the immunosupression of gliomas by combining immunostimulants with other forms of immunotherapy like passive antibody treatment, active immunotherapy, or adoptive immunotherapy strategies. Several recent reviews have addressed this topic in the larger context of various types of immunotherapy.[7,52,119–124]

## REFERENCES

1. Stupp R, Mason WP, van den Bent MJ, et al. Radiotherapy plus concomitant and adjuvant temozolomide for glioblastoma. N Engl J Med 2005; 352(10):987–96.
2. Stewart LA. Chemotherapy in adult high-grade glioma: a systematic review and meta-analysis of individual patient data from 12 randomised trials. Lancet 2002;359(9311):1011–8.
3. Fine HA, Dear KB, Loeffler JS, et al. Meta-analysis of radiation therapy with and without adjuvant chemotherapy for malignant gliomas in adults. Cancer 1993;71(8):2585–97.
4. Kruger C, Greten TF, Korangy F. Immune-based therapies in cancer. Histol Histopathol 2007;22(6): 687–96.
5. Kushen MC, Sonabend AM, Lesniak MS. Current immunotherapeutic strategies for central nervous

system tumors. Surg Oncol Clin N Am 2007;16(4): 987–1004.

6. Ksendzovsky A, Feinstein D, Zengou R, et al. Investigation of immunosuppressive mechanisms in a mouse glioma model. J Neurooncol 2009;93(1): 107–14.

7. Mitchell DA, Fecci PE, Sampson JH. Immunotherapy of malignant brain tumors. Immunol Rev 2008;222:70–100.

8. Mahaley MS Jr, Aronin PA, Michael AJ, et al. Prevention of glioma induction in rats by simultaneous intracerebral inoculation of avian sarcoma virus plus bacillus Calmette-Guerin cell wall preparation. Surg Neurol 1983;19(5):453–5.

9. Jaeckle KA, Mittelman A, Hill FH. Phase II trial of Serratia marcescens extract in recurrent malignant astrocytoma. J Clin Onco 1990;8(8):1408–18.

10. Marras C, Mendola C, Legnani FG, et al. Immunotherapy and biological modifiers for the treatment of malignant brain tumors. Curr Opin Oncol 2003; 15(3):204–8.

11. Constam DB, Philipp J, Malipiero UV, et al. Differential expression of transforming growth factor-beta 1, -beta 2, and -beta 3 by glioblastoma cells, astrocytes, and microglia. J Immunol 1992;148(5):1404–10.

12. Hao C, Parney IF, Roa WH, et al. Cytokine and cytokine receptor mRNA expression in human glioblastomas: evidence of Th1, Th2 and Th3 cytokine dysregulation. Acta Neuropathol 2002;103(2): 171–8.

13. Zou JP, Yamamoto N, Fujii T, et al. Systemic administration of rIL-12 induces complete tumor regression and protective immunity: response is correlated with a striking reversal of suppressed IFN-gamma production by anti-tumor T cells. Int Immunol 1995;7(7):1135–45.

14. Leonard JP, Sherman ML, Fisher GL, et al. Effects of single-dose interleukin-12 exposure on interleukin-12-associated toxicity and interferon-gamma production. Blood 1997;90(7):2541–8.

15. Benedetti S, Bruzzone MG, Pollo B, et al. Eradication of rat malignant gliomas by retroviral-mediated, in vivo delivery of the interleukin 4 gene. Cancer Res 1999;59(3):645–52.

16. Glick RP, Lichtor T, Mogharbel A, et al. Intracerebral versus subcutaneous immunization with allogeneic fibroblasts genetically engineered to secrete interleukin-2 in the treatment of central nervous system glioma and melanoma. Neurosurgery 1997;41(4):898–906 [discussion: 906–7].

17. Kikuchi T, Joki T, Abe T, et al. Antitumor activity of killer cells stimulated with both interleukin-2 and interleukin-12 on mouse glioma cells. J Immunother 1999;22(3):245–50.

18. Nagai M, Arai T. Clinical effect of interferon in malignant brain tumours. Neurosurg Rev 1984; 7(1):55–64.

19. Packer RJ, Prados M, Phillips P, et al. Treatment of children with newly diagnosed brain stem gliomas with intravenous recombinant beta-interferon and hyperfractionated radiation therapy: a children's cancer group phase I/II study. Cancer 1996; 77(10):2150–6.

20. Piguet V, Carrel S, Diserens AC, et al. Heterogeneity of the induction of HLA-DR expression by human immune interferon on glioma cell lines and their clones. J Natl Cancer Inst 1986;76(2):223–8.

21. Yu JS, Wei MX, Chiocca EA, et al. Treatment of glioma by engineered interleukin 4-secreting cells. Cancer Res 1993;53(13):3125–8.

22. Ehtesham M, Kabos P, Kabosova A, et al. The use of interleukin 12-secreting neural stem cells for the treatment of intracranial glioma. Cancer Res 2002; 62(20):5657–63.

23. Liu Y, Ehtesham M, Samoto K, et al. In situ adenoviral interleukin 12 gene transfer confers potent and long-lasting cytotoxic immunity in glioma. Cancer Gene Ther 2002;9(1):9–15.

24. Fathallah-Shaykh HM, Zhao LJ, Kafrouni AI, et al. Gene transfer of IFN-gamma into established brain tumors represses growth by antiangiogenesis. J Immunol 2000;164(1):217–22.

25. Ehtesham M, Kabos P, Gutierrez MA, et al. Induction of glioblastoma apoptosis using neural stem cell-mediated delivery of tumor necrosis factor-related apoptosis-inducing ligand. Cancer Res 2002;62(24):7170–4.

26. Saleh M, Jonas NK, Wiegmans A, et al. The treatment of established intracranial tumors by in situ retroviral IFN-gamma transfer. Gene Ther 2000; 7(20):1715–24.

27. Lee J, Hampl M, Albert P, et al. Antitumor activity and prolonged expression from a TRAIL-expressing adenoviral vector. Neoplasia 2002;4(4):312–23.

28. Kuppner MC, Hamou MF, Sawamura Y, et al. Inhibition of lymphocyte function by glioblastoma-derived transforming growth factor beta 2. J Neurosurg 1989;71(2):211–7.

29. Siepl C, Bodmer S, Frei K, et al. The glioblastoma-derived T cell suppressor factor/transforming growth factor-beta 2 inhibits T-cell growth without affecting the interaction of interleukin-2 with its receptor. Eur J Immunol 1988;18(4):593–600.

30. Gansbacher B, Zier K, Daniels B, et al. Interleukin-2 gene transfer into tumor cells abrogates tumorigenicity and induces protective immunity. J Exp Med 1990;172(4):1217–24.

31. Saris SC, Rosenberg SA, Friedman RB, et al. Penetration of recombinant interleukin-2 across the blood–cerebrospinal fluid barrier. J Neurosurg 1988;69(1):29–34.

32. Barba D, Saris SC, Holder C, et al. Intratumoral LAK cell and interleukin-2 therapy of human gliomas. J Neurosurg 1989;70(2):175–82.

33. Vaquero J, Martinez R, Oya S, et al. Intratumoural injection of autologous lymphocytes plus human lymphoblastoid interferon for the treatment of glioblastoma. Acta Neurochir [Wien] 1989;98:35–41.

34. Merchant RE, McVicar DW, Merchant LH, et al. Treatment of recurrent malignant glioma by repeated intracerebral injections of human recombinant interleukin-2 alone or in combination with systemic interferon-alpha. Results of a phase I clinical trial. J Neurooncol 1992;12(1):75–83.

35. Lesniak MS, Sampath P, DiMeco F, et al. Comparative analysis of paracrine immunotherapy in experimental brain tumors. Neurosurg Focus 2000;9(6):e4.

36. Ewend MG, Thompson RC, Anderson R, et al. Intracranial paracrine interleukin-2 therapy stimulates prolonged antitumor immunity that extends outside the central nervous system. J Immunother 2000; 23(4):438–48.

37. Sampath P, Hanes J, DiMeco F, et al. Paracrine immunotherapy with interleukin-2 and local chemotherapy is synergistic in the treatment of experimental brain tumors. Cancer Res 1999;59(9): 2107–14.

38. Hanes J, Sills A, Zhao Z, et al. Controlled local delivery of interleukin-2 by biodegradable polymers protects animals from experimental brain tumors and liver tumors. Pharm Res 2001;18(7): 899–906.

39. Colombo F, Barzon L, Franchin E, et al. Combined HSV-TK/IL-2 gene therapy in patients with recurrent glioblastoma multiforme: biological and clinical results. Cancer Gene Ther 2005;12(10):835–48.

40. Dillman RO, Duma CM, Schiltz PM, et al. Intracavitary placement of autologous lymphokine-activated killer (LAK) cells after resection of recurrent glioblastoma. J Immunother 2004;27(5):398–404.

41. Giezeman-Smits KM, Okada H, Brissette-Storkus CS, et al. Cytokine gene therapy of gliomas: induction of reactive CD4+ T cells by interleukin-4-transfected 9L gliosarcoma is essential for protective immunity. Cancer Res 2000;60(9):2449–57.

42. Okada H, Giezeman-Smits KM, Tahara H, et al. Effective cytokine gene therapy against an intracranial glioma using a retrovirally transduced IL-4 plus HSVtk tumor vaccine. Gene Ther 1999;6(2): 219–26.

43. Benedetti S, Pirola B, Pollo B, et al. Gene therapy of experimental brain tumors using neural progenitor cells. Nat Med 2000;6(4):447–50.

44. Benedetti S, Pirola B, Poliani PL, et al. Dexamethasone inhibits the antitumor effect of interleukin-4 on rat experimental gliomas. Gene Ther 2003;10(2): 188–92.

45. Weiss JM, Subleski JJ, Wigginton JM, et al. Immunotherapy of cancer by IL-12-based cytokine combinations. Expert Opin Biol Ther 2007;7(11): 1705–21.

46. DiMeco F, Rhines LD, Hanes J, et al. Paracrine delivery of IL-12 against intracranial 9L gliosarcoma in rats. J Neurosurg 2000;92(3):419–27.

47. Tahara H, Zitvogel L, Storkus WJ, et al. Effective eradication of established murine tumors with IL-12 gene therapy using a polycistronic retroviral vector. J Immunol 1995;154(12):6466–74.

48. Kikuchi T, Akasaki Y, Abe T, et al. Vaccination of glioma patients with fusions of dendritic and glioma cells and recombinant human interleukin 12. J Immunother 2004;27(6):452–9.

49. de Vries IJ, Eggert AA, Scharenborg NM, et al. Phenotypical and functional characterization of clinical grade dendritic cells. J Immunother 2002;25(5):429–38.

50. Herrlinger U, Kramm CM, Johnston KM, et al. Vaccination for experimental gliomas using GM-CSF-transduced glioma cells. Cancer Gene Ther 1997;4(6):345–52.

51. Sedegah M, Weiss W, Sacci JB Jr, et al. Improving protective immunity induced by DNA-based immunization: priming with antigen and GM-CSF-encoding plasmid DNA and boosting with antigen-expressing recombinant poxvirus. J Immunol 2000;164(11): 5905–12.

52. Yamanaka R. Cell- and peptide-based immunotherapeutic approaches for glioma. Trends Mol Med 2008;14(5):228–35.

53. Enderlin M, Kleinmann EV, Struyf S, et al. TNF-alpha and the IFN-gamma-inducible protein 10 (IP-10/CXCL-10) delivered by parvoviral vectors act in synergy to induce antitumor effects in mouse glioblastoma. Cancer Gene Ther 2009;16(2):149–60.

54. Villeneuve J, Tremblay P, Vallieres L. Tumor necrosis factor reduces brain tumor growth by enhancing macrophage recruitment and microcyst formation. Cancer Res 2005;65(9):3928–36.

55. Ali S, King GD, Curtin JF, et al. Combined immunostimulation and conditional cytotoxic gene therapy provide long-term survival in a large glioma model. Cancer Res 2005;65(16):7194–204.

56. Miller G, Pillarisetty VG, Shah AB, et al. Murine Flt3 ligand expands distinct dendritic cells with both tolerogenic and immunogenic properties. J Immunol 2003;170(7):3554–64.

57. Daga A, Orengo AM, Gangemi RM, et al. Glioma immunotherapy by IL-21 gene-modified cells or by recombinant IL-21 involves antibody responses. Int J Cancer 2007;121(8):1756–63.

58. Lamprecht B, Kreher S, Anagnostopoulos I, et al. Aberrant expression of the Th2 cytokine IL-21 in Hodgkin lymphoma cells regulates STAT3 signaling and attracts Treg cells via regulation of MIP-3alpha. Blood 2008;112(8):3339–47.

59. Brandes AA, Scelzi E, Zampieri P, et al. Phase II trial with BCNU plus alpha-interferon in patients with recurrent high-grade gliomas. Am J Clin Oncol 1997;20(4):364–7.

60. Buckner JC, Brown LD, Kugler JW, et al. Phase II evaluation of recombinant interferon alpha and BCNU in recurrent glioma. J Neurosurg 1995;82(3):430–5.

61. Rajkumar SV, Buckner JC, Schomberg PJ, et al. Phase I evaluation of radiation combined with recombinant interferon alpha-2a and BCNU for patients with high-grade glioma. Int J Radiat Oncol Biol Phys 1998;40(2):297–302.

62. Yung WK, Steck PA, Kelleher PJ, et al. Growth inhibitory effect of recombinant alpha and beta interferon on human glioma cells. J Neurooncol 1987;5(4):323–30.

63. Hiroishi K, Tuting T, Tahara H, et al. Interferon-alpha gene therapy in combination with CD80 transduction reduces tumorigenicity and growth of established tumor in poorly immunogenic tumor models. Gene Ther 1999;6(12):1988–94.

64. Buckner JC, Schomberg PJ, McGinnis WL, et al. A phase III study of radiation therapy plus carmustine with or without recombinant interferon-alpha in the treatment of patients with newly diagnosed high-grade glioma. Cancer 2001;92(2):420–33.

65. Olson JJ, McKenzie E, Skurski-Martin M, et al. Phase I analysis of BCNU-impregnated biodegradable polymer wafers followed by systemic interferon alfa-2b in adults with recurrent glioblastoma multiforme. J Neurooncol 2008;90(3):293–9.

66. Makar TK, Wilt S, Dong Z, et al. IFN-beta gene transfer into the central nervous system using bone marrow cells as a delivery system. J Interferon Cytokine Res 2002;22(7):783–91.

67. Mahaley MS Jr, Dropcho EJ, Bertsch L, et al. Systemic beta-interferon therapy for recurrent gliomas: a brief report. J Neurosurg 1989;71(5 Pt 1):639–41.

68. Allen J, Packer R, Bleyer A, et al. Recombinant interferon beta: a phase I-II trial in children with recurrent brain tumors. J Clin Oncol 1991;9(5):783–8.

69. Fetell MR, Housepian EM, Oster MW, et al. Intratumor administration of beta-interferon in recurrent malignant gliomas. A phase I clinical and laboratory study. Cancer 1990;65(1):78–83.

70. Wakabayashi T, Kayama T, Nishikawa R, et al. A multicenter phase I trial of interferon-beta and temozolomide combination therapy for high-grade gliomas (INTEGRA Study). Jpn J Clin Oncol 2008;38(10):715–8.

71. Sethna MP, Lampson LA. Immune modulation within the brain: recruitment of inflammatory cells and increased major histocompatability antigen expression following intracerebral injection of interferon-gamma. J Neuroimmunol 1991;34:121–32.

72. Glick RP, Lichtor T, Kim TS, et al. Fibroblasts genetically engineered to secrete cytokines suppress tumor growth and induce antitumor immunity to a murine glioma in vivo. Neurosurgery 1995;36(3):548–55.

73. Ehtesham M, Samoto K, Kabos P, et al. Treatment of intracranial glioma with in situ interferon-gamma and tumor necrosis factor-alpha gene transfer. Cancer Gene Ther 2002;9(11):925–34.

74. Lichtor T, Glick RP, Kim TS, et al. Prolonged survival of mice with glioma injected intracerebrally with double cytokine-secreting cells. J Neurosurg 1995;83(6):1038–44.

75. Wolff JE, Wagner S, Reinert C, et al. Maintenance treatment with interferon-gamma and low-dose cyclophosphamide for pediatric high-grade glioma. J Neurooncol 2006;79(3):315–21.

76. Lotfi R, Schrezenmeier H, Lotze MT. Immunotherapy for cancer: promoting innate immunity. Front Biosci 2009;14:818–32.

77. Ehrchen JM, Sunderkotter C, Foell D, et al. The endogenous Toll-like receptor 4 agonist S100A8/S100A9 (calprotectin) as innate amplifier of infection, autoimmunity, and cancer. J Leukoc Biol 2009;86(3):557–66.

78. Mariani CL, Rajon D, Bova FJ, et al. Nonspecific immunotherapy with intratumoral lipopolysaccharide and zymosan A but not GM-CSF leads to an effective antitumor response in subcutaneous RG-2 gliomas. J Neurooncol 2007;85(3):231–40.

79. Wolska A, Lech-Maranda E, Robak T. Toll-like receptors and their role in carcinogenesis and anti-tumor treatment. Cell Mol Biol Lett 2009;14(2):248–72.

80. Tsan MF. Toll-like receptors, inflammation and cancer. Semin Cancer Biol 2006;16(1):32–7.

81. Jack CS, Arbour N, Manusow J, et al. TLR signaling tailors innate immune responses in human microglia and astrocytes. J Immunol 2005;175(7):4320–30.

82. Ito A, Matsuoka F, Honda H, et al. Heat shock protein 70 gene therapy combined with hyperthermia using magnetic nanoparticles. Cancer Gene Ther 2003;10(12):918–25.

83. Ito A, Shinkai M, Honda H, et al. Heat shock protein 70 expression induces antitumor immunity during intracellular hyperthermia using magnetite nanoparticles. Cancer Immunol Immunother 2003;52(2):80–8.

84. Kirsch M, Fischer H, Schackert G. Activated monocytes kill malignant brain tumor cells in vitro. J Neurooncol 1994;20(1):35–45.

85. Wu A, Oh S, Gharagozlou S, et al. In vivo vaccination with tumor cell lysate plus CpG oligodeoxynucleotides eradicates murine glioblastoma. J Immunother 2007;30(8):789–97.

86. Grauer O, Poschl P, Lohmeier A, et al. Toll-like receptor triggered dendritic cell maturation and IL-12 secretion are necessary to overcome T-cell inhibition by glioma-associated TGF-beta2. J Neurooncol 2007;82(2):151–61.

87. Carpentier AF, Meng Y. Recent advances in immunotherapy for human glioma. Curr Opin Oncol 2006;18(6):631–6.

88. Meng Y, Carpentier AF, Chen L, et al. Successful combination of local CpG-ODN and radiotherapy in malignant glioma. Int J Cancer 2005;116(6):992–7.

89. Carpentier AF, Xie J, Mokhtari K, et al. Successful treatment of intracranial gliomas in rat by oligodeoxynucleotides containing CpG motifs. Clin Cancer Res 2000;6(6):2469–73.

90. Carpentier AF, Chen L, Maltonti F, et al. Oligodeoxynucleotides containing CpG motifs can induce rejection of a neuroblastoma in mice. Cancer Res 1999;59(21):5429–32.

91. Carpentier A, Laigle-Donadey F, Zohar S, et al. Phase 1 trial of a CpG oligodeoxynucleotide for patients with recurrent glioblastoma. Neuro Oncol 2006;8(1):60–6.

92. Talmadge JE, Adams J, Phillips H, et al. Immunomodulatory effects in mice of polyinosinic-polycytidylic acid complexed with poly-L-lysine and carboxymethylcellulose. Cancer Res 1985;45(3):1058–65.

93. Levy HB, Lvovsky E, Riley F, et al. Immune modulating effects of poly ICLC. Ann N Y Acad Sci 1980;350:33–41.

94. Hubbell HR, Liu RS, Maxwell BL. Independent sensitivity of human tumor cell lines to interferon and double-stranded RNA. Cancer Res 1984;44(8):3252–7.

95. Black PL, Hartmann D, Pennington R, et al. Effect of tumor burden and route of administration on the immunotherapeutic properties of polyinosinic-polycytidylic acid stabilized with poly-L-lysine in carboxymethyl cellulose [Poly(I, C)-LC]. Int J Immunopharmacol 1992;14(8):1341–53.

96. Dick RS, Hubbell HR. Sensitivities of human glioma cell lines to interferons and double-stranded RNAs individually and in synergistic combinations. J Neurooncol 1987;5(4):331–8.

97. Rosenblum MG, Yung WK, Kelleher PJ, et al. Growth inhibitory effects of interferon-beta but not interferon-alpha on human glioma cells: correlation of receptor binding, 2',5'-oligoadenylate synthetase and protein kinase activity. J Interferon Res 1990;10(2):141–51.

98. Strayer DR, Weisband J, Carter WA, et al. Growth of astrocytomas in the human tumor clonogenic assay and sensitivity to mismatched dsRNA and interferons. Am J Clin Oncol 1987;10(4):281–4.

99. Droller MJ. Immunotherapy of metastatic renal cell carcinoma with polyinosinic–polycytidylic acid. J Urol 1987;137(2):202–6.

100. Hawkins MJ, Levin L, Borden EC. An Eastern Cooperative Oncology Group phase I-II pilot study of polyriboinosinic–polyribocytidylic acid poly-L-lysine complex in patients with metastatic malignant melanoma. J Biol Response Mod 1985;4(6):664–8.

101. Krown SE, Kerr D, Stewart WE 2nd, et al. Phase I trials of poly(I, C) complexes in advanced cancer. J Biol Response Mod 1985;4(6):640–9.

102. Nakamura O, Shitara N, Matsutani M, et al. Phase I-II trials of poly(ICLC) in malignant brain tumor patients. J Interferon Res 1982;2(1):1–4.

103. Rettenmaier MA, Berman ML, DiSaia PJ. Treatment of advanced ovarian cancer with polyinosinic-polycytidylic lysine carboxymethylcellulose poly[ICLC]. Gynecol Oncol 1986;24(3):359–61.

104. Theriault RL, Hortobagyi GN, Buzdar AU, et al. Evaluation of polyinosinic-polycytidylic and poly-L-lysine in metastatic breast cancer. Cancer Treat Rep 1986;70(11):1341–2.

105. Talmadge JE, Herberman RB, Chirigos MA, et al. Hyporesponsiveness to augmentation of murine natural killer cell activity in different anatomical compartments by multiple injections of various immunomodulators including recombinant interferons and interleukin 2. J Immunol 1985;135(4):2483–91.

106. Ewel CH, Urba WJ, Kopp WC, et al. Polyinosinic–polycytidylic acid complexed with poly-L-lysine and carboxymethylcellulose in combination with interleukin 2 in patients with cancer: clinical and immunological effects. Cancer Res 1992;52(11):3005–10.

107. Black KL, Chen K, Becker DP, et al. Inflammatory leukocytes associated with increased immunosuppression by glioblastoma. J Neurosurg 1992;77(1):120–6.

108. Levy HB. Historical overview of the use of polynucleotides in cancer. J Biol Response Mod 1985;4(5):475–80.

109. Levy HB, Levine AS. Antitumor effects of interferon and poly ICLC, and their possible utility as antineoplastic agents in man. Tex Rep Biol Med 1981;41:653–62.

110. Matsumoto M, Seya T. TLR3: Interferon induction by double-stranded RNA including poly(I: C). Adv Drug Deliv Rev 2008;60(7):805–12.

111. Kim H, Yang E, Lee J, et al. Double-stranded RNA mediates interferon regulatory factor 3 activation and interleukin-6 production by engaging Toll-like receptor 3 in human brain astrocytes. Immunology 2008;124(4):480–8.

112. Salazar AM, Levy HB, Ondra S, et al. Long-term treatment of malignant gliomas with intramuscularly administered polyinosinic–polycytidylic acid stabilized with polylysine and carboxymethylcellulose: an open pilot study. Neurosurgery 1996;38(6):1096–103 [discussion: 1103–4].

113. Stupp R, Dietrich PY, Ostermann Kraljevic S, et al. Promising survival for patients with newly diagnosed glioblastoma multiforme treated with concomitant radiation plus temozolomide followed by adjuvant temozolomide. J Clin Oncol 2002;20(5):1375–82.

114. Chong G, Morse MA. Combining cancer vaccines with chemotherapy. Expert Opin Pharmacother 2005;6(16):2813–20.
115. Wheeler CJ, Das A, Liu G, et al. Clinical responsiveness of glioblastoma multiforme to chemotherapy after vaccination. Clin Cancer Res 2004; 10(16):5316–26.
116. van der Most RG, Currie A, Robinson BW, et al. Cranking the immunologic engine with chemotherapy: using context to drive tumor antigen cross-presentation towards useful antitumor immunity. Cancer Res 2006;66(2):601–4.
117. Zhu X, Nishimura F, Sasaki K, et al. Toll like receptor-3 ligand poly-ICLC promotes the efficacy of peripheral vaccinations with tumor antigen-derived peptide epitopes in murine CNS tumor models. J Transl Med 2007;5:10.
118. Wong ET, Hess KR, Gleason MJ, et al. Outcomes and prognostic factors in recurrent glioma patients enrolled onto phase II clinical trials. J Clin Oncol 1999;17(8):2572–8.
119. Okada H, Pollack IF. Cytokine gene therapy for malignant glioma. Expert Opin Biol Ther 2004; 4(10):1609–20.
120. Selznick LA, Shamji MF, Fecci P, et al. Molecular strategies for the treatment of malignant glioma—genes, viruses, and vaccines. Neurosurg Rev 2008;31(2):141–55 [discussion: 155].
121. Sehgal A, Berger MS. Basic concepts of immunology and neuroimmunology. Neurosurg Focus 2000;9(6):e1.
122. Tanriover N, Ulu MO, Sanus GZ, et al. The effects of systemic and intratumoral interleukin-12 treatment in C6 rat glioma model. Neurol Res 2008;30(5):511–7.
123. Grauer OM, Molling JW, Bennink E, et al. TLR ligands in the local treatment of established intracerebral murine gliomas. J Immunol 2008;181(10):6720–9.
124. Everson RG, Graner MW, Gromeier M, et al. Immunotherapy against angiogenesis-associated targets: evidence and implications for the treatment of malignant glioma. Expert Rev Anticancer Ther 2008;8(5):717–32.

# Passive Antibody-Mediated Immunotherapy for the Treatment of Malignant Gliomas

Siddhartha Mitra, PhD, Gordon Li, MD*,
Griffith R. Harsh IV, MD

## KEYWORDS

- Monoclonal antibody
- Epidermal growth factor receptor variant III
- Epidermal growth factor receptor
- Tenascin-C • Bevacizumab • Glioblastoma multiforme

Malignant gliomas are the most common primary intracranial tumors and among the most lethal of solid and hematopoietic cancers.[1] Their ruthless malignant progression invades and destroys normal brain tissue, resists traditional therapies, and causes death for sure. Infiltration throughout the brain is a prominent feature of high-grade gliomas and is the principal basis for refractoriness to local therapies, including surgery.[1] Although in most cases, recurrent tumor is first noted radiographically near or within several centimeters of the resection cavity, the tumor has already infiltrated widely by that time.[2] Invasion of tumor cells within normal brain structures makes normal brain function vulnerable to therapies, which do not discriminate between neoplastic and normal cells. Potential for such discrimination arises, however, from differences between tumor and normal cells, in the protein-carbohydrate complexes on their surface.[3] Immunotherapeutic approaches selectively target tumor cells by exploiting these differences in cell surface molecules. This strategy has the dual benefit of increasing efficacy against the tumor cells and decreasing toxicity to nonneoplastic cells. Although many immunotherapeutic approaches are being investigated, this article focuses on monoclonal antibodies (mAbs), or serotherapies, that have progressed to clinical trials against malignant gliomas.

## MONOCLONAL ANTIBODIES

mAbs, made in large numbers outside the body, are considered agents of passive immunotherapy, which does not require the patient's immune system to take an active role in fighting the cancer.[4,5] The first mAbs were produced by hybridoma cells formed by fusing a mouse myeloma cell with a mouse B cell making a specific antibody.[6] Because the antibodies, which are all identical, are made from a single (mono) hybridoma clone, they are called monoclonal antibodies. mAbs can be used in treating malignant gliomas either alone or attached to a cytotoxic or radioactive agent.[7] Repeated treatments with murine mAbs frequently trigger allergic reactions and human antimouse antibody responses in patients. This is prevented by humanizing the mAbs by linking the murine antibody variable region to human IgG constant regions.[8,9] Human antibodies should have even less immunogenicity.[10] Yang and colleagues[11] reported generation of mAb E7.6.3, a human anti-EGF (epidermal

Authors contributed equally to the manuscript.

Department of Neurosurgery, Stanford University School of Medicine, 300 Pasteur Drive, Edwards Building Room 200, Stanford, CA 94305, USA

* Corresponding author.

E-mail address: gordonli@stanford.edu (G. Li).

Neurosurg Clin N Am 21 (2010) 67–76

doi:10.1016/j.nec.2009.08.010

growth factor) receptor IgG2 mAb from humanized transgenic mice.

The antineoplastic activity of mAbs could have multiple mechanisms: (1) opsonization of cancer cells and subsequent activation of immune effector mechanisms,[12] (2) disruption of cellular signaling,[13,14] and (3) inducing antibody-dependent cellular cytotoxicity (ADCC) or complement-dependent cellular cytotoxicity, whereby an effector cell of the immune system lyses a target cell by releasing granzymes, porforins, tumor necrosis factor α, and interferon-γ.[15–17] Bleeker and colleagues[18] showed that anti-EGF receptor antibodies cause cell death by compromising EGF-induced signaling and inducing ADCC. Several EGF receptor mAbs have shown promise in vitro and in murine xenograft models.[19–26]

## TARGET DETERMINATION OF PASSIVE ANTIBODY IMMUNOTHERAPY

Effective mAb therapy requires that the targeted tumor-specific antigen has stable cell surface expression (ie, low turnover time) of at least $1 \times 10^5$ molecules per tumor cell.[27] Glioblastoma multiformes (GBMs) overexpress many different antigens, including EGF receptor, melanoma associated antigen, Her2/neu, tyrosinase, Trp-1, Trp-2, gp100, IL-13Rα2, survivin,[28] and EphA2.[29] Treatment targeting these antigens is potentially toxic as they are also expressed on cells of normal tissue. Targeting a novel epitope unique to cancer cells would be preferable. EGF receptor variant III (EGFRvIII), the most common genetic alteration of the EGF receptor, is such a protein.[30–34]

An alternative mAb strategy targets a ligand/receptor pair essential for tumor proliferation or maintenance. An example includes vascular endothelial growth factor (VEGF) and its receptor, which stimulate the extensive vascularization of high-grade gliomas. One final method is the targeting of tenascin-C, an extracellular matrix protein, which drives tumor cell invasion of normal tissue.

## ANTI-EGFR THERAPY

The EGF receptor is overexpressed, mutated, or both in many solid tumors, notably high-grade gliomas, where it is overexpressed in 40% to 50% of cases.[35] Cetuximab is a human:mouse chimeric mAb that binds with high specificity to the extracellular domain of EGF receptor and prevents receptor dimerization and signaling.[36] Crystal structural studies showed that binding of the cetuximab antigen-binding fragment (Fab) to domain III of the receptor prevents growth factor binding. Ferguson[37] showed that the heavy-chain

($V_H$) region of the antibody sterically prevents domain I of the EGF receptor from adopting the conformation required for the dimerization essential for preventing potential ligand-independent modes of EGF receptor activation. In preclinical studies, cetuximab inhibits growth and increases apoptosis in GBM cell lines. There are conflicting data regarding whether EGF receptor amplification imparts cetuximab sensitivity.[38,39]

These preclinical studies have led to multiple human clinical trials (**Table 1**). Seventeen patients with pathologically confirmed GBM underwent standard postoperative radiation and temozolomide treatment followed by weekly infusions of cetuximab in a phase 1/2 trial, "Radiochemotherapy with Temozolomide and Cetuximab in patients with primary GBM (GERT trial)".[40] Median follow-up was 13 months in 17 patients, of whom 7 received gross total resection, 7 had subtotal resection, and 3 had biopsy only. This study concluded that the combination of radiation, temozolomide, and cetuximab is safe and well tolerated. At 6 months, 81% of patients were free of tumor progression, and at 12 months, 87% of patients were still alive. Methylated methyl guanine methyl transferase (MGMT) was not associated with longer overall or progression-free survival, and analysis of EGF receptor status is ongoing.[40]

Single-agent cetuximab has been tried in patients with recurrent high-grade glioma after surgery, radiotherapy, and chemotherapy.[41] Patients were stratified into 2 treatment arms according to the amplification status of the EGF receptor gene as determined by fluorescence in situ hybridization. A total of 55 patients underwent treatment with cetuximab (28 with and 27 without an increased EGF receptor copy number). The EGF receptor mAb was generally well tolerated, the median duration of progression-free survival was 1.9 months, and the median duration of overall survival was 5.0 months. The rates of 6-month progression-free survival and overall survival were 10% and 40%, respectively. Although progression-free survival lasted less than 5 months in most ($n = 49$) patients, 5 patients survived without tumor progression for at least 9 months (range, 9.5 to >16.5). No significant correlation was found between response, duration of survival, and EGF receptor copy number.[41]

Cetuximab has also been tried in a phase 2 trial that combined cetuximab, bevacizumab, and irinotecan for patients with primary GBMs following tumor progression after radiation therapy and temozolomide treatment.[42] The mean duration of overall survival was 29 weeks, and the mean time to tumor progression was 24 weeks. Thirty

**Table 1**
**Summary of clinical trials using anti-EGF receptor mAbs**

| Treatment | Patients Evaluated | Number of Patients | Results | Secondary Result |
|---|---|---|---|---|
| Cetuximab (phase 1/2) | Newly diagnosed GBM after surgical treatment and standard postoperative radiation and temozolomide | 17 (7 gross total resection, 7 subtotal resection, 3 biopsy only) | OS = 87% at 12 months PFS = 81% at 6 months | MGMT not associated with longer survival. EGF status analysis ongoing |
| Cetuximab (phase 2) | Recurrent GBM | 55 (28 with increased EGF copy number, 27 without) | PFS = 1.9 months OS = 5 months 6 month PFS = 10% 6 month OS = 40% | No correlation between response and EGF receptor copy number |
| Cetuximab with bevacizumab and irinotecan (phase 2) | Recurrent GBM | 43 | OS = 29 weeks 6 month PFS = 30.2% Mean TTP = 24 wk | 6-month PFS for responders was 72.7% when compared to 23.8% for nonresponders |
| Nimotuzumab (phase 1/2) | Newly diagnosed GBM or anaplastic astrocytoma after surgical treatment and standard postoperative radiation and temozolomide | 28 (16 GBM, 12 anaplastic astrocytoma) | Response rate was 37.9% Median OS, 22.17 months | |
| $^{125}$I-mAb 425 (phase 2) | Newly diagnosed patients with GBM or astrocytoma with anaplastic foci after surgery, postoperative radiation $\pm$ chemotherapy | 180 | OS GBM = 13.4 months OS astrocytoma with anaplastic foci = 50.9 months | |

*Abbreviations:* MGMT, methyl guanine methyl transferase; OS, overall survival; PFS, progression-free survival; TTP, time to progression.

percent of patients were free of tumor progression at 6 months.

Nimotuzumab (h-R3) is a humanized mAb that targets the extracellular domain of the EGF receptor. It has both antiangiogenic and proapoptotic effects. A phase 1/2 trial using nimotuzumab and radiation in 28 individuals with newly diagnosed high-grade gliomas (16 with GBM and 12 with anaplastic astrocytoma) found an objective response rate (defined in this study as either a complete or partial response) of 7.9%. Median duration of overall survival was 22.17 months with a median follow-up of 29 months.[43]

EGF receptor mAbs attached to cytotoxic agents have also been evaluated in clinical trials. mAb 425, a murine mAb raised against human A431 carcinoma cells (which have very high levels of EGF receptor on the cell surface), conjugated with iodine 125,[44] has been used to treat high-grade gliomas in a phase 2 study[45] of 180 patients with either GBM or astrocytomas with anaplastic foci (AAF). When radiolabeled mAb 425 was administered after surgery and radiation therapy, with or without chemotherapy, the median durations of overall survival of patients with GBM and AAF were 13.4 and 50.9 months, respectively.

## ANTI-EGFRVIII THERAPY

EGFRvIII, the most common genetic variation of the EGF receptor, is expressed only in cancer tissue and is thus an ideal immunotherapeutic target.[46] This variant is missing 801 coding bases, a deletion which includes exons 2 to 7 of the wt receptor.[47] The deletion of amino acids 6 to 273 from the extracellular domain of the wild-type protein is accompanied by the encoding of a novel glycine residue at the fusion junction (**Fig. 1**). EGFRvIII was initially discovered in GBM, where it is expressed in approximately 40% of cases.

Among the EGFRvIII mAbs generated against this antigen, mAb 806 is the most tumor-specific.[48,49] Treatment with mAb 806 significantly decreased tumor volume and prolonged the survival of mice with xenografts from EGFRvIII expressing U87 glioma cells.[50]

Y10 is an IgG2a murine mAb. Although Y10 is generated towards an artificially created murine homolog of human EGFRvIII,[51] it recognizes human and murine equivalents of this tumor-specific antigen. Y10 inhibits DNA synthesis and cellular proliferation in vitro and induces autonomous complement-mediated and antibody-dependent cell-mediated cytotoxicity. Intratumoral injection of Y10 in an intracranial B16 melanoma expressing EGFRvIII increased the median duration of survival by 286%. A human chimeric antibody based on Y10 has been developed for clinical use. It induces lysis of human EGFRvIII-expressing malignant glioma cells autonomously and in the presence of activated human macrophages.[52]

One drawback of EGFRvIII serotherapy is that mAbs binding EGFRvIII are rapidly internalized at ambient temperatures.[48,53–55] This disadvantage has been mitigated by modified labeling methods, which has resulted in EGFRvIII mAbs successfully targeting radioisotopes in the radioimmunotherapy of tumors in rodent models.[53,54,56] Despite this preclinical work, mAbs targeting EGFRvIII have not been tested clinically. Clinical trials evaluating a peptide vaccine targeting this unique tumor antigen[57] are underway.

## ANTIANGIOGENESIS THERAPIES

Microvascular proliferation is a histopathologic hallmark of GBMs and an independent prognostic factor for adult gliomas.[58,59] Increasing evidence suggests that tumor angiogenesis is not an adaptive response to tumor-induced hypoxia, but

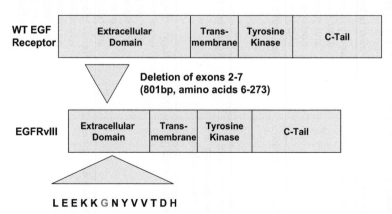

**Fig. 1.** EGFRvIII. An in-frame deletion of exons 2 to 7 of the EGF receptor permits fusion of exon 1 and exon 8, which generates a novel glycine.

rather a result of decisive genetic mutations that activate an angiogenic transcriptional program which is further modified by the regional tumor oxygen status. Antiangiogenic therapies are being developed in hopes that disrupting the tumor vasculature will lead to regression of the tumor. The most successful therapy from this approach is serotherapy against VEGF and its cognate receptor.[60–62]

Bevacizumab is a humanized mAb that binds to circulating VEGF-A (the most common isoform in GBMs). Treatment with bevacizumab in combination with irinotecan (CPT-11), a topoisomerase-1 inhibitor, resulted in increased duration of survival in patients with metastatic colorectal cancer and has subsequently received approval for treatment of other solid tumors, including lung and breast cancers.[63,64] Bevacizumab and irinotecan were first used for patients with malignant glioma when a medical oncologist, Dr Stark-Vance, who had success treating patients with colorectal cancer, applied this regimen to 21 patients with recurrent GBM and saw a response rate of 43% (1 patient with complete response and 8 patients with partial response using MacDonald's criteria).[65] Prompted by these exciting results, Vredenburgh and colleagues[60,61] treated 32 patients with recurrent malignant gliomas in a prospective trial with bevacizumab and irinotecan and saw dramatic rates of radiographic response (61% in GBM and 67% in anaplastic glioma) and a near doubling of the rate of 6-month progression-free survival of 30% for GBM and 56% for anaplastic gliomas, compared with historical controls of 15% and 31%, respectively. Long-term follow-up of these patients revealed that they lived no longer than historical controls.[66] Norden and colleagues[67] published similar results from Dana Farber Cancer Institute after using bevacizumab and irinotecan treatment for 33 patients with recurrent GBM and 21 patients with recurrent anaplastic glioma. This study showed that patients who failed treatment with bevacizumab and irinotecan were unlikely to respond favorably to subsequent cytotoxic chemotherapy or other novel therapeutics. They were likely to have very rapid disease progression and clinical deterioration.

The 2 earlier studies did not evaluate the incremental benefit of adding irinotecan to bevacizumab. Fine[68] treated 79 patients with recurrent GBM in a phase 2 study with bevacizumab alone. The response rate was 60%, and the rate of 6-month progression-free survival was 30% (similar to the other 2 studies), suggesting that irinotecan treatment is not necessary. Moreover, the toxicity of bevacizumab in the Fine study was less than that of the other 2 studies. Preliminary results of

a Genentech study of patients with recurrent GBM randomized between bevacizumab alone or bevacizumab in combination with irinotecan[65] showed a response rate and progression-free survival rate of 28% and 42.6% in patients receiving bevacizumab monotherapy versus 37.8% and 50.3% in patients receiving the combination therapy; this suggests that irinotecan adds benefit to bevacizumab treatment. The median duration of overall survival for patients receiving bevacizumab alone was 9.2 months, and for the combination group, it was 8.7 months. Neither of these numbers is significantly different from those of historical controls.

Although the superior rates of radiographic response and 6-month progression-free survival from the bevacizumab trials are enticing, many clinicians question bevacizumab's benefit, given the lack of improvement in overall survival. Although the magnetic resonance imaging (MRI) shows decreased volume of contrast enhancement (**Fig. 2**), bevacizumab may simply be normalizing tumor blood vessels to decrease leakage of gadolinium and may have no real antitumor affect. Laboratory studies and randomized trials are seeking to resolve this issue. Meanwhile, patients with newly diagnosed GBM are being treated with bevacizumab immediately after surgery and radiation in ongoing clinical trials.

## SEROTHERAPY AGAINST EXTRACELLULAR MATRIX PROTEINS

Tenascin-C is an extracellular matrix protein expressed in more than 90% of gliomas but not in the normal brain; its presence increases with increasing tumor grade.[69–72] Although the function of tenascin-C is debated, the protein seems to be important for cellular processes including adhesion, migration, and proliferation. Several anti-tenascin-C antibodies have been generated.[73–75] The tenascin-C mAb 81C6, a murine IgG2b that targets an isoform of tenascin-C expressed in malignant gliomas,[73,76] has been used in most clinical studies. This antibody does not cross-react with normal brain and has been used in conjugation with $^{131}$I radioisotope.

$^{131}$I-labeled mAb 81C6 injected into the tumor resection cavity to deliver a target dose of 44 Gy was evaluated in 10 human GBM trials. Newly diagnosed GBM patients treated with surgery, postoperative radiotherapy, temozolomide, and $^{131}$I-labeled mAb 81C6 in the phase 2 trial had a median duration of overall survival of 91 weeks.[77–79] A further analysis after 231 weeks of median follow-up revealed an average time to

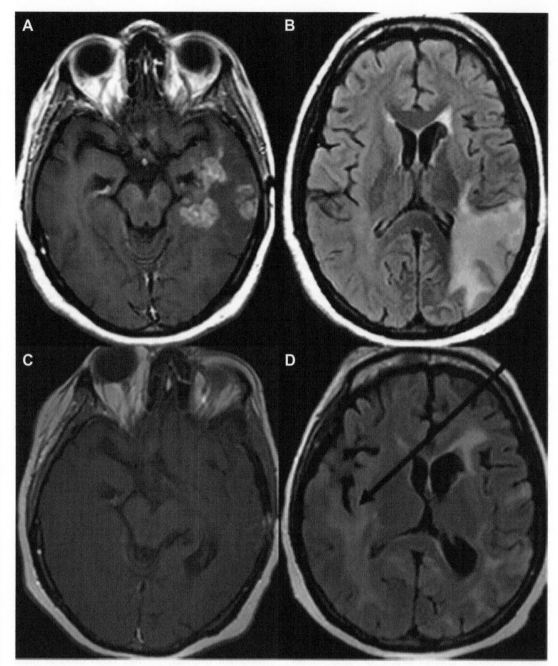

**Fig. 2.** MRI images from a patient with recurrent GBM before and after bevacizumab treatment showing significant radiographic response. Pretreatment axial T1 with contrast (*A*) and axial FLAIR (fast fluid attenuated inversion recovery) (*B*). Posttreatment axial T1 with contrast (*C*) and axial FLAIR (*D*). *Arrow* points to interval white matter change that may indicate new tumor.

progression of 77.3 weeks (17.8 months) and an overall survival duration of 102.1 weeks (*n* = 14). These data are the basis of a randomized phase 3 trial, which is currently recruiting patients to either the control treatment arm of surgery and postoperative radiochemotherapy or the treatment arm of surgery, postoperative radiochemotherapy, and $^{131}$I-conjugated 81C6 mAb.

## DISCUSSION

mAbs are widely accepted as standard-of-care agents for several solid and hematopoietic cancers. They afford high target specificity, relatively low toxicity, and efficacy based on target inhibition and immune enhancement. The authors optimistically await completion of randomized trials evaluating mAbs such as bevacizumab, cetuximab, and [131]I-labeled mAb 81C6 for malignant gliomas and of preclinical studies of newer mAbs against other targets.

There are many ways to improve mAb therapy. Clinical testing and use of newer agents will require the humanization of mouse mAbs to reduce the risk of infusion and allergic reactions. This involves cloning the immunoglobulin light and heavy chains from an established hybridoma and directed amino acid substitution. Alternatively, antibodies could be created in mice that are genetically engineered to produce fully human antibodies. Alteration of either the mAb's Fc protein or its glycosylation may enhance ADCC, which should improve tumor lysis. Even single-residue substitutions and/or minor changes in glycosylation may enhance binding of the Fc portion of the antibody to the Fc receptor gamma. This improves opsonization of target-expressing tumor cells for cell killing by ADCC.

The need for brain tumor therapeutic agents to traverse the blood-brain barrier has prompted development and testing of smaller antibody fragments, such as diabodies, minibodies, Fab fragments, single-chain Fv domains, and single-chain antibodies derived from camels and llamas.[80–82] These antibody fragments range in size from 15 to 60 kD; they become distributed throughout the tumor more quickly and homogeneously when compared to full mAbs but have more limited tumor retention, serum half-life, and ADCC functionality. Tumor retention, however, can be improved with multivalent constructs.[4,83,84]

Many investigators believe that the initiation and maintenance of malignant gliomas, and particularly their early and aggressive recurrence, depend on limited numbers of highly tumorigenic stem cells.[85–87] mAbs directed against epitopes unique to brain tumor stem cells theoretically hold special promise. CD133 has been identified as 1 stem cell marker for malignant gliomas.[88–90] However, CD133 is also shared by neural/hematopoietic stem cells, and therapy directed indiscriminately against this stem cell marker may cause significant side effects. Therapy directed against CD33, the marker shared by acute myeloid leukemia cancer stem cells and hematopoietic stem cells, causes myelosuppression and neutropenia.[91] To avoid such toxicity, identification of markers highly specific for tumor progenitor cells will likely be required. Screening of glioma cells for expression of such cell surface markers is being pursued.

Identification of a tumor-specific marker unique to brain tumor stem cells would permit development of mAbs that would selectively target the cells of a tumor that are critical to its self-renewing proliferation and resistance to therapy. Success would validate the stem cell hypothesis of cancer, the mAb strategy of therapy, and the hope for a cure of malignant brain tumors.

## REFERENCES

1. Furnari FB, Fenton T, Bachoo RM, et al. Malignant astrocytic glioma: genetics, biology, and paths to treatment. Genes Dev 2007;21:2683–710.
2. Lefranc F, Brotchi J, Kiss R. Possible future issues in the treatment of glioblastomas: special emphasis on cell migration and the resistance of migrating glioblastoma cells to apoptosis. J Clin Oncol 2005;23: 2411–22.
3. Bolesta E, Kowalczyk A, Wierzbicki A, et al. DNA vaccine expressing the mimotope of GD2 ganglioside induces protective GD2 cross-reactive antibody responses. Cancer Res 2005;65:3410–8.
4. Adams GP, Weiner LM. Monoclonal antibody therapy of cancer. Nat Biotechnol 2005;23:1147–57.
5. Farah RA, Clinchy B, Herrera L, et al. The development of monoclonal antibodies for the therapy of cancer. Crit Rev Eukaryot Gene Expr 1998;8:321–56.
6. Kohler G, Milstein C. Continuous cultures of fused cells secreting antibody of predefined specificity. Nature 1975;256:495–7.
7. Diaz Miqueli A, Rolff J, Lemm M, et al. Radiosensitisation of U87MG brain tumours by anti-epidermal growth factor receptor monoclonal antibodies. Br J Cancer 2009;100:950–8.
8. Leonard DS, Hill AD, Kelly L, et al. Anti-human epidermal growth factor receptor 2 monoclonal antibody therapy for breast cancer. Br J Surg 2002;89: 262–71.
9. Mendelsohn J, Baselga J. The EGF receptor family as targets for cancer therapy. Oncogene 2000;19: 6550–65.
10. van Dijk MA, van de Winkel JG. Human antibodies as next generation therapeutics. Curr Opin Chem Biol 2001;5:368–74.
11. Yang XD, Jia XC, Corvalan JR, et al. Development of ABX-EGF, a fully human anti-EGF receptor monoclonal antibody, for cancer therapy. Crit Rev Oncol Hematol 2001;38:17–23.
12. Nadler LM, Stashenko P, Hardy R, et al. Serotherapy of a patient with a monoclonal antibody directed against a human lymphoma-associated antigen. Cancer Res 1980;40:3147–54.
13. Cragg MS, French RR, Glennie MJ. Signaling antibodies in cancer therapy. Curr Opin Immunol 1999;11:541–7.

14. Glennie MJ. Signaling antibodies for the treatment of neoplastic disease. Dis markers 2000;16:63.

15. Eisenthal A, Cameron RB, Rosenberg SA. Induction of antibody-dependent cellular cytotoxicity in vivo by IFN-alpha and its antitumor efficacy against established B16 melanoma liver metastases when combined with specific anti-B16 monoclonal antibody. J Immunol 1990;144:4463–71.

16. Eisenthal A, McIntosh JK. Effect of recombinant human tumor necrosis factor alpha on the induction of antibody-dependent cellular cytotoxicity in the treatment of established B16 melanoma liver nodules. Cancer Immunol Immunother 1990;31:243–9.

17. Shiloni E, Eisenthal A, Sachs D, et al. Antibody-dependent cellular cytotoxicity mediated by murine lymphocytes activated in recombinant interleukin 2. J Immunol 1987;138:1992–8.

18. Bleeker WK, Lammerts van Bueren JJ, van Ojik HH, et al. Dual mode of action of a human anti-epidermal growth factor receptor monoclonal antibody for cancer therapy. J Immunol 2004;173:4699–707.

19. Baselga J, Mendelsohn J. Receptor blockade with monoclonal antibodies as anti-cancer therapy. Pharmacol Ther 1994;64:127–54.

20. Goldstein NI, Prewett M, Zuklys K, et al. Biological efficacy of a chimeric antibody to the epidermal growth factor receptor in a human tumor xenograft model. Clin Cancer Res 1995;1:1311–8.

21. Gutowski MC, Briggs SL, Johnson DA. Epidermal growth factor receptor-reactive monoclonal antibodies: xenograft antitumor activity alone and as drug immunoconjugates. Cancer Res 1991;51:5471–5.

22. Masui H, Kawamoto T, Sato JD, et al. Growth inhibition of human tumor cells in athymic mice by anti-epidermal growth factor receptor monoclonal antibodies. Cancer Res 1984;44:1002–7.

23. Mendelsohn J. Epidermal growth factor receptor inhibition by a monoclonal antibody as anticancer therapy. Clin Cancer Res 1997;3:2703–7.

24. Mendelsohn J, Baselga J. Epidermal growth factor receptor targeting in cancer. Semin Oncol 2006;33:369–85.

25. Modjtahedi H, Eccles S, Box G, et al. Immunotherapy of human tumor xenografts over expressing the EGF receptor with rat antibodies that block growth factor-receptor interaction. Br J Cancer 1993;67:254–61.

26. Modjtahedi H, Eccles SA, Box G, et al. Antitumor activity of combinations of antibodies directed against different epitopes on the extracellular domain of the human EGF receptor. Cell Biophys 1993;22:129–46.

27. Wikstrand CJ, Cokgor I, Sampson JH, et al. Monoclonal antibody therapy of human gliomas: current status and future approaches. Cancer Metastasis Rev 1999;18:451–64.

28. Prins RM, Liau LM. Cellular immunity and immunotherapy of brain tumors. Front Biosci 2004;9:3124–36.

29. Wykosky J, Gibo DM, Stanton C, et al. EphA2 as a novel molecular marker and target in glioblastoma multiforme. Mol Cancer Res 2005;3:541–51.

30. Bigner SH, Burger PC, Wong AJ, et al. Gene amplification in malignant human gliomas: clinical and histopathologic aspects. J Neuropathol Exp Neurol 1988;47:191–205.

31. Bigner SH, Humphrey PA, Wong AJ, et al. Characterization of the epidermal growth factor receptor in human glioma cell lines and xenografts. Cancer Res 1990;50:8017–22.

32. Garcia de Palazzo IE, Adams GP, Sundareshan P, et al. Expression of mutated epidermal growth factor receptor by non-small cell lung carcinomas. Cancer Res 1993;53:3217–20.

33. Humphrey PA, Gangarosa LM, Wong AJ, et al. Deletion-mutant epidermal growth factor receptor in human gliomas: effects of type II mutation on receptor function. Biochem Biophys Res Commun 1991;178:1413–20.

34. Humphrey PA, Wong AJ, Vogelstein B, et al. Amplification and expression of the epidermal growth factor receptor gene in human glioma xenografts. Cancer Res 1988;48:2231–8.

35. Ekstrand AJ, James CD, Cavenee WK, et al. Genes for epidermal growth factor receptor, transforming growth factor alpha, and epidermal growth factor and their expression in human gliomas in vivo. Cancer Res 1991;51:2164–72.

36. Harding J, Burtness B. Cetuximab: an epidermal growth factor receptor chimeric human-murine monoclonal antibody. Drugs Today (Barc) 2005;41:107–27.

37. Ferguson KM. Active and inactive conformations of the epidermal growth factor receptor. Biochem Soc Trans 2004;32:742–5.

38. Eller JL, Longo SL, Hicklin DJ, et al. Activity of anti-epidermal growth factor receptor monoclonal antibody C225 against glioblastoma multiforme. Neurosurgery 2002;51:1005–13 [discussion: 1013–4].

39. Eller JL, Longo SL, Kyle MM, et al. Anti-epidermal growth factor receptor monoclonal antibody cetuximab augments radiation effects in glioblastoma multiforme in vitro and in vivo. Neurosurgery 2005;56:155–62 [discussion: 162].

40. Combs SE, Schulz-Ertner D, Hartmann C, et al. Phase I/II study of cetuximab plus temozolomide as radiochemotherapy for primary glioblastoma (GERT). J Clin Oncol 2008;26. May 20 Suppl; abstr 2077.

41. Neyns B, Sadones J, Joosens E, et al. A multicenter stratified phase II study of cetuximab for the treatment of patients with recurrent high-grade glioma. J Clin Oncol 2008;26. May 20 Suppl; abstr 2017.

42. Hasselbalch B, Lassen U, Soerensen M, et al. A phase 2 trial with cetuximab, bevacizumab and irinotecan for patients with primary glioblastomas and progression after radiation therapy and temozolomide. Neuro-oncology 10 Abstract: Society of Neuro-Oncology Annual Meeting 2008. Las Vegas, Nevada, November 21–23, 2008.

43. Casaco A, Lopez G, Garcia I, et al. Phase I single-dose study of intracavitary-administered Nimotuzumab labeled with 188 Re in adult recurrent high-grade glioma. Cancer Biol Ther 2008;7:333–9.

44. Bender H, Takahashi H, Adachi K, et al. Immunotherapy of human glioma xenografts with unlabeled, 131I-, or 125I-labeled monoclonal antibody 425 to epidermal growth factor receptor. Cancer Res 1992;52:121–6.

45. Quang TS, Brady LW. Radioimmunotherapy as a novel treatment regimen: 125I-labeled monoclonal antibody 425 in the treatment of high-grade brain gliomas. Int J Radiat Oncol Biol Phys 2004;58: 972–5.

46. Humphrey PA, Wong AJ, Vogelstein B, et al. Anti-synthetic peptide antibody reacting at the fusion junction of deletion-mutant epidermal growth factor receptors in human glioblastoma. Proc Natl Acad Sci U S A 1990;87:4207–11.

47. Wong AJ, Ruppert JM, Bigner SH, et al. Structural alterations of the epidermal growth factor receptor gene in human gliomas. Proc Natl Acad Sci U S A 1992;89:2965–9.

48. Johns TG, Stockert E, Ritter G, et al. Novel monoclonal antibody specific for the de2-7 epidermal growth factor receptor (EGFR) that also recognizes the EGFR expressed in cells containing amplification of the EGFR gene. Int J Cancer 2002;98: 398–408.

49. Jungbluth AA, Stockert E, Huang HJ, et al. A monoclonal antibody recognizing human cancers with amplification/over expression of the human epidermal growth factor receptor. Proc Natl Acad Sci U S A 2003;100:639–44.

50. Perera RM, Narita Y, Furnari FB, et al. Treatment of human tumor xenografts with monoclonal antibody 806 in combination with a prototypical epidermal growth factor receptor-specific antibody generates enhanced antitumor activity. Clin Cancer Res 2005; 11:6390–9.

51. Sampson JH, Crotty LE, Lee S, et al. Unarmed, tumor-specific monoclonal antibody effectively treats brain tumors. Proc Natl Acad Sci U S A 2000;97:7503–8.

52. Mitchell DA, Fecci PE, Sampson JH. Immunotherapy of malignant brain tumors. Immunol Rev 2008;222: 70–100.

53. Reist CJ, Archer GE, Kurpad SN, et al. Tumor-specific anti-epidermal growth factor receptor variant III monoclonal antibodies: use of the tyramine-cellobiose radioiodination method enhances cellular retention and uptake in tumor xenografts. Cancer Res 1995;55:4375–82.

54. Reist CJ, Archer GE, Wikstrand CJ, et al. Improved targeting of an anti-epidermal growth factor receptor variant III monoclonal antibody in tumor xenografts after labeling using N-succinimidyl 5-iodo-3-pyridinecarboxylate. Cancer Res 1997;57:1510–5.

55. Reist CJ, Batra SK, Pegram CN, et al. In vitro and in vivo behavior of radiolabeled chimeric anti-EGFRvIII monoclonal antibody: comparison with its murine parent. Nucl Med Biol 1997;24:639–47.

56. Kuan CT, Reist CJ, Foulon CF, et al. 125I-labeled anti-epidermal growth factor receptor-vIII single-chain Fv exhibits specific and high-level targeting of glioma xenografts. Clin Cancer Res 1999;5:1539–49.

57. Li G, Wong A. EGF receptor variant III as a target antigen for tumor immunotherapy. Expert Rev Vaccines 2008;7:977–85.

58. Birlik BCS, Ozer E. Tumour vascularity is of prognostic significance in adult, but not paediatric astrocytomas. Neuropathol Appl Neurobiol 2006;32:532–8.

59. Leon S, Folkerth R, Black P. Microvessel density is a prognostic indicator for patients with astroglial brain tumors. Cancer 1996;77.

60. Vredenburgh JJ, Desjardins A, Herndon JE 2nd, et al. Phase II trial of bevacizumab and irinotecan in recurrent malignant glioma. Clin Cancer Res 2007;13:1253–9.

61. Vredenburgh JJ, Desjardins A, Herndon JE 2nd, et al. Bevacizumab plus irinotecan in recurrent glioblastoma multiforme. J Clin Oncol 2007;25:4722–9.

62. Winkler F, Kozin SV, Tong RT, et al. Kinetics of vascular normalization by VEGFR2 blockade governs brain tumor response to radiation: role of oxygenation, angiopoietin-1, and matrix metalloproteinases. Cancer Cell 2004;6:553–63.

63. Hurwitz H. Integrating the anti-VEGF-A humanized monoclonal antibody bevacizumab with chemotherapy in advanced colorectal cancer. Clin Colorectal Cancer 2004;4(Suppl 2):S62–8.

64. Hurwitz H, Fehrenbacher L, Novotny W, et al. Bevacizumab plus irinotecan, fluorouracil, and leucovorin for metastatic colorectal cancer. N Engl J Med 2004; 350:2335–42.

65. de Groot JF, Yung WK. Bevacizumab and irinotecan in the treatment of recurrent malignant gliomas. Cancer J 2008;14:279–85.

66. Wagner SA, Desjardins A, Reardon DA, et al. Vredenburgh update on survival from the original phase 2 trial of bevacizumab and irinotecan in recurrent malignant gliomas. J Clin Oncol 2008;26. May 20 Suppl: abst 2021.

67. Norden AD, Young GS, Setayesh K, et al. Bevacizumab for recurrent malignant gliomas: efficacy, toxicity, and patterns of recurrence. Neurology 2008;70:779–87.

68. Fine HA. Promising new therapies for malignant gliomas. Cancer J 2007;13:349–54.

69. Behrem S, Zarkovic K, Eskinja N, et al. Distribution pattern of tenascin-C in glioblastoma: correlation with angiogenesis and tumor cell proliferation. Pathol Oncol Res 2005;11:229–35.

70. Jallo GI, Friedlander DR, Kelly PJ, et al. Tenascin-C expression in the cyst wall and fluid of human brain tumors correlates with angiogenesis. Neurosurgery 1997;41:1052–9.

71. Leins A, Riva P, Lindstedt R, et al. Expression of tenascin-C in various human brain tumors and its relevance for survival in patients with astrocytoma. Cancer 2003;98:2430–9.

72. Sarkar S, Nuttall RK, Liu S, et al. Tenascin-C stimulates glioma cell invasion through matrix metalloproteinase-12. Cancer Res 2006;66: 11771–80.

73. Brack SS, Silacci M, Birchler M, et al. Tumor-targeting properties of novel antibodies specific to the large isoform of tenascin-C. Clin Cancer Res 2006; 12:3200–8.

74. He X, Archer GE, Wikstrand CJ, et al. Generation and characterization of a mouse/human chimeric antibody directed against extracellular matrix protein tenascin. J Neuroimmunol 1994;52:127–37.

75. Silacci M, Brack SS, Spath N, et al. Human monoclonal antibodies to domain C of tenascin-C selectively target solid tumors in vivo. Protein Eng Des Sel 2006;19:471–8.

76. Reardon DA, Zalutsky MR, Bigner DD. Antitenascin-C monoclonal antibody radioimmunotherapy for malignant glioma patients. Expert Rev Anticancer Ther 2007;7:675–87.

77. Reardon DA, Akabani G, Coleman RE, et al. Phase II trial of murine (131)I-labeled antitenascin monoclonal antibody 81C6 administered into surgically created resection cavities of patients with newly diagnosed malignant gliomas. J Clin Oncol 2002; 20:1389–97.

78. Reardon DA, Akabani G, Coleman RE, et al. Salvage radioimmunotherapy with murine iodine-131-labeled antitenascin monoclonal antibody 81C6 for patients with recurrent primary and metastatic malignant brain tumors: phase II study results. J Clin Oncol 2006;24:115–22.

79. Reardon DA, Quinn JA, Akabani G, et al. Novel human IgG2b/murine chimeric antitenascin monoclonal antibody construct radiolabeled with 131I and administered into the surgically created resection cavity of patients with malignant glioma: phase I trial results. J Nucl Med 2006;47:912–8.

80. Omidfar K, Rasaee MJ, Kashanian S, et al. Studies of thermostability in Camelus bactrianus (Bactrian camel) single-domain antibody specific for the mutant epidermal-growth-factor receptor expressed by Pichia. Biotechnol Appl Biochem 2007;46:41–9.

81. Omidfar K, Rasaee MJ, Modjtahedi H, et al. Production and characterization of a new antibody specific for the mutant EGF receptor, EGFRvIII, in Camelus bactrianus. Tumour Biol 2004;25:179–87.

82. Omidfar K, Rasaee MJ, Modjtahedi H, et al. Production of a novel camel single-domain antibody specific for the type III mutant EGFR. Tumour Biol 2004;25:296–305.

83. Adams GP, Weiner LM. Intracellular single-chain Fv antibodies–a knockout punch for neoplastic cells? Gynecol Oncol 1995;59:6–7.

84. Schaedel O, Reiter Y. Antibodies and their fragments as anti-cancer agents. Curr Pharm Des 2006;12:363–78.

85. Clarke MF, Dick JE, Dirks PB, et al. Cancer stem cells–perspectives on current status and future directions: AACR workshop on cancer stem cells. Cancer Res 2006;66:9339–44.

86. Dirks PB. Brain tumor stem cells. Biol Blood Marrow Transplant 2005;11:12–3.

87. Dirks PB. Cancer: stem cells and brain tumours. Nature 2006;444:687–8.

88. Galli R, Binda E, Orfanelli U, et al. Isolation and characterization of tumorigenic, stem-like neural precursors from human glioblastoma. Cancer Res 2004; 64:7011–21.

89. Singh SK, Clarke ID, Terasaki M, et al. Identification of a cancer stem cell in human brain tumors. Cancer Res 2003;63:5821–8.

90. Singh SK, Hawkins C, Clarke ID, et al. Identification of human brain tumour initiating cells. Nature 2004; 432:396–401.

91. Larson RA, Le Beau MM. Therapy-related myeloid leukaemia: a model for leukemogenesis in humans. Chem Biol Interact 2005;153-154:187–95.

# Interferon-gamma in Brain Tumor Immunotherapy

Ari Kane, BA, Isaac Yang, MD*

**KEYWORDS**

- Interferon gamma • Gliomas • Immunotherapy
- Cytokines • Brain tumors • Gene transcription
- Tumor angiogenesis

Each year, approximately 17,000 new patients in the United States are diagnosed with uniformly fatal, malignant glioblastoma.[1] Over the past several decades there have been only marginal gains in treatment. The median survival and five-year survival for the most common type of primary brain tumor, malignant glioma, remains less than 1 year and 2% respectively.[2–4] Current treatment modalities are largely unsuccessful in altering patients' mortality and are also associated with adverse side effects. During tumor genesis, neoplasms acquire several characteristics including the ability to evade the host immune response, proliferate, and recruit a vascular supply. Novel approaches using immunotherapy offer the potential to specifically target neoplasms, their unique characteristics, and decrease adverse effects.[5,6]

Interferon-gamma (IFNγ) is a cytokine that acts on cell-surface receptors, activating transcription of genes that offer treatment potential by increasing tumor immunogenicity, disrupting proliferative mechanisms, and inhibiting tumor angiogenesis. However, abnormally low levels of IFNγ are produced by tumor cells and local T cells in the glioma microenvironment.[7,8] Current investigations into the immunomodulating effects of IFNγ suggest that IFNγ has the potential to be used clinically in the treatment of brain tumors and as a promising adjunct to other immunotherapeutic modalities. Here the authors review the published literature that highlights the potential role of IFNγ in the treatment and immunotherapy of malignant gliomas.

## INTERFERON-GAMMA AND THE CELL CYCLE

IFNγ has numerous effects on transcriptional gene regulation involving the cell cycle. Several lines of evidence demonstrate the utility of IFNγ to inhibit actively dividing cells and induce apoptosis. IFNγ has significant cytotoxic effects on actively dividing neural cells, but much less on immature cells, and no apparent effect on mature cells.[9] IFNγ preferentially disrupts the cell cycle of proliferating cells by causing a delay in the G1/S-phase transition.[9–12] Discrete mechanisms by which IFNγ can cause cell cycle arrest have recently been further characterized (**Fig. 1**). Horiuchi and colleagues[9] demonstrated a reversal of IFNγ-induced cell growth inhibition by partially inhibiting the MEK-mitogen-activated protein kinase and extracellular signal regulated kinase (ERK) pathway. This finding supported the postulation that IFNγ induces a transient increase in ERK activity which has downstream effects of inhibiting G1/S transition. Kominksy and colleagues[11,12] have presented evidence that IFNγ has antiproliferative effects on glioblastoma cells by way of the p21 pathway, although having little effect on normal human astrocyte cell proliferation. They have reported that the percent inhibition across glioma cell lines is directly proportional to the level of p21 expression post-IFNγ exposure.

Department of Neurological Surgery, University of California at San Francisco, 505 Parnassus Avenue, San Francisco, CA 94143, USA
* Corresponding author.
*E-mail address:* Yangi@neurosurg.ucsf.edu (I. Yang).

Neurosurg Clin N Am 21 (2010) 77–86
doi:10.1016/j.nec.2009.08.011

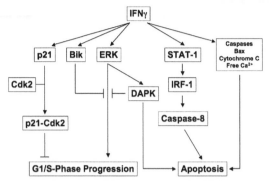

**Fig. 1.** IFNγ disrupts proliferative mechanisms in gliomas by several mechanisms. p21 is upregulated by IFNγ which binds cdk2 inactivating cdk2 and arresting cell cycle progression. IFNγ upregulates ERK and Bik. Bik blocks ERK's proliferative effects, while ERK increases death associated protein kinase activity leading to apoptosis. IFNγ induces apoptosis through further activation of capsases and downstream mediators of STAT-1.

Additionally, the level of p21 expression directly correlates with the level of cyclin dependent kinase 2 (cdk2) bound to p21 and subsequently the inhibition of cdk2 activity. Janardhanan and colleagues[10] have also reported their findings that IFNγ inhibits cdk2. These experiments collectively suggest the potential ability of IFNγ to arrest cell cycle progression at the G/S1-phase transition by way of ERK and p21 signaling and act as an antiproliferative agent in the potential treatment of malignant glioma.

IFNγ has also been shown to promote apoptosis by way of the mechanism of signal transducer and activator of transcription 1 (STAT-1) and caspase activity. IFNγ has been demonstrated by several studies to be a potent inducer of STAT-1 activity,[9,13–15] which subsequently induces transcription of interferon regulatory factor 1, promoting caspase-8 activity.[14] This mechanism has been further validated in that inhibition of STAT-1 blocks the proapoptotic effects of IFNγ and the increase in caspase-8 activity.[14] In addition, other laboratory investigations have found that IFNγ also causes the upregulation of caspase-1, -3, -8, and -9[10,13,16] and is associated with increased Bax/Bcl-2 ratio, cytochrome C, and free intracellular calcium.[13]

### INTERFERON-GAMMA SIGNALING

IFNγ is encoded by a gene on chromosome 12.[17] It is a homodimer in its functionally active state. The IFNγ membrane receptor is called the type II interferon receptor and is composed of the distinct subunits IFNGR1 and IFNGR2, which are constitutively associated with Janus Kinases (JAK) 1 and 2

respectively.[17–21] The IFNγ homodimer binds to two IFNGR1 subunits causing dimerization and recruitment of two IFNGR2 subunits.[18] This interaction results in the cytoplasmic domain autophosphorylation of the associated JAK creating a docking site for STAT-1.[18,19,21] Two free STAT-1 molecules localize to the cytoplasmic binding site, are phosphorylated by the kinases, and associate with each other to form a homodimer. The homodimer then translocates to the cell nucleus and can interact with other coactivator proteins. These oligomers bind IFNγ-activated sites (GAS) in the promoter region of IFNγ-inducible genes and stimulate the transcription of various types of proteins including transcription factors, adaptor proteins, enzymes, and numerous other classes of molecules.[17–19]

The genetic products include proapoptotic elements, such as death-associated proteins.[18,19] Immunogencity is increased by production of proteasomes and major histocompatibility complex (MHC) subunits that increase antigen processing, loading, and presentation.[20] Antiproliferative transcripts result in p21, p27, p38, repressor activator protein 1 (RAS1) and RAS, which are involved in controlling the cell cycle.[17–21] More complex cascades are initiated by inducing transcription factors, such as interferon regulatory factors and class II transactivator (CIITA).[20,21]

More recently it has become clear that IFNγ signaling involves more than the well-described JAK-STAT pathway. Studies suggest that interferon receptors can form higher order complexes and that other molecules have influential control on the interferon signaling pathway. Candidate molecules include PI3-K, protein kinase C, MyD88, and c-Cbl.[17,21] Upon activation of interferon receptors these interacting molecules can initiate independent signaling pathways, such as the MEK-ERK, mammalian target of rapamycin (MTOR), and peroxisome proliferator-activated receptor (PPAR) pathways, or augment the STAT1 pathways.[17,21]

### MAJOR HISTOCOMPATIBILITY COMPLEX REGULATION BY INTERFERON-GAMMA

MHC molecules are proteins that display peptide antigens on the cell surface and are crucial to the cellular immune response.[22–24] MHC class I molecules are found on all nucleated cells and function to present to cytotoxic T lymphocytes (CD8), whereas MHC class II molecules are more commonly found on antigen presenting cells (APC) and present to T helper cells (CD4).[24] MHC class I is expressed, but at low levels in malignant gliomas[24–28] and other forms of neoplasms.[29–31]

MHC class II molecules are expressed at varying levels on malignant gliomas[25,27,32–35] and infiltrating APC.[35–37] IFNγ has the ability to upregulate surface expression of class I and II MHC molecules (**Fig. 2**).[24,38–40]

Increasing MHC class I expression on glioma cells could potentially increase the immunogenicity of the glioma and elicit a tumor-specific CD8 cytotoxic response.[24] Findings in animal and human studies indicate that IFNγ upregulates MHC class I expression in gliomas[24,25,27,28,41–44] and other neoplasms.[40,45] In addition, IFNγ may alter antigen processing allowing for better antigen quality control,[39] presentation, and increased expression of tumor-specific peptide antigens.[24] The upregulation of MHC class I molecules also promotes tumor-cell apoptosis by CD8 T cell interactions and has been shown to decrease mortality in animal models.[25,42,44,46] These effects can be abrogated by MHC class I antibody, which inhibit the MHC molecule.[25,42] Additional evidence also suggests that tumors that survive in the presence of IFNγ administration may have preferential mutations causing resistance to IFNγ-induction.[29]

Increasing MHC class II expression on glioma cells and local infiltrating APC may serve to increase immunogenicity by way of a tumor-specific CD4 helper T-cell response. Findings in animal and human studies indicate that IFNγ upregulates MHC class II expression in gliomas[47–50] and infiltrating APC.[35,36,41,47,51] IFNγ also induces STAT-1α expression concurrently with MHC class II upregulation.[48] STAT-1α in turn induces MHC CIITA, a regulator of MHC class II expression, by way of two CIITA promoters.[48–50] STAT-1α inhibitors have been demonstrated to block IFNγ-induced upregulation of MHC class II molecules. These potential mechanisms suggest that IFNγ may elicit malignant glioma cells to process and present MHC II associated native antigen to CD4 helper T cells.[50] IFNγ treatment has also been shown to be associated with an increase in APC MHC Class II expression and an increase in infiltrating tumor-specific APC.[35,36,41,51] One recent study reported a concomitant increase in survival with an associated increase in infiltrating APC with MHC class II molecules on glioma cells.[51]

## GENE THERAPY USING INTERFERON-GAMMA TRANSFECTION

Gene therapy offers another potential therapeutic approach to use IFNγ and to induce its possible antitumor effects in the micro environment surrounding gliomas. Several studies have demonstrated the efficacy and feasibility of using IFNγ gene treatment as either monotherapy or as an adjuvant therapy against gliomas and other neoplasms.[52–64] Various methods have been devised to transfect IFNγ genes into cells; however, only several general systems-based approaches have been investigated and explored in gliomas. IFNγ expression has been accomplished in vitro and in vivo by transfecting APC, T cells, and glioma tumor cells. These reports demonstrate the feasibility and potential for durable IFNγ expression[52] along with inhibition of tumor growth,[52,60,65–67] increased T-cell infiltration and T cell-mediated killing,[25,56,57,60,61,66–68] decreased tumor size,[52,66] prolonged survival,[52,61–63,65,66,68,69] and in some cases tumor eradication.[65,68,69] Nishihara and colleagues[57] reported that the level of IFNγ expression in their study correlated with the level of CD8-mediated tumoricidal activity, and that these tumoricidal

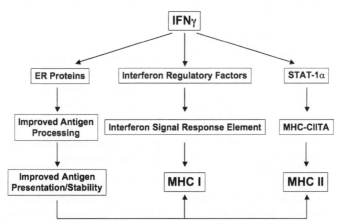

**Fig. 2.** IFNγ alters endoplasmic reticulum regulatory proteins to improve antigen processing and stability of MHC complexes. Further through Interferon regulatory factors and STAT-1α, IFNγ upregulates expression of both MHC class I and class II molecules increasing the immunogenicity of gliomas to CD4 and CD8 T cells.

processes could be inhibited with the administration of IFNγ-antibody, further suggesting a mechanism that specifically implicates the involvement of the IFNγ pathway in an antitumor effect.

Regardless of the cell type, transfection of the IFNγ gene causes specific changes in the phenotypic status of the tumor and its interaction with immune cells. First, the expression of cell-surface proteins is altered to induce antitumor effects and immunogenic pathways. Paul and colleagues[67] and Ehtesham and colleagues[66] have recently demonstrated modification of cell-surface proteins with the upregulation of MHC class I and II molecules on glioma cells modified to express IFNγ. Mizuno and colleagues[70] have reported that the insertion of an IFNγ gene induces expression of intercellular adhesion molecule 1 (ICAM-1) and FAS antigen, and they also report that enhanced CD8-mediated killing was blocked by ICAM-1 antibody. In another recent animal study, Saleh and colleagues[68] have reported their investigation where all animals who have IFNγ-modified glioma survived to an arbitrary endpoint of 3 months compared with 14 days for their control counterpoints. Pathologic examination of these animals who have IFNγ-modified tumor reportedly revealed eradication of the tumor with normal-appearing brain tissue remaining.

## INTERFERON-GAMMA INHIBITS TUMOR ANGIOGENESIS

Inhibiting tumor angiogenesis is another potential mechanism for limiting tumor growth and metastasis.[71–75] IFNγ is one of several cytokines that has been reported to effectively inhibit angiogenesis in tumors.[76–79] Several potential mechanisms have been shown to be associated with this vascular inhibition (**Fig. 3**). Friesel and colleagues[80] have demonstrated that IFNγ causes a decrease in vascular endothelial proliferation. Furthermore, IFNγ enhances the release of antiangiogenic chemokines, such as CXC chemokine, γ-IFN, monokine induced by gamma interferon (MIG), and IFN-inducible protein 10.[81–84] IFNγ has also been shown to down-regulate platelet endothelial cell-adhesion molecule 1 (PECAM-1),[85,86] a molecule constitutively expressed at vascular endothelial cell junctions. Ruegg and colleagues[87] has also recently reported that IFNγ down-regulates integrin alphaVbeta3, an adhesion receptor that plays a key role in tumor angiogenesis. This alteration may lead to decreased endothelial cell adhesion, survival, detachment, and apoptosis of angiogenic endothelial cells in tumors.

Elegant experiments also support the antiangiogenic potential of IFNγ in gliomas. Saleh and

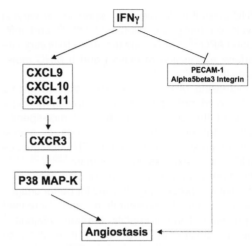

**Fig. 3.** IFNγ inhibits tumor angiogenesis through chemokines and cell surface proteins involved in neovascularization. IFNγ induces CXCL9, CXCL10, and CXCL11 which act through their receptor, CXCR3, via MAP-K pathway to promote angiostasis. Additionally, IFNγ promotes angiostasis by downregulating proangiogenic PECAM-1 and alpha5beta3 integrin.

colleagues[68] treated established rodent gliomas with in situ retroviral IFNγ cDNA. This treatment resulted in dramatically increased survival and eradication of glioma tissue in this animal glioma model. Anti-PECAM antibody stains revealed significantly reduced numbers of tumor vessels, decreased vessel caliber, and thinner vascular walls. In another animal study, Fathallah-Shaykh and colleagues[69] transfected established glioma cells in vivo with IFNγ or beta-galactosidase and compared the effects on animal survival and tumor pathology. They found that the animals that received IFNγ had significantly prolonged survival, and on pathologic examination 38% rejected the tumor with resultant cavity formation. They also showed that the tumors exhibited decreased hemoglobin content and spheroid growth (as opposed to linear in the control) in a gelatinous protein mixture assay in vivo. Furthermore, they report that the transfected cells inhibited neovascularization of tumor cells and induced apoptosis of endothelial cells.

## INTERFERON-GAMMA IN COMBINED IMMUNOTHERAPY

Combined therapy offers the advantage of disrupting multiple oncogenic pathways thereby simultaneously promoting discreet yet synergistic therapeutic mechanisms. As the effects of IFNγ are further elucidated, other agents could be used in combination to specifically augment parts of the IFNγ pathway to increase its antitumor efficacy. IFNγ has been used in combination in gene transfer models and recombinant form in addition to other forms of immuno- and chemotherapy including granulocyte-macrophage colony-stimulating factor (GM-CSF),[88] retinoid compounds, and inducible nitric oxide synthase (iNOS) inhibitors.

The importance of GM-CSF and IFNγ in regulating antitumor surveillance has been demonstrated as double-knockout mice spontaneously develop tumors.[89] Additionally, in other tumor lines combination therapy has demonstrated antitumor effects.[90,91] Relevant to antitumor strategies, GM-CSF encourages development of APC and T cells, which may subsequently have their antitumor effects enhanced by IFNγ.[92–94] As described, IFNγ has the capability to augment T cell-mediated tumor killing, thus combining a leukocyte growth and differentiation stimulating agent could serve to augment the local effects of IFNγ on tumor cytolysis and phagocytosis. Indeed, Smith and colleagues[88,92] have demonstrated this in an established glioma rodent model. They administered GM-CSF gene-modified glioma cells and recombinant IFNγ into established intracranial gliomas and found not only tumor volume reduction and increased lymphocytic infiltration but an 88% tumor eradication rate. Furthermore, they demonstrated that combination therapy was associated with increases in CD4 and CD8 counts, an increase in IFNγ-producing T cells, and rejection of tumors upon rechallenge post-initial eradication.

IFNγ is a potent inducer of iNOS that results in dramatic increases in Nitric oxide (NO).[95,96] NO itself has immunosuppressive effects including suppression of lymphocyte proliferation and lymphocyte-derived chemokines.[97–99] Thus, although IFNγ has many potent antitumor and immunogenic effects, it may also be paradoxically engaging immunosuppressive mechanisms. Medot-Pirenne and colleagues[100] established that inhibiting NO could augment antitumor cytotoxic T lymphocyte activity. Demonstrating the feasibility of this therapy in an animal glioma model, Badn and colleagues[101] showed that iNOS inhibitors administered concurrently with IFNγ transduced glioma cells in rat intracerebral tumors lead to prolonged survival over IFNγ-modified glioma cells alone.

The theory of combining retinoid compounds with IFNγ is based on the concept that chemo-immunotherapy could simultaneously reduce tumor burden and overcome immune resistance. All-trans retinoic acid (ATRA) has been shown in vitro and in vivo to induce differentiation and

suppress proliferation by arresting the G1 phase of the cell cycle and down regulating telomerase activity.[13,102,103] Combination therapy in human glioma demonstrates that ATRA causes differentiation, decreased proliferation, and down regulation of telomerase, thus sensitizing tumor cells to IFNγ activity leading to increased apoptosis compared with IFNγ alone.[13,102,103] Another retinoid compound, N-(4-Hydroxphenyl)retinamide, used in combination with IFNγ has shown similar results.[10]

## CLINICAL TRIALS

There has been few clinical trials using IFNγ as therapy for gliomas, and all have thus far used recombinant IFNγ (rIFNγ) as the form of delivery. Although rIFNγ has been shown to decrease cell viability, proliferation, and migration while increasing cell death in human glioma cell lines, clinical trials have not yet been proven successful.[104] One recent trial[105] followed 14 subjects given an intravenous dose between IFNγ twice weekly for 8 weeks. Evidence of CT response was only observed in one subject with stabilization between 12 to 86 weeks. Additionally, side effects potentially attributable to rIFNγ administration were observed. In another study,[106] 31 subjects were randomized to receive either intravenous or subcutaneous rIFNγ in escalating triweekly doses over 4 weeks plus adjuvant radiotherapy. Although the treatment was tolerated well, there was no difference between the groups in tumor progression or survival. The most recent study[107] treated 40 subjects who had pediatric glioma with induction radiation and chemotherapy followed by increasing daily doses of rIFNγ for 7 weeks. Although a historical control was used as a comparison group, no difference in the median survival was observed with this treatment in these subjects who had pediatric glioma.

## SUMMARY

Treatment gains have been significant for a variety of neoplastic processes. However, malignant gliomas remain seemingly impervious to the range of current clinical therapeutic modalities. Evidence is accumulating that IFNγ has the potential to overcome this barrier by simultaneously targeting multiple mechanisms that typically render gliomas treatment resistant. Research demonstrates that IFNγ interrupts glioma proliferation, induces apoptosis, enhances tumor immunogenicity, and inhibits glioma neovascularization. The diverse array of intra- and extracellular signaling cascades that IFN$\gamma$ influences continues to be discovered, particularly in relevance to its antitumor properties.

Although clinical trials have been disappointing, scientific insight into IFN$\gamma$ antitumor effects continues to progress. There remains a huge opportunity to devise improved methods of treatment and expand clinical trials to larger populations. As with any therapeutic intervention, immunotherapy with IFN$\gamma$ requires establishing durable treatment, refining delivery techniques, optimizing the pharmacokinetic and pharmacodynamic parameters, reducing systemic toxicity, and devising appropriate clinical selection criteria. Initial clinical trials involved small numbers of patients and used only recombinant systemic delivery. Newer technologies allowing for effective gene transfer, local delivery systems, and multi-agent therapies all hold promise to facilitate the efficacious use of IFN$\gamma$ as immunotherapy for malignant gliomas.

## REFERENCES

1. Greenlee RT, Hill-Harmon MB, Murray T, et al. Cancer statistics, 2001. CA Cancer J Clin 2001; 51(1):15–36.
2. Burton EC, Prados MD. Malignant gliomas. Curr Treat Options Oncol 2000;1(5):459–68.
3. Nieder C. Treatment of newly diagnosed glioblastoma multiforme. J Clin Oncol 2002;20(14): 3179–80 [author reply 3181–2].
4. Surawicz TS, Davis F, Freels S, et al. Brain tumor survival: results from the National Cancer Data Base. J Neurooncol 1998;40(2):151–60.
5. Jaeckle KA. Immunotherapy of malignant gliomas. Semin Oncol 1994;21(2):249–59.
6. Prins RM, Liau LM. Cellular immunity and immunotherapy of brain tumors. Front Biosci 2004;9: 3124–36.
7. Zisakis A, Piperi C, Themistocleous MS, et al. Comparative analysis of peripheral and localised cytokine secretion in glioblastoma patients. Cytokine 2007;39(2):99–105.
8. Hao C, Parney IF, Roa WH, et al. Cytokine and cytokine receptor mRNA expression in human glioblastomas: evidence of Th1, Th2 and Th3 cytokine dysregulation. Acta Neuropathol 2002;103(2): 171–8.
9. Horiuchi M, Itoh A, Pleasure D, et al. MEK-ERK signaling is involved in interferon-gamma-induced death of oligodendroglial progenitor cells. J Biol Chem 2006;281(29):20095–106.
10. Janardhanan R, Banik NL, Ray SK. N-(4-Hydroxyphenyl)retinamide induced differentiation with repression of telomerase and cell cycle to increase interferon-gamma sensitivity for apoptosis in

11. Kominsky S, Johnson HM, Bryan G, et al. IFN-gamma inhibition of cell growth in glioblastomas correlates with increased levels of the cyclin dependent kinase inhibitor p21WAF1/CIP1. Oncogene 1998;17(23):2973–9.
12. Kominsky SL, Subramaniam PS, Johnson HM, et al. Inhibitory effects of IFN-gamma and acyclovir on the glioblastoma cell cycle. J Interferon Cytokine Res 2000;20(5):463–9.
13. Das A, Banik NL, Ray SK. Molecular mechanisms of the combination of retinoid and interferon-gamma for inducing differentiation and increasing apoptosis in human glioblastoma T98G and U87MG cells. Neurochem Res 2008.
14. Fulda S, Debatin KM. IFNgamma sensitizes for apoptosis by upregulating caspase-8 expression through the Stat1 pathway. Oncogene 2002; 21(15):2295–308.
15. Sluder G. Two-way traffic: centrosomes and the cell cycle. Nat Rev Mol Cell Biol 2005;6(9): 743–8.
16. Choi C, Jeong E, Benveniste EN. Caspase-1 mediates Fas-induced apoptosis and is up-regulated by interferon-gamma in human astrocytoma cells. J Neurooncol 2004;67(1–2):167–76.
17. Platanias LC. Mechanisms of type-I- and type-II-interferon-mediated signaling. Nat Rev Immunol 2005;5(5):375–86.
18. Boehm U, Klamp T, Groot M, et al. Cellular responses to interferon-gamma. Annu Rev Immunol 1997;15:749–95.
19. Stark GR, Kerr IM, Williams BR, et al. How cells respond to interferons. Annu Rev Biochem 1998; 67:227–64.
20. Schroder K, Hertzog PJ, Ravasi T, et al. Interferon-gamma: an overview of signals, mechanisms and functions. J Leukoc Biol 2004;75(2):163–89.
21. Gough DJ, Levy DE, Johnstone RW, et al. IFNgamma signaling-does it mean JAK-STAT? Cytokine Growth Factor Rev 2008;19(5–6):383–94.
22. Jensen PE. Recent advances in antigen processing and presentation. Nat Immunol 2007;8(10): 1041–8.
23. Trombetta ES, Mellman I. Cell biology of antigen processing in vitro and in vivo. Annu Rev Immunol 2005;23:975–1028.
24. Yang I, Kremen TJ, Giovannone AJ, et al. Modulation of major histocompatibility complex Class I molecules and major histocompatibility complex-bound immunogenic peptides induced by interferon-alpha and interferon-gamma treatment of human glioblastoma multiforme. J Neurosurg 2004;100(2):310–9.
25. Read SB, Kulprathipanja NV, Gomez GG, et al. Human alloreactive CTL interactions with gliomas

and with those having upregulated HLA expression from exogenous IFN-gamma or IFN-gamma gene modification. J Interferon Cytokine Res 2003; 23(7):379–93.

26. Ito A, Shinkai M, Honda H, et al. Augmentation of MHC class I antigen presentation via heat shock protein expression by hyperthermia. Cancer Immunol Immunother 2001;50(10):515–22.

27. Parney IF, Farr-Jones MA, Chang LJ, et al. Human glioma immunobiology in vitro: implications for immunogene therapy. Neurosurgery 2000;46(5): 1169–77 [discussion: 1177–8].

28. Oshiro S, Fukushima T, Tomonaga M, et al. Response of MHC class-1 antigen on rat glioma cells to cytokines. Anticancer Res 2000;20(1C): 605–10.

29. Garcia-Lora A, Algarra I, Gaforio JJ, et al. Immunoselection by T lymphocytes generates repeated MHC class I-deficient metastatic tumor variants. Int J Cancer 2001;91(1):109–19.

30. Garrido F, Ruiz-Cabello F, Cabrera T, et al. Implications for immunosurveillance of altered HLA class I phenotypes in human tumours. Immunol Today 1997;18(2):89–95.

31. Restifo NP, Kawakami Y, Marincola F, et al. Molecular mechanisms used by tumors to escape immune recognition: immunogenetherapy and the cell biology of major histocompatibility complex class I. J Immunother Emphasis Tumor Immunol 1993;14(3):182–90.

32. Piguet V, Carrel S, Diserens AC, et al. Heterogeneity of the induction of HLA-DR expression by human immune interferon on glioma cell lines and their clones. J Natl Cancer Inst 1986;76(2): 223–8.

33. Rossi ML, Hughes JT, Esiri MM, et al. Immunohistological study of mononuclear cell infiltrate in malignant gliomas. Acta Neuropathol 1987;74(3): 269–77.

34. Saito T, Tanaka R, Yoshida S, et al. Immunohistochemical analysis of tumor-infiltrating lymphocytes and major histocompatibility antigens in human gliomas and metastatic brain tumors. Surg Neurol 1988;29(6):435–42.

35. Schartner JM, Haqar AR, Van Handel M, et al. Impaired capacity for upregulation of MHC class II in tumor-associated microglia. Glia 2005;51(4): 279–85.

36. Dutta T, Spence A, Lampson LA. Robust ability of IFN-gamma to upregulate class II MHC antigen expression in tumor bearing rat brains. J Neurooncol 2003;64(1–2):31–44.

37. Tran CT, Wolz P, Egensperger R, et al. Differential expression of MHC class II molecules by microglia and neoplastic astroglia: relevance for the escape of astrocytoma cells from immune surveillance. Neuropathol Appl Neurobiol 1998;24(4):293–301.

38. Lampson LA. Interpreting MHC class I expression and class I/class II reciprocity in the CNS: reconciling divergent findings. Microsc Res Tech 1995; 32(4):267–85.

39. Fromm SV, Ehrlich R. IFN-gamma affects both the stability and the intracellular transport of class I MHC complexes. J Interferon Cytokine Res 2001; 21(4):199–208.

40. Ljunggren G, Anderson DJ. Cytokine induced modulation of MHC class I and class II molecules on human cervical epithelial cells. J Reprod Immunol 1998;38(2):123–38.

41. Wen PY, Lampson MA, Lampson LA. Effects of gamma-interferon on major histocompatibility complex antigen expression and lymphocytic infiltration in the 9L gliosarcoma brain tumor model: implications for strategies of immunotherapy. J Neuroimmunol 1992;36(1):57–68.

42. Schiltz PM, Gomez GG, Read SB, et al. Effects of IFN-gamma and interleukin-1beta on major histocompatibility complex antigen and intercellular adhesion molecule-1 expression by 9L gliosarcoma: relevance to its cytolysis by alloreactive cytotoxic T lymphocytes. J Interferon Cytokine Res 2002; 22(12):1209–16.

43. Yin D, Kondo S, Takeuchi J, et al. Interferon-gamma induces a decrease in the susceptibility of human glioma cells to lysis by lymphokine-activated killer cells. Neurosurgery 1994;35(1):113–8.

44. Oshiro S, Liu Y, Fukushima T, et al. Modified immunoregulation associated with interferon-gamma treatment of rat glioma. Neurol Res 2001;23(4): 359–66.

45. Abril E, Mendez RE, García A, et al. Characterization of a gastric tumor cell line defective in MHC class I inducibility by both alpha- and gamma-interferon. Tissue Antigens 1996;47(5):391–8.

46. Tang J, Flomenberg P, Harshyne L, et al. Glioblastoma patients exhibit circulating tumor-specific CD8+ T cells. Clin Cancer Res 2005;11(14): 5292–9.

47. Gresser O, Hein A, Riese S, et al. Tumor necrosis factor alpha and interleukin-1 alpha inhibit through different pathways interferon-gamma-induced antigen presentation, processing and MHC class II surface expression on astrocytes, but not on microglia. Cell Tissue Res 2000;300(3):373–82.

48. Lee YJ, Benveniste EN. Stat1 alpha expression is involved in IFN-gamma induction of the class II transactivator and class II MHC genes. J Immunol 1996;157(4):1559–68.

49. Moses H, Sasaki A, Ting JP. Identification of an interferon-gamma-responsive element of a class II major histocompatibility gene in rat type 1 astrocytes. J Neuroimmunol 1991;31(3):273–8.

50. Soos JM, Krieger JI, Stüve O, et al. Malignant glioma cells use MHC class II transactivator (CIITA)

promoters III and IV to direct IFN-gamma-inducible CIITA expression and can function as nonprofessional antigen presenting cells in endocytic processing and CD4(+) T-cell activation. Glia 2001; 36(3):391–405.

51. Oshiro S, Fukushima T, Tomonaga M, et al. Antitumor activity and modified immunoregulation associated with IFN-gamma treatment of RG2 gliomas. Anticancer Res 1999;19(6B):5029–36.

52. Wu A, Oh S, Ericson K, et al. Transposon-based interferon gamma gene transfer overcomes limitations of episomal plasmid for immunogene therapy of glioblastoma. Cancer Gene Ther 2007;14(6): 550–60.

53. Gansbacher B, Bannerji R, Daniels B, et al. Retroviral vector-mediated gamma-interferon gene transfer into tumor cells generates potent and long lasting antitumor immunity. Cancer Res 1990;50(24):7820–5.

54. Howard B, Burrascano M, McCallister T, et al. Retrovirus-mediated gene transfer of the human gamma-IFN gene: a therapy for cancer. Ann N Y Acad Sci 1994;716:167–87.

55. King GD, Curtin JF, Candolfi M, et al. Gene therapy and targeted toxins for glioma. Curr Gene Ther 2005;5(6):535–57.

56. Miyatake S, Nishihara K, Kikuchi H, et al. Efficient tumor suppression by glioma-specific murine cytotoxic T lymphocytes transfected with interferon-gamma gene. J Natl Cancer Inst 1990;82(3): 217–20.

57. Nishihara K, Miyatake S, Sakata T, et al. Augmentation of tumor targeting in a line of glioma-specific mouse cytotoxic T-lymphocytes by retroviral expression of mouse gamma-interferon complementary DNA. Cancer Res 1988;48(17):4730–5.

58. Porgador A, Bannerji R, Watanabe Y, et al. Antimetastatic vaccination of tumor-bearing mice with two types of IFN-gamma gene-inserted tumor cells. J Immunol 1993;150(4):1458–70.

59. Watanabe Y. Transfection of interferon-gamma gene in animal tumors–a model for local cytokine production and tumor immunity. Semin Cancer Biol 1992;3(1):43–6.

60. Pan J, Zhang M, Wang J, et al. Intratumoral injection of interferon-gamma gene-modified dendritic cells elicits potent antitumor effects: effective induction of tumor-specific CD8+ CTL response. J Cancer Res Clin Oncol 2005;131(7):468–78.

61. Ma YH, Yu JB, Yao HP, et al. Treatment of intracerebral glioblastomas with G422 tumour cell vaccine in a mouse model. J Int Med Res 2008;36(2):308–13.

62. Lichtor T, Glick RP. Cytokine immuno-gene therapy for treatment of brain tumors. J Neurooncol 2003; 65(3):247–59.

63. Lichtor T, Glick RP, Kim TS, et al. Prolonged survival of mice with glioma injected intracerebrally with double cytokine-secreting cells. J Neurosurg 1995;83(6):1038–44.

64. Siesjo P, Visse E, Sjogren HO. Cure of established, intracerebral rat gliomas induced by therapeutic immunizations with tumor cells and purified APC or adjuvant IFN-gamma treatment. J Immunother Emphasis Tumor Immunol 1996;19(5):334–45.

65. Visse E, Siesjö P, Widegren B, et al. Regression of intracerebral rat glioma isografts by therapeutic subcutaneous immunization with interferon-gamma, interleukin-7, or B7-1-transfected tumor cells. Cancer Gene Ther 1999;6(1):37–44.

66. Ehtesham M, Samoto K, Kabos P, et al. Treatment of intracranial glioma with in situ interferon-gamma and tumor necrosis factor-alpha gene transfer. Cancer Gene Ther 2002;9(11):925–34.

67. Paul DB, Read SB, Kulprathipanja NV, et al. Gamma interferon transduced 9L gliosarcoma. Cytokine gene therapy and its relevance to cellular therapy with alloreactive cytotoxic T lymphocytes. J Neurooncol 2003;64(1–2):89–99.

68. Saleh M, Jonas NK, Wiegmans A, et al. The treatment of established intracranial tumors by in situ retroviral IFN-gamma transfer. Gene Ther 2000; 7(20):1715–24.

69. Fathallah-Shaykh HM, Zhao LJ, Kafrouni AI, et al. Gene transfer of IFN-gamma into established brain tumors represses growth by antiangiogenesis. J Immunol 2000;164(1):217–22.

70. Mizuno M, Yoshida J, Takaoka T, et al. Reinforced cytotoxicity of lymphokine-activated killer cells toward glioma cells by transfection of the killer cells with the gamma-interferon gene. Jpn J Cancer Res 1995;86(1):95–100.

71. Claffey KP, Brown LF, del Aguila LF, et al. Expression of vascular permeability factor/vascular endothelial growth factor by melanoma cells increases tumor growth, angiogenesis, and experimental metastasis. Cancer Res 1996;56(1):172–81.

72. Folkman J. The role of angiogenesis in tumor growth. Semin Cancer Biol 1992;3(2):65–71.

73. Folkman J, Ingber D. Inhibition of angiogenesis. Semin Cancer Biol 1992;3(2):89–96.

74. Hanahan D, Folkman J. Patterns and emerging mechanisms of the angiogenic switch during tumorigenesis. Cell 1996;86(3):353–64.

75. Wang RF. Human tumor antigens: implications for cancer vaccine development. J Mol Med 1999; 77(9):640–55.

76. Beatty G, Paterson Y. IFN-gamma-dependent inhibition of tumor angiogenesis by tumor-infiltrating CD4+ T cells requires tumor responsiveness to IFN-gamma. J Immunol 2001;166(4):2276–82.

77. Coughlin CM, Salhany KE, Gee MS, et al. Tumor cell responses to IFNgamma affect tumorigenicity and response to IL-12 therapy and antiangiogenesis. Immunity 1998;9(1):25–34.

78. Maheshwari RK, Srikantan V, Bhartiya D, et al. Differential effects of interferon gamma and alpha on in vitro model of angiogenesis. J Cell Physiol 1991;146(1):164–9.

79. Sidky YA, Borden EC. Inhibition of angiogenesis by interferons: effects on tumor- and lymphocyte-induced vascular responses. Cancer Res 1987; 47(19):5155–61.

80. Friesel R, Komoriya A, Maciag T. Inhibition of endothelial cell proliferation by gamma-interferon. J Cell Biol 1987;104(3):689–96.

81. Arenberg DA, Kunkel SL, Polverini PJ, et al. Interferon-gamma-inducible protein 10 (IP-10) is an angiostatic factor that inhibits human non-small cell lung cancer (NSCLC) tumorigenesis and spontaneous metastases. J Exp Med 1996;184(3):981–92.

82. Sgadari C, Angiolillo AL, Tosato G. Inhibition of angiogenesis by interleukin-12 is mediated by the interferon-inducible protein 10. Blood 1996;87(9): 3877–82.

83. Sgadari C, Farber JM, Angiolillo AL, et al. Mig, the monokine induced by interferon-gamma, promotes tumor necrosis in vivo. Blood 1997; 89(8):2635–43.

84. Strieter RM, Polverini PJ, Arenberg DA, et al. The role of CXC chemokines as regulators of angiogenesis. Shock 1995;4(3):155–60.

85. Romer LH, McLean NV, Yan HC, et al. IFN-gamma and TNF-alpha induce redistribution of PECAM-1 (CD31) on human endothelial cells. J Immunol 1995;154(12):6582–92.

86. Stewart RJ, Kashour TS, Marsden PA. Vascular endothelial platelet endothelial adhesion molecule-1 (PECAM-1) expression is decreased by TNF-alpha and IFN-gamma. Evidence for cytokine-induced destabilization of messenger ribonucleic acid transcripts in bovine endothelial cells. J Immunol 1996;156(3):1221–8.

87. Rüegg C, Yilmaz A, Bieler G, et al. Evidence for the involvement of endothelial cell integrin alphaVbeta3 in the disruption of the tumor vasculature induced by TNF and IFN-gamma. Nat Med 1998; 4(4):408–14.

88. Smith KE, Janelidze S, Visse E, et al. Synergism between GM-CSF and IFNgamma: enhanced immunotherapy in mice with glioma. Int J Cancer 2007;120(1):75–80.

89. Enzler T, Gillessen S, Manis JP, et al. Deficiencies of GM-CSF and interferon gamma link inflammation and cancer. J Exp Med 2003;197(9):1213–9.

90. Yoon SJ, Lee JC, Kang JO, et al. Anti-tumor effect associated with down-regulation of MHC class 1 antigen after co-transfection of GM-CSF and IFN-gamma genes in CT26 tumor cells. Anticancer Res 2001;21(6A):4031–9.

91. Yoon SJ, Heo DS, Kang JO, et al. Synergistic anti-tumor effects with co-expression of GM-CSF and IFN-gamma in murine tumors. Int J Cancer 1998; 77(6):907–12.

92. Smith KE, Fritzell S, Badn W, et al. Cure of established GL261 mouse gliomas after combined immunotherapy with GM-CSF and IFNgamma is mediated by both CD8+ and CD4+ T-cells. Int J Cancer 2009;124(3):630–7.

93. Inaba K, Inaba M, Romani N, et al. Generation of large numbers of dendritic cells from mouse bone marrow cultures supplemented with granulocyte/macrophage colony-stimulating factor. J Exp Med 1992;176(6):1693–702.

94. Basak SK, Harui A, Stolina M, et al. Increased dendritic cell number and function following continuous in vivo infusion of granulocyte macrophage-colony-stimulating factor and interleukin-4. Blood 2002;99(8):2869–79.

95. Dalton DK, Pitts-Meek S, Keshav S, et al. Multiple defects of immune cell function in mice with disrupted interferon-gamma genes. Science 1993; 259(5102):1739–42.

96. Huang S, Hendriks W, Althage A, et al. Immune response in mice that lack the interferon-gamma receptor. Science 1993;259(5102):1742–5.

97. Albina JE, Henry WL Jr. Suppression of lymphocyte proliferation through the nitric oxide synthesizing pathway. J Surg Res 1991;50(4):403–9.

98. Allione A, Bernabei P, Bosticardo M, et al. Nitric oxide suppresses human T lymphocyte proliferation through IFN-gamma-dependent and IFN-gamma-independent induction of apoptosis. J Immunol 1999;163(8):4182–91.

99. Bauer H, Jung T, Tsikas D, et al. Nitric oxide inhibits the secretion of T-helper 1- and T-helper 2-associated cytokines in activated human T cells. Immunology 1997;90(2):205–11.

100. Medot-Pirenne M, Heilman MJ, Saxena M, et al. Augmentation of an antitumor CTL response In vivo by inhibition of suppressor macrophage nitric oxide. J Immunol 1999;163(11):5877–82.

101. Badn W, Hegardt P, Fellert MA, et al. Inhibition of inducible nitric oxide synthase enhances antitumour immune responses in rats immunized with IFN-gamma-secreting glioma cells. Scand J Immunol 2007;65(3):289–97.

102. Haque A, Das A, Hajiaghamohseni LM, et al. Induction of apoptosis and immune response by all-trans retinoic acid plus interferon-gamma in human malignant glioblastoma T98G and U87MG cells. Cancer Immunol Immunother 2007;56(5):615–25.

103. Haque A, Banik NL, Ray SK. Emerging role of combination of all-trans retinoic acid and interferon-gamma as chemoimmunotherapy in the management of human glioblastoma. Neurochem Res 2007;32(12):2203–9.

104. Knupfer MM, Knüpfer H, Jendrossek V, et al. Interferon-gamma inhibits growth and migration of A172

human glioblastoma cells. Anticancer Res 2001; 21(6A):3989–94.

105. Mahaley MS Jr, Bertsch L, Cush S, et al. Systemic gamma-interferon therapy for recurrent gliomas. J Neurosurg 1988;69(6):826–9.

106. Farkkila M, Jääskeläinen J, Kallio M, et al. Rando-mised, controlled study of intratumoral recombinant gamma-interferon treatment in newly diagnosed glioblastoma. Br J Cancer 1994;70(1): 138–41.

107. Wolff JE, Wagner S, Reinert C, et al. Maintenance treatment with interferon-gamma and low-dose cyclophosphamide for pediatric high-grade glioma. J Neurooncol 2006;79(3):315–21.

# The Epidermal Growth Factor Variant III Peptide Vaccine for Treatment of Malignant Gliomas

Gordon Li, MD, Siddhartha Mitra, PhD, Albert J. Wong, MD*

## KEYWORDS

- Epidermal growth factor receptor variant III
- Epidermal growth factor receptor • Cancer vaccine
- Immunotherapy • Glioblastoma multiforme

## MALIGNANT GLIOMAS AND PEPTIDE VACCINATION

There have been significant advances in the understanding of the molecular and cellular biology of malignant gliomas in recent years. Unfortunately, the median survival of patients who have newly diagnosed glioblastoma multiforme (GBM) still remains 14.6 months after surgery followed by postoperative radiation therapy and temozolomide.[1] Despite several different therapeutic approaches, at the clinical and preclinical stage, the median overall survival of these patients has not changed significantly and current standard of care treatment results in toxic side effects to normal brain and hematopoietic function. One of the main difficulties in the treatment of this tumor is its highly invasive and diffuse spread through the brain parenchyma. Under these circumstances local therapies are ineffective and systemic therapies are limited by the blood brain barrier and lack of specificity. New systemic therapies are needed and unique approaches from immunotherapy have emerged over the past two decades with promising results. Immunotherapy has the advantage of being tumor specific and systemic in delivery. Examples of immunotherapeutic approaches include treatment with tumor-specific monoclonal antibodies (MAb)

alone, MAb attached to cytotoxic agents, or vaccination with tumor-associated antigens. One of the main challenges to immunotherapy, however, has been finding the ideal tumor associated antigen and overcoming the tumor's ability to downregulate the surrounding immune microenvironment. In this article, the authors discuss a peptide vaccination strategy developed around the tumor-associated antigen epidermal growth factor variant III (EGFRvIII).

Peptide vaccines are chemically synthesized based on the sequence of tumor-associated antigens and are injected subcutaneously or intravenously into patients who have cancer to stimulate a tumor-specific immune response. This delivery method is safe, inexpensive, and the peptide itself is easy to produce and store. Peptide vaccination strategies for cancer therapy have been studied since the early 1990s with the identification of MAGE-1, the first human cancer associated gene, which encodes melanoma-specific antigens.[2] That discovery was followed by the description of the first human tumor-specific peptide, which was nine amino acids long and restricted by HLA-A1.[3] Since then there have been many clinical trials using peptide-based vaccines for the treatment of a variety of cancer types. The exact mechanism of immune activation

Albert Wong is a shareholder and consultant to Celldex Therapeutics, and a co-inventor of the EGFRvIII sequence and EGFRvIII peptide vaccine and receives royalties related to these patents.
Department of Neurosurgery, Stanford University School of Medicine, 300 Pasteur Drive, Edwards Building Room 213, Stanford, CA 94305, USA
* Corresponding author.
*E-mail address:* ajwong@stanford.edu (A. Wong).

Neurosurg Clin N Am 21 (2010) 87–93
doi:10.1016/j.nec.2009.08.004
1042-3680/09/$ – see front matter © 2010 Elsevier Inc. All rights reserved.

after peptide vaccination is not known, but theoretically the peptides are processed by antigen-presenting cells and presented to T cells in the context of major histocompatibility complex (MHC) molecules.

## EPIDERMAL GROWTH FACTOR VARIANT III

The epidermal growth factor (EGF) receptor is a transmembrane tyrosine kinase growth factor receptor that belongs to a family of four related receptors: EGF receptor (ErbB-1), ErbB2/Neu/Her2, ErbB3/Her3, and ErbB4/Her4.[4] Ligand binding to the monomeric receptor leads to dimerization, resulting in activation of cytoplasmic catalytic function and subsequent autophosphorylation.[5] Following autophosphorylation, numerous intracellular signaling pathways are activated with a multitude of downstream effects ranging from cell division and migration to adhesion, differentiation, and apoptosis.[6] Aspects of EGF-receptor signaling have been implicated in the pathogenesis of many human cancers as many tumor types exhibit over expression or aberrant activity of the EGF receptor[7,8] leading to unregulated growth and malignant transformation. Cetuximab and panitumumab, two monoclonal antibodies against the EGF receptor, and erlotinib and gefitinib, two EGF receptor tyrosine kinase small molecule inhibitors, are examples of EGF receptor antagonists that have been approved by the US Food and Drug Administration. They are currently available for treatment of metastatic non-small cell lung cancer, squamous cell carcinoma of the head and neck, colorectal cancer, and pancreatic cancer[9] and are now being investigated in many clinical trials for a variety of tumor types including malignant gliomas. However, EGF receptors have wide expression in normal tissues and therapeutics directed against it theoretically could lead to unwanted toxic effects. An antigen present only in tumor tissue would be a more ideal target.

There are at least ten classes of EGF receptor genomic variants described in gliomas. EGFRvIII is the most common variant of the EGF receptor and is present in 24% to 67% of GBM where it was first identified,[10,11] but has not been observed in normal brain. This mutant receptor has subsequently been detected in many other solid tumors including medulloblastomas, breast, colon, ovarian, metastatic prostate, head and neck, and non-small cell lung carcinomas.[12–18] There is debate over the prognostic significance of this mutant receptor in malignant gliomas, but the most recent and largest study indicated that EGFRvIII is a negative prognostic indicator when considering long-term GBM survivors only.[19–21]

EGFRvIII results from an in-frame deletion corresponding to exons 2 to 7 of the EGF receptor gene resulting in the fusion of exon 1 to exon 8 and deletion of a large portion of the extracellular domain (Fig. 1). This deletion removes amino acids 6 to 273 and generates a novel glycine at the junction. This novel epitope is at the amino terminus of the extracellular domain of the truncated receptor resulting in a protein of 145 kDa compared with the wild-type EGF receptor, which is 170 kDa. Although it does not bind ligand, EGFRvIII is constitutively active and can lead directly to cancer phenotypes because of its oncogenic properties.[22] The molecular mechanism by which this mutant receptor acts is not completely known. Constitutive activity of phosphatidylinositol 3 kinase and c-Jun N-terminal kinase have been implicated.[23,24] EGFRvIII is an attractive target for malignant gliomas because it is not expressed in the normal brain and because cells producing EGFRvIII have an enhanced capacity for unregulated growth, survival, invasion, and angiogenesis. It is an especially valuable target for immunotherapeutic approaches because the juxtaposition of ordinarily distant amino acids plus the unique glycine at the junction produces a highly immunogenic and novel epitope. Tumor antigens are generally over-expressed self-antigens that have triggered immune tolerance. Peptide vaccination with these tumor antigens carries the risk of either an autoimmune response or a muted immune

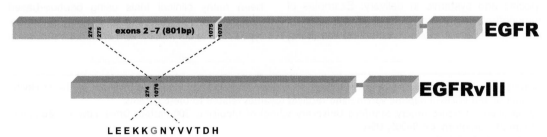

**Fig. 1.** EGFRvIII is an alternatively spliced form of the EGF receptor that is the result of the deletion of exons 2 to 7 removing 801 base pairs from the extracellular domain of the receptor. The fusion on exons 1 to 8 results in a novel glycine.

response because of tolerance. EGFRvIII is seen only on tumor cells and therefore has a less likely risk of autoimmunity or muted response because of immune tolerance.

## PRECLINICAL TRIALS STUDYING ACTIVE IMMUNIZATION WITH EPIDERMAL GROWTH FACTOR VARIANT III

The unique extracellular peptide sequence of the EGFRvIII junction can be used to raise polyclonal and monoclonal antibodies that specifically recognize EGFRvIII[10,25] but not wild-type EGF receptor. The ability of this peptide to elicit a humoral response in rabbits suggested that a vaccine based on this novel antigen could be used against tumors, although evidence of a T-cell reaction was also needed for full antitumor response. Moreover, Purev and colleagues[16] evaluated the serum of subjects who had EGFRvIII-expressing breast cancer and found EGFRvIII-specific antibodies and an EGFRvIII-specific lymphoproliferative response suggesting that patients may benefit from vaccination against EGFRvIII by boosting existing immune responses.

Moscatello and colleagues[26] were the first to demonstrate the possibility of using a peptide derived from EGFRvIII as an antitumor vaccine in mouse models. For this study, the 14 amino acid peptide corresponding to the exon 1 to exon 8 junction (LEEKKGNYVVTDHC, where the terminal cysteine was added for conjugation) was conjugated to keyhole limpet hemocyanin (KLH) and used as the peptide vaccine. KLH is a well-established carrier protein for conjugated peptide vaccines that increase peptide half-life, provides strong CD4 T helper response, and activates antigen-presenting cells.[27] NIH Swiss mice or Fischer 344 rats were pre-immunized with peptide-KLH conjugate and subsequently injected subcutaneously with NIH3T3 cells transformed by the overexpression of human EGFRvIII. Pre-immunization with this peptide vaccine significantly decreased tumor incidence when compared with controls, and the antitumor effect was long lasting as seven animals that had successfully rejected the original tumor were rechallenged 6 to 12 months later and showed no tumor growth. This peptide conjugate was also able to mediate the rejection of established tumors in mice, a paradigm for the treatment of human disease. The magnitude of the regression was significant where tumors of up to 4 cm$^3$ completely involuted within 3 weeks. In a few of the mice treated, a secondary tumor recurred approximately 40 to 50 days later. Upon analysis, four of five tumors no longer expressed EGFRvIII demonstrating that the vaccine

treatment successfully targeted cells expressing the antigen. Immunologic studies revealed that the tumor regression was dependent on an EGFRvIII-specific CD8+ T lymphocyte mediated cytotoxic response that did not recognize cells expressing wild-type EGF receptor.

In a subsequent study, mice pre-immunized with the identical peptide vaccine as the prior study, which they called pep-3-KLH,[28] were challenged subcutaneously or intracerebrally with murine melanoma cells expressing artificially generated mouse EGFRvIII. A significant antitumor effect was also noticed in the pre-immunized mice. They noted a significant humoral response in these vaccinated mice, but not a cytotoxic T-cell response. Passive transfer of sera from immunized mice to non-immunized mice protected against tumor development suggesting that antibodies were responsible for the response. Depletion studies showed that the CD8+ T cells and natural killer cells were important for the antitumor effect, and in vitro assays showed that macrophages could lyse target tumor cells with serum from the pep-3–KLH–vaccinated mice raising speculation that these were effector cells for antibodies. Another group of mice that had been injected intracerebrally were also vaccinated after tumor inoculation. Mice with established intracerebral tumors injected with the pep-3-KLH exhibited a 26% increase in survival. As had been seen by Moscatello and colleagues, 80% of recurrent tumors in this study no longer expressed EGFRvIII.

In a variation to the vaccine, Ciesielski and colleagues[29] created a homo-chimeric peptide vaccine with multiple copies of the EGFRvIII epitope linked together by a lysine bridge (MAP). In rats pre-immunized with MAP, the authors demonstrated attenuated tumorigenesis of EGFRvIII expressing cells but not wild-type EGF-receptor expressing tumor cells. Moreover, the median survival of pre-immunized rats was increased 72% more than unvaccinated controls injected with intracerebral EGFRvIII expressing tumor cells. Supplementation with granulocyte-macrophage colony-stimulating factor (GM-CSF) led to increased titer of EGFRvIII-specific antibodies and increased recruitment of CD4+ and CD8+ T cells at the tumor site. Splenocytes and CD8+ T cells from vaccinated rats produced IFN-γ in vitro in response to stimulation by rat glioma cells expressing EGFRvIII, but not by those expressing wild-type EGF receptor, suggesting a role for cell mediated immunity in the antitumor response.

Heimberger and colleagues attempted an additional method of EGFRvIII antigen presentation by way of dendritic cells (DC). Mice pre-immunized with DC mixed with pep-3-KLH and then intracerebrally challenged with melanoma cells expressing EGFRvIII had an approximately 600% increase in median survival time compared with unvaccinated controls.[30] Pre-immunized mice that survived tumor challenge were reinjected 100 days later in the contralateral hemisphere and survived showing long-lasting protection, confirming the results of Moscatello and colleagues.[26]

Using a bioinformatic and combinatorial peptide approach to find a peptide that could evoke superior immune response, Wu and colleagues[31] screened the EGFRvIII peptide sequence with two software programs to predict candidate epitopes restricted by the MHC class 1 subtype HLA-A0201, which is the predominant subtype in most ethnic groups. Three peptides were predicted, synthesized, and then subsequently loaded into mature human DC from peripheral blood monocytes. Autologous CD8+ T cells were then stimulated in vitro with DC mixed with the peptides. As demonstrated by IFN$\gamma$ production and cytotoxicity against HLA-A0201+ EGFRvIII transfected U87 glioma cells, one of the three peptides was found to induce an EGFRvIII-specific cytotoxic T lymphocyte response. The difference between peptide one (LEEKKGNYV), which was the successful peptide, and peptide two (LEEKKGNYVV) was only one amino acid.

## CLINICAL TRIALS STUDYING ACTIVE IMMUNIZATION WITH EPIDERMAL GROWTH FACTOR VARIANT III

Encouraging results from these preclinical studies have resulted in clinical trials evaluating active immunization with the EGFRvIII peptide as defined by Moscatello and colleagues.[26] The first Phase I trial was performed by the Southwestern Oncology Group (protocol S0114)[32] for subjects who had prostate and ovarian cancer. The study evaluated the safety of vaccinating patients who have the EGFRvIII peptide administered with KLH and GM-CSF intradermally once every month for 6 months. There were no serious adverse events among the 10 subjects who enrolled. The next trial was Vaccine for Intra-Cranial Tumors I, a Phase I clinical trial for subjects who had newly diagnosed malignant gliomas (World Health Organization grade III or IV) to determine the safety of vaccinating with mature DC loaded with the 500 µg of vaccine conjugate. Twenty subjects were enrolled, but four of these subjects did not qualify for the vaccine. Beginning 2 weeks after surgical resection and postoperative radiotherapy, subjects were vaccinated 2 weeks apart for a total of three vaccinations. There was a lack of

delayed-type hypersensitivity reaction to KLH or the EGFRvIII peptide before vaccination, but after vaccination 16 out of 16 subjects (3 grade III, 13 GBM) reacted to KLH, and 10 out of 16 (62.5%) reacted to the peptide. There was a detectable humoral response although all subjects tested had significantly higher antigen-specific T-cell proliferation in vitro after vaccination in response to peptide and KLH. Of the two subjects who did not undergo gross total resection, one subject who had glioblastoma presently remains alive 6.2 years later and had a complete response after vaccination, whereas the other subject who had anaplastic astrocytoma is alive and progression-free 5.4 years later. Two of the three subjects who had grade III tumors are alive and with evidence of recurrence at 66.2 and 123.7 months after vaccination, whereas one subject recurred 47.7 months after vaccination. For subjects who had GBM, the median survival time was 775.6 days, significantly higher compared with published trials evaluating subjects who were newly diagnosed with GBM.[33,34]

A third clinical trial, A Complementary Trial of an Immunotherapy Vaccine Against Tumor-specific EGFRvIII (ACTIVATE), was a Phase 2 trial that evaluated the efficacy of the peptide vaccine conjugate for 23 subjects who had newly diagnosed EGFRvIII-expressing GBM as assayed by immunohistochemistry or polymerase chain reaction. To be included, the subjects must have undergone gross total resection followed by conformal radiation and concurrent temozolomide (75 mg/m$^2$/d) but not have shown tumor recurrence. Intradermal vaccine inoculation was done concurrently with GM-CSF in 2-week intervals for three doses followed by monthly injections until tumor progression.[34–36] The vaccination resulted in an EGFRvIII-specific humoral response with minimal toxicity. Using an immunoassay developed by Schmittling and colleagues,[37] the authors were able to detect increased levels of anti-EGFRvIII and anti-KLH antibodies in the serum of subjects in this trial after vaccination. Moreover, there was an induction of CD8+ IFN$\gamma$ EGFRvIII-specific T cells as a result of vaccination. The median time to progression was 64.5 weeks and the median survival was 126.1 weeks. Historically matched controls had a median time to progression of 28.5 weeks and median survival of 56 weeks. Similar to the preclinical studies, recurrent tumors from subjects after vaccination no longer expressed EGFRvIII.

Although the ACTIVATE study was ongoing, results were published from a randomized trial in subjects who had newly diagnosed GBM, which showed radiotherapy plus continuous daily temozolomide[1] followed by six cycles of adjuvant temozolomide demonstrated prolonged median survival of 14.6 months when compared with 12.1 months for subjects receiving radiotherapy alone. Because the standard of care for newly diagnosed patients who have GBM has now become radiotherapy with concurrent temozolomide followed by six cycles of adjuvant temozolomide, the ACTIVATE II trial was initiated with 21 subjects who were newly diagnosed with GBM and underwent gross total resection followed by concurrent radiotherapy and temozolomide. Currently, the vaccine for this and subsequent trials is now produced by Celldex Therapeutics and is called CDX-110. CDX-110 vaccination is given on day 21 of the 28-day temozolomide cycle when the immune system has theoretically recovered from the temozolomide-induced immune suppression. Many chemotherapeutic agents, including temozolomide, induce pronounced lymphopenia that prevents an effective combined immunotherapeutic approach. However, chemotherapy can be integrated well with tumor vaccines by taking advantage of their pharmacodynamic properties.[38] Results from this trial demonstrated no diminution of the EGFRvIII-specific immune response after co-administration of temozolomide with EGFRvIII vaccination. Although the trial has not reached final median survival, the preliminary data reveals median time to progression of 16.6 months and median overall survival of 33.1 months when compared with historical matched controls that had a median time to progression of 6.4 months and median survival of 14.3 months.[36,39]

Currently, patients who are newly diagnosed with EGFRvIII-positive glioblastoma are being enrolled into ACT III, a phase II/III randomized multicenter nationwide clinical trial sponsored by Celldex Therapeutics. Subjects were randomized 2:1 into a treatment group including gross total resection followed by radiation, chemotherapy and CDX-110 vaccination, or the control group receiving gross total resection followed by radiation and chemotherapy without vaccination. A recent amendment to the trial will enroll all eligible subjects into the vaccine arm.[40]

## DISCUSSION

Among the many tumor-specific mutations found in brain tumors, those with unique extracellular epitopes are the most useful practically for therapeutic purposes. EGFRvIII is an ideal target antigen for immunotherapy because it is a unique epitope that is expressed only in cancer cells. Several preclinical studies have focused on understanding and the targeting of this mutant EGF receptor. Therapeutic approaches have included the use of unarmed MAb, immunoliposomes, radiolabelled MAb, MAb conjugated to immunotoxins or boronated dendrimers, and small molecule inhibitors. However, active immunization with the peptide vaccine is the only strategy that has shown the most promise and has successfully made it to clinical trials. The use of EGFRvIII extracellular peptide sequence elicits specific immune response. Data from early clinical trials have been extremely promising, especially given the poor prognosis of patients who express EGFRvIII.

The ongoing, randomized clinical trial evaluating CDX-110 is highly pivotal. If successful, this will be the first randomized trial demonstrating the efficacy of CDX-110 and the first trial demonstrating a successful cancer peptide vaccine. Should the vaccine be effective in prolonging overall survival in patients who have newly diagnosed GBM, the vaccine could be extended to other tumor types that express this target. As discussed earlier, the two largest challenges to immunotherapy are finding the appropriate target antigen and overcoming the local tumor immune suppression. GBM downregulate or express defective HLA antigens[41] and alter MHC class II expression of nearby microglia and macrophages.[42] The overall number of T cells is decreased in patients who have GBM with a decrease of effector T cells and an increase in the T-regulatory cells.[43] Combining EGFRvIII targeted therapies with an immune modulator may help the immune system to mount a larger response against the tumor. One such immune modulator was studied by Hussain and colleagues[44] who showed that signal transducers and activators of transcription 3 blockade by a novel small molecule can reverse immune tolerance in patients who have GBM.

Malignant neoplasms are complex and have a heterogeneous group of genetic alterations. A single targeted approach is unlikely to cure patients. As seen in the preclinical trials and the early clinical trials with the EGFRvIII vaccine, recurrences occur even after successful vaccination. The tumors that recur are no longer expressing EGFRvIII, suggesting that recurrent tumors find an alternative mechanism of tumorigenesis. Trials involving a combinatorial approach, such as that proposed by Huang and colleagues,[45] will likely be evaluated in future studies. Targeting of multiple pathways may prove to be more effective than targeting a single antigen. With advancing technologies and increasing knowledge, the hope is that we will one day be able to resect a tumor, analyze the tumor, and treat patients with targeted therapies directed specifically to the biology of that specific tumor.

## REFERENCES

1. Stupp R, Mason WP, van den Bent MJ, et al. Radiotherapy plus concomitant and adjuvant temozolomide for glioblastoma. N Engl J Med 2005;352(10):987–96.
2. van der BP, Traversari C, Chomez P, et al. A gene encoding an antigen recognized by cytolytic T lymphocytes on a human melanoma. Science 1991;254(5038):1643–7.
3. Kanodia S, Kast WM. Peptide-based vaccines for cancer: realizing their potential. Expert Rev Vaccines 2008;7(10):1533–45.
4. Salomon DS, Brandt R, Ciardiello F, et al. Epidermal growth factor-related peptides and their receptors in human malignancies. Crit Rev Oncol Hematol 1995;19(3):183–232.
5. Citri A, Yarden Y. EGF-ERBB signaling: towards the systems level. Nat Rev Mol Cell Biol 2006;7(7):505–16.
6. Hynes NE, Lane HA. ERBB receptors and cancer: the complexity of targeted inhibitors. Nat Rev Cancer 2005;5(5):341–54.
7. Wong AJ, Bigner SH, Bigner DD, et al. Increased expression of the epidermal growth factor receptor gene in malignant gliomas is invariably associated with gene amplification. Proc Natl Acad Sci U S A 1987;84(19):6899–903.
8. Libermann TA, Nusbaum HR, Razon N, et al. Amplification, enhanced expression and possible rearrangement of EGF receptor gene in primary human brain tumours of glial origin. Nature 1985;313(5998):144–7.
9. Ciardiello F, Tortora G. EGFR antagonists in cancer treatment. N Engl J Med 2008;358(11):1160–74.
10. Humphrey PA, Wong AJ, Vogelstein B, et al. Antisynthetic peptide antibody reacting at the fusion junction of deletion-mutant epidermal growth factor receptors in human glioblastoma. Proc Natl Acad Sci U S A 1990;87(11):4207–11.
11. Wong AJ, Ruppert JM, Bigner SH, et al. Structural alterations of the epidermal growth factor receptor gene in human gliomas. Proc Natl Acad Sci U S A 1992;89(7):2965–9.
12. Moscatello DK, Holgado-Madruga M, Godwin AK, et al. Frequent expression of a mutant epidermal growth factor receptor in multiple human tumors. Cancer Res 1995;55(23):5536–9.
13. Garcia de Palazzo IE, Adams GP, Sundareshan P, et al. Expression of mutated epidermal growth factor receptor by non-small cell lung carcinomas. Cancer Res 1993;53(14):3217–20.
14. Cunningham MP, Essapen S, Thomas H, et al. Coexpression, prognostic significance and predictive value of EGFR, EGFRvIII and phosphorylated EGFR in colorectal cancer. Int J Oncol 2005;27(2):317–25.
15. Ge H, Gong X, Tang CK. Evidence of high incidence of EGFRvIII expression and coexpression with EGFR in human invasive breast cancer by laser capture microdissection and immunohistochemical analysis. Int J Cancer 2002;98(3):357–61.
16. Purev E, Cai D, Miller E, et al. Immune responses of breast cancer patients to mutated epidermal growth factor receptor (EGF-RvIII, Delta EGF-R, and de2-7 EGF-R). J Immunol 2004;173(10):6472–80.
17. Sok JC, Coppelli FM, Thomas SM, et al. Mutant epidermal growth factor receptor (EGFRvIII) contributes to head and neck cancer growth and resistance to EGFR targeting. Clin Cancer Res 2006;12(17):5064–73.
18. Olapade-Olaopa EO, Moscatello DK, MacKay EH, et al. Evidence for the differential expression of a variant EGF receptor protein in human prostate cancer. Br J Cancer 2000;82(1):186–94.
19. Heimberger AB, Hlatky R, Suki D, et al. Prognostic effect of epidermal growth factor receptor and EGFRvIII in glioblastoma multiforme patients. Clin Cancer Res 2005;11(4):1462–6.
20. Heimberger AB, Suki D, Yang D, et al. The natural history of EGFR and EGFRvIII in glioblastoma patients. J Transl Med 2005;3:38.
21. Pelloski CE, Ballman KV, Furth AF, et al. Epidermal growth factor receptor variant III status defines clinically distinct subtypes of glioblastoma. J Clin Oncol 2007;25(16):2288–94.
22. Fernandes H, Cohen S, Bishayee S. Glycosylation-induced conformational modification positively regulates receptor-receptor association: a study with an aberrant epidermal growth factor receptor (EGFRvIII/DeltaEGFR) expressed in cancer cells. J Biol Chem 2001;276(7):5375–83.
23. Antonyak MA, Moscatello DK, Wong AJ. Constitutive activation of c-Jun N-terminal kinase by a mutant epidermal growth factor receptor. J Biol Chem 1998;273(5):2817–22.
24. Moscatello DK, Holgado-Madruga M, Emlet DR, et al. Constitutive activation of phosphatidylinositol 3-kinase by a naturally occurring mutant epidermal growth factor receptor. J Biol Chem 1998;273(1):200–6.
25. Wikstrand CJ, Hale LP, Batra SK, et al. Monoclonal antibodies against EGFRvIII are tumor specific and react with breast and lung carcinomas and malignant gliomas. Cancer Res 1995;55(14):3140–8.
26. Moscatello DK, Ramirez G, Wong AJ. A naturally occurring mutant human epidermal growth factor receptor as a target for peptide vaccine immunotherapy of tumors. Cancer Res 1997;57(8):1419–24.
27. Harris JR, Markl J. Keyhole limpet hemocyanin (KLH): a biomedical review. Micron 1999;30(6):597–623.
28. Heimberger AB, Crotty LE, Archer GE, et al. Epidermal growth factor receptor VIII peptide

vaccination is efficacious against established intra-cerebral tumors. Clin Cancer Res 2003;9(11): 4247–54.

29. Ciesielski MJ, Kazim AL, Barth RF, et al. Cellular anti-tumor immune response to a branched lysine multiple antigenic peptide containing epitopes of a common tumor-specific antigen in a rat glioma model. Cancer Immunol Immunother 2005;54(2): 107–19.

30. Heimberger AB, Archer GE, Crotty LE, et al. Dendritic cells pulsed with a tumor-specific peptide induce long-lasting immunity and are effective against murine intracerebral melanoma. Neurosurgery 2002;50(1):158–64.

31. Wu AH, Xiao J, Anker L, et al. Identification of EGFR-vIII-derived CTL epitopes restricted by HLA A0201 for dendritic cell based immunotherapy of gliomas. J Neurooncol 2006;76(1):23–30.

32. Li G, Wong AJ. EGF receptor variant III as a target antigen for tumor immunotherapy. Expert Rev Vaccines 2008;7(7):977–85.

33. Archer G, Bigner D, Friedman A, et al. Dendritic cell vaccine for intracranial tumors 1 (DC VICTORI Trial) [abstract]. Presented at the 2004 Society of Neuro-oncology Meeting. Toronto, Ontario, Canada, November 18–21, 2004.

34. Sampson JH, Archer GE, Mitchell DA, et al. Tumor-specific immunotherapy targeting the EGFRvIII mutation in patients with malignant glioma. Semin Immunol 2008;20:267–75.

35. Heimberger AB, Hussain SF, Aldape K, et al. Tumor-specific peptide vaccination in newly-diagnosed patients with GBM. 2006 ASCO Annual Meeting Proceedings. J Clin Oncol 2006;24(Suppl 18): S2529.

36. Sampson JH, Aldape K, Gilbert S, et al. Temozolo-mide as a vaccine adjuvant in GBM. 2007 ASCO Annual Meeting Proceedings Part 1. J Clin Oncol 2007;25(S18):2020.

37. Schmittling RJ, Archer GE, Mitchell DA, et al. Detection of humoral response in patients with glioblas-toma receiving EGFRvIII-KLH vaccines. J Immunol Methods 2008;339(1):74–81.

38. Emens LA, Reilly RT, Jaffee EM. Cancer vaccines in combination with multimodality therapy. Cancer Treat Res 2005;123:227–45.

39. Sampson JH, Archer GE, Bigner DD, et al. Effect of EGFRvIII-targeted vaccine (CDX-110) on immune response and TTP when given with simultaneous standard and continuous temozolomide in patients with GBM [abstract]. J Clin Oncol 2008;26(Suppl): 2011.

40. Sonabend AM, Dana K, Lesniak MS. Targeting epidermal growth factor receptor variant III: a novel strategy for the therapy of malignant glioma. Expert Rev Anticancer Ther 2007;7(Suppl 12):S45–50.

41. Facoetti A, Nano R, Zelini P, et al. Human leukocyte antigen and antigen processing machinery compo-nent defects in astrocytic tumors. Clin Cancer Res 2005;11(23):8304–11.

42. Schartner JM, Hagar AR, Van Handel M, et al. Impaired capacity for upregulation of MHC class II in tumor-associated microglia. Glia 2005;51(4):279–85.

43. Fecci PE, Mitchell DA, Whitesides JF, et al. Increased regulatory T-cell fraction amidst a dimin-ished CD4 compartment explains cellular immune defects in patients with malignant glioma. Cancer Res 2006;66(6):3294–302.

44. Hussain SF, Kong LY, Jordan J, et al. A novel small molecule inhibitor of signal transducers and activa-tors of transcription 3 reverses immune tolerance in malignant glioma patients. Cancer Res 2007; 67(20):9630–6.

45. Huang PH, Mukasa A, Bonavia R, et al. Quantitative analysis of EGFRvIII cellular signaling networks reveals a combinatorial therapeutic strategy for glio-blastoma. Proc Natl Acad Sci U S A 2007;104(31): 12867–72.

# Clinical Applications of a Peptide-Based Vaccine for Glioblastoma

Charles W. Kanaly, MD[a], Dale Ding, BS[b],
Amy B. Heimberger, MD[c],
John H. Sampson, MD, PhD, MHSc[d],*

**KEYWORDS**

- Brain neoplasms • Glioblastoma • Immunotherapy
- Epidermal growth factor receptor • Neoplasm antigens
- Immune system

Glioblastoma multiforme (GBM) is the most common primary malignant tumor in the adult central nervous system.[1] Current therapy for this disease usually includes surgical resection, radiation, and the administration of temozolomide chemotherapy. It is a devastating diagnosis, because even with this standard treatment, median survival is less than 15 months.[2] Additionally, most current therapies are not selective for tumor cells; and therefore, large amounts of normal healthy tissue are injured as collateral damage while treating these tumors. This is a problem for most types of cancer, and particularly GBM, as it is highly infiltrative.

The ideal treatment for GBM needs to be selective enough to accurately discriminate between normal tissue and tumor cells and be able to reach across the blood brain barrier, while being potent enough to kill all of the tumor cells. The immune system certainly has this capability as evidenced by its ability to fight infections within the central nervous system (CNS). Therefore, the immune system could be an ideal candidate for an effective GBM therapy as well. Although it would appear that the immune system inherently possesses the ability to recognize and eliminate GBMs, the fact that GBMs are able to proliferate in these patients suggests that without intervention, the immune system is not an effective check against this disease. The reasons for this failure are likely multifactorial, including the immune-privileged status of the CNS and immunosuppressive effects of the tumor. As there is clearly a significant need for more effective treatment options against GBM, attempting to direct the immune system to attack this disease is a promising area of active research.

## IMMUNOTHERAPY

Multiple different approaches are being used to activate the immune system against the tumor. To provoke the immune system into being stimulated against tumor cells, attempts have included injections of peptides, proteins, DNA, RNA, viruses

[a] Division of Neurosurgery, Department of Surgery, Duke University Medical Center, Box 3050, 220 Sands Building, Research Drive, Durham, NC 27710, USA
[b] School of Medicine, Duke University, DUMC Box 3050, 220 Sands Building, Research Drive, Durham, NC 27710, USA
[c] Department of Neurosurgery, University of Texas, M.D. Anderson Cancer Center, Unit 442, 1400 Holcombe Boulevard, FC7.2000, Houston, TX 77030-4009, USA
[d] Division of Neurosurgery, Department of Surgery, The Preston Robert Tisch Brain Tumor Center at Duke, Box 3050, 220 Sands Building, Research Drive, Duke University Medical Center, Durham, NC 27710, USA
* Corresponding author.
*E-mail address:* john.sampson@duke.edu (J.H. Sampson).

Neurosurg Clin N Am 21 (2010) 95–109
doi:10.1016/j.nec.2009.09.001
1042-3680/09/$ – see front matter © 2010 Elsevier Inc. All rights reserved.

encoding cancer antigens, viruslike particles, whole tumor cells or their lysates, altered tumor cells that express cytokines, heat shock proteins, pulsed dendritic cells (DCs), and anti-idiotype antibodies.[3,4] Other methods are directed at overcoming tumor-related immune suppression by blocking the effect of inhibitory cells of the immune system or by blocking the effect of inhibitory molecules secreted by tumors like transforming growth factor-β (TGF-β). Administration of cytokines that promote lymphocyte expansion have led to some cases of dramatic tumor regression. For example interleukin-2 (IL-2) has been studied in the treatment of renal cancer, metastatic melanoma, and non-Hodgkin's lymphoma with some important treatment successes.[5–8]

The two main approaches for immunotherapy can be grouped into (active) vaccine therapy or (passive or adoptive) cell-transfer therapy (**Fig. 1**).[9]

To be successful, both approaches require the patient to develop lymphocytes that are activated against tumor cell antigens. Vaccine therapy in general follows the principle that injections of various substances that ultimately result in the presentation of tumor peptides to the patient's immune system will sensitize lymphocytes against an antigen of interest, and then these lymphocytes migrate to the tumor and cause cell killing. Vaccines typically are derived from cancer cells, cancer cell lysates, or specific peptides or proteins that encode cancer antigens. These can be pulsed onto antigen-presenting cells (APCs), which are then injected, or can be administered by themselves with adjuvants or cytokines that stimulate the immune system in a nonspecific manner.[10]

In contrast, cell-transfer therapy involves removing lymphocytes from the patient, expanding those lymphocytes, usually T cells,

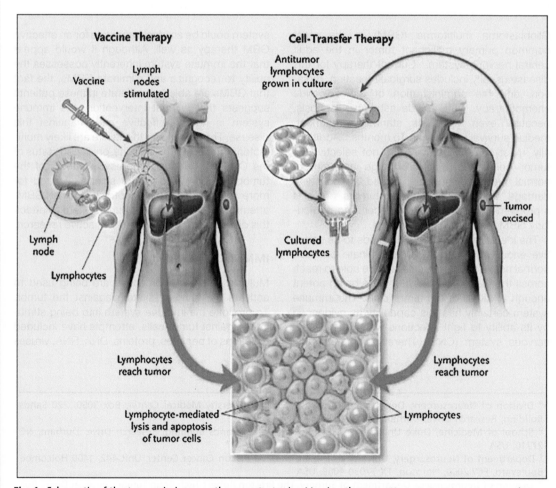

**Fig. 1.** Schematic of the two main immunotherapy strategies. Vaccine therapy attempts to generate an antitumor response by activating the immune system of the patient in vivo. Cell-Transfer Therapy removes lymphocytes from the patient, activates them in vitro against the tumor, then infuses them back into the patient. (*From* Rosenberg SA. Shedding light on immunotherapy for cancer. N Engl J Med 2004;350(14):1462; with permission.) Copyright © 2004, Massachusetts Medical Society.

that demonstrate activity against the tumor antigens, and then reintroducing that expanded and enriched cell population back into the same patient so they can migrate to the tumor and cause cell killing. In one form of cell-transfer therapy, T cells that are able to respond to defined cancer antigens are harvested from resected tumors and are termed tumor-infiltrating lymphocytes (TILs). Importantly, ex vivo cell transfer therapy allows one to directly manipulate both the lymphocytes outside of the body and the host immune system itself before infusion. It is thought that these manipulations before infusion are beneficial because they allow for stimulation and expansion of the cells at the time of reinfusion and also correction of the host environment to make it more hospitable for the infused, activated cells to be able to attack the tumor.[10] In fact, such host manipulations have recently enhanced the success of cell transfer therapy significantly and revolutionized this approach.

## IMMUNE SYSTEM COMPONENTS

The role of the immune system is basically to discriminate between self and non-self, and thereby defend the body from foreign attack. This role is critical for defense from microorganisms and other pathogens, but also prunes the body's own cells, causing removal of those cells that are no longer viable or exhibit a number of different warning signals to the immune system. The immune system is traditionally divided into two main arms, the innate and adaptive systems. The innate system is composed of macrophages/monocytes, neutrophils, natural killer cells, basophils, and eosinophils. The complement system is also a component of the innate system. The innate system is so named because it is present from birth, and it provides the initial line of defense, but it is not as specific as the adaptive system and does not have any memory of the protein previously defended against.[11]

In contrast, the adaptive immune system is able to refine its response to improve its ability to detect and respond against a specific offender particularly if it has defended against this foreigner previously. The main components of the adaptive immune system are T and B lymphocytes, and both cell types are able to adapt their response to foreign antigens and microorganisms. T cells are named because of their maturation in the thymus. Mature T cells are mainly divided into CD8$^+$ cytotoxic and CD4$^+$ helper cell types. Both types possess a T-cell receptor, and through this they bind to and recognize foreign antigens that are presented on the surface of tumor cells

or cells infected by viruses. These antigens are small peptide fragments that are presented in the groove of human leukocyte antigen (HLA) molecules that are present on almost all cells in the human body. CD8$^+$ cells recognize HLA class I molecules, and the peptide antigens presented on these molecules are typically 8 to 10 amino acids in length. These peptides come from intracellular proteins that are broken down in the proteasome. When activated, CD8$^+$ cells typically cause cell-mediated killing. CD4$^+$ cells, in contrast, recognize HLA class II molecules, and these molecules present peptides that are typically 13 amino acids in length. These peptides that are presented on class II molecules arise from the digestion of extracellular proteins that were taken into the cell via endocytosis. After activation, CD4$^+$ cells modulate the immune response by secreting different cytokines, and in general adjust the response of other cells of the immune system.[11] Most cells in the body express HLA class I molecules, but HLA class II expression is limited to antigen presenting cells.

B cells are named because of their derivation from precursor cells in the bone marrow. They are a component of the adaptive response, and they secrete antibodies in response to foreign antigens. Antibodies are secreted in five main types: IgG, IgM, IgE, IgD, and IgA.[12] Antibodies bind to specific antigens through protein-protein noncovalent biding, and this can lead to destruction of the offending cell or microorganism through a variety of means. In theory at least, each antibody recognizes a single antigen, but the wide diversity of antibodies that is created allows them as a whole to recognize a large number of antigens. When cells become abnormal from infection, mutation, or other danger to the host, they can change their surface protein expression. These altered or unique proteins can become antigens that can then be bound by antibodies, which leads to immune detection and subsequent killing of these cells by natural killer cells. This is called antibody-dependent cell-mediated cytotoxicity (ADCC).

## CENTRAL NERVOUS SYSTEM IMMUNE PRIVILEGE

It was classically believed that a few areas of the body, including the CNS, are privileged from standard surveillance by the immune system. Early studies by Medawar[13] in 1948 suggested that tissue grafts transplanted into the brain and other sites were not rejected, suggesting that these areas were not under immune surveillance. This idea has been supported by numerous findings specific to the CNS, including the decreased amount of HLA antigen presentation, the lack of conventional antigen presenting cells, the lack of a conventional lymphatic drainage system, and the existence of the blood brain barrier (BBB), which helps to block entry into the CNS. However, the reality is much more complicated and cells of the immune system are able to enter and interact with the CNS to a great extent. Furthermore, HLA antigen presentation does occur on astrocytes, microglia, endothelial cells, and in the choroid plexus, and microglia in particular may be the predominant antigen presenting cells within the CNS.[12,14,15] Although traditional lymphatics are not present in the CNS, it has been suggested that cervical lymph nodes do receive lymphatic drainage from the brain and that an immune response can be generated against antigens in the brain via this pathway.[16]

Antibody penetration across the BBB has generally been thought to be poor, as there is a low level of immunoglobulin in the CNS as compared with serum levels. Importantly, antibody permeability can drastically increase in certain conditions such as widespread inflammation. Furthermore, antibodies have been shown to penetrate the CNS, although at 0.1% to 10.0% of the peripheral blood levels.[14]

Early results from our group proved in humans that a radiolabeled monoclonal antibody against the extracellular matrix antigen tenascin was able to reach intracerebral tumor when given via intravenous administration, although only 0.0006% to 0.0043% of the total injected dose was measured at the tumor site.[17] Despite the low dose, this demonstrates that antibody is able to reach intracerebral tumors. However, it also suggests that in order to achieve clinical benefits, it may be necessary to give higher or more sustained doses of antibody, or more specific antibodies that do not exhibit systemic binding.

Later studies using antibodies recognizing epitopes restricted to the CNS have confirmed that antibodies can localize to the site of an intracerebral glioma after systemic administration, as **Fig. 2** depicts.[18] In this study, monoclonal antibody 806 was used, which recognizes the tumor-specific antigen, epidermal growth factor receptor variant III (EGFRvIII). This antibody was radiolabeled with Indium-111, and after a single dose was administered, imaging verified that the radiolabeled antibody localized to the intracerebral tumor site with no evidence of uptake in normal tissues. Localization of antibody to subcutaneous tumor xenografts in mice has also been published.[19] When an antibody is highly specific for the tumor and does not cross-react with systemic antigens, the lack of systemic binding may make it possible to get a much higher percentage of antibody penetration into the CNS and to the tumor site.

Moreover, the existence of paraneoplastic syndromes conclusively demonstrates that antibodies can penetrate the CNS at clinically significant levels. In this spectrum of disorders, antibodies directed against systemic tumor antigens have cross-reactivity with neuronal cells and therefore provoke an immune response in the CNS that leads to significant clinical morbidity.[20] Numerous antibodies arising from a variety of different cancers have been detected, including anti-Hu, anti-Yo, anti-Ri, anti-CV2, anti-Ma, anti-Tr, anti-amphiphysin, voltage gated potassium channel (VGKC) antibodies, anti–voltage gated calcium channel (anti-VGCC) antibodies, and antibodies to the N-methyl-D-aspartate (NMDA) receptor.[21–23] Many of these antibodies can also be detected in the cerebrospinal fluid (CSF) of affected individuals. Along with antibodies, T-cell responses in the CNS are also seen and it is thought that both responses contribute to the neuronal injury seen in these diseases.[22,24] Often, in addition to treatment of the underlying tumor, immune suppression is used to control the CNS immune response.[25–28]

Although it appears that antibody responses may be a more predominant aspect of the response against CNS antigens than cell-mediated responses, all aspects of the immune response are able to be generated in the CNS.[14] Prior experiments have shown that activated T cells can readily cross an intact BBB.[29] When these activated T cells are specific to myelin basic protein, they can cause normal rats to undergo lethal experimental autoimmune encephalitis (EAE).[30] Numerous adhesion molecules and chemotactic factors have been implicated in this process. Naïve T cells are not believed to cross the normal BBB, however.

As an acknowledgment to the limitations caused by the BBB, there have also been attempts to bypass it via direct drug delivery to the brain. Some of the more promising of these methods include transnasal drug delivery and convection-enhanced delivery (CED). Transnasal drug delivery can theoretically bypass the blood brain barrier and achieve drug levels in the CNS, although this method has largely failed when it has been studied in humans.[31,32] Another important method that may be successful in the future is convection-enhanced delivery (CED), where drug is delivered via catheters directly to the tumor site under a steady pressure.[33] This method permits better drug distribution than simple diffusion, and should distribute drug over much greater areas in a more

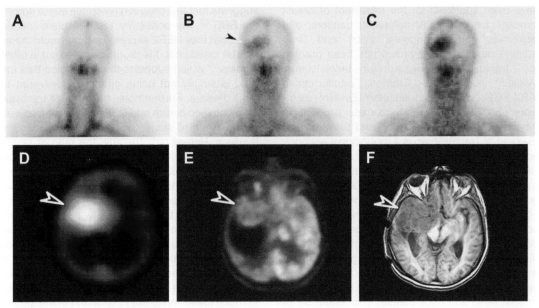

**Fig. 2.** Localization of a radiolabeled, tumor-specific monoclonal antibody against a CNS glioma. A monoclonal antibody, ch806, which recognizes a tumor-specific mutation in the epidermal growth factor receptor (EGFRvIII) was radiolabeled with Indium-111 and infused into a patient with an anaplastic astrocytoma. *A* to *C* all depict gamma camera images of the head, with *A* representing day 0 of infusion, *B* representing day 3, and *C* representing day 7 after infusion. Over time, increased radioactivity at the right temporal tumor site can be seen. *Black arrowhead* in *B* illustrates the first visualization of radiolabeled antibody at the tumor site. *D* is single-photon emission computed tomography (SPECT) imaging that demonstrates antibody uptake at the right temporal tumor site. *E* demonstrates tumor localization with $^{18}$F-fluorodeoxyglucose positron emission tomography (FDG-PET), and *F* is an axial MRI slice at the equivalent level that demonstrates that the right temporal tumor is in the same location as the antibody uptake. *White arrowheads* in *D* to *F* point to the tumor region. (*From* Scott AM, Lee FT, Tebbutt N, et al. A phase I clinical trial with monoclonal antibody ch806 targeting transitional state and mutant epidermal growth factor receptors. Proc Natl Acad Sci U S A 2007;104(10):4073; with permission.) Copyright © 2007, National Academy of Sciences, USA.

homogeneous fashion.[34] This method has been successfully used by our group and others in humans for targeted treatment of GBM.[35–37] Research is ongoing in all of these areas, and much more work still needs to be done to validate these various delivery techniques.

## TUMOR-RELATED IMMUNE SUPPRESSION

Tumors appear to be accompanied by immune suppression both locally and systemically. This is likely multifactorial in nature, and multiple immuno-suppressive molecules have been implicated in addition to the important role suggested by inhibitory cells of the immune system. For example, TGF-β, a cytokine secreted by many tumor cells appears to be an important component of this immunosuppression.[38] Fas ligand, a protein on the surface of many tumor cells that is capable of killing T cells directly, may also be important in inhibiting the immune response.[39] Many other molecules have also been implicated and may play important roles, including IL-10, prostaglandin

$E_2$, and NF-κB.[40,41] Regulatory T cells are a subset of CD4+ cells and generally function as inhibitory cells of the immune system.[14,42–44] They have been shown to be an increased fraction of lymphocyte counts in patients with GBMs,[45] and their depletion has been shown to improve antitumor responses.[41] Also, the inhibitory T-cell receptor CTLA-4 is likely involved, as it has been shown that blockade of this receptor improves antitumor immune response.[46] Tumors are also known to have immune evasion techniques, including decreased amount of antigen presentation molecules.[41] It will undoubtedly be critical to understand and overcome the immune suppression and evasion techniques in order to develop an effective immunotherapy.

## MONOCLONAL ANTIBODIES AS THERAPEUTICS

There have been numerous clinical trials verifying the passive administration of monoclonal antibodies as a viable treatment for cancer. Antibodies have been approved for the treatment of breast cancers, lung cancers, colorectal cancers, and leukemias and lymphomas. Food and Drug Administration (FDA) approval has been granted for trastuzumab (Herceptin), bevacizumab (Avastin), cetuximab (Erbitux), panitumumab (ABX-EGF), ibritumomab tiuxetan (Zevalin), alemtuzumab (Campath), gemtuzumab ozogamicin (Mylotarg), rituximab (Rituxan), and tositumomab (Bexxar).[40] Trastuzumab is a monoclonal antibody against the HER2 receptor and is approved for HER2-positive breast cancer. Bevacizumab is a monoclonal antibody against vascular endothelial growth factor and is approved for the treatment of non–small-cell lung cancer, breast cancer, colorectal cancer, and very recently recurrent GBM. Cetuximab and panitumumab are both directed against the epidermal growth factor receptor, and both are approved for colorectal cancer, whereas cetuximab also has approval against head and neck cancer. The remainder of the listed antibodies are directed against cell surface antigens and are approved for the treatment of leukemias and lymphomas.

Bevacizumab has also demonstrated efficacy against metastatic renal cancer[47] and in combination with irinotecan, it has shown efficacy against recurrent GBM.[48] The mechanism of this synergistic effect may be due to slowing tumor growth by slowing angiogenesis, or it possibly may allow for improved delivery of chemotherapy to the tumor by normalizing tumor vasculature. Further studies with bevacizumab against GBM are ongoing, and it recently obtained approval for treatment of recurrent GBM. Interestingly, bevacizumab has also demonstrated efficacy against pituitary adenomas in a mouse model,[49] and newer antibodies that block vascular endothelial growth factor in both humans and mice have also been developed.[50]

Trastuzumab has become an important component of HER2-positive breast cancer therapy,[51] and because of the high prevalence of metastases to the CNS in this disease, there have been a number of studies with data related to the CNS. It has been shown that patients with HER2-overexpressing breast cancer have a greater risk of developing CNS metastases than other breast cancer patients.[52,53] There is also an increased incidence of CNS metastases in those HER2-positive patients who are undergoing treatment with trastuzumab, but because of the improved control of extracranial disease, there is still improved survival of these patients when compared with unselected breast cancer patients.[53–56] Another study showed that despite a survival benefit from trastuzumab therapy, there was no delay in onset of CNS metastases, which

suggests that this drug is having little effect across the BBB.[57] The possibility that the brain metastases lost their HER2 expression (and would therefore be resistant to the drug) was ruled out in other studies,[58] which supports the conclusion that the drug is simply not being effectively delivered to CNS disease. Furthermore, the ratio of trastuzumab between serum and CSF has been measured during different stages of treatment and disease burdens. Before radiotherapy, the ratio of serum to CSF was 420:1, but this improves to 76:1 after radiotherapy, and after radiotherapy with meningeal carcinomatosis this ratio is 49:1.[59] Other authors have reported in a patient with meningeal carcinomatosis that this ratio was 300:1,[60] but others have also reported on possible treatment benefits of trastuzumab for meningeal carcinomatosis despite these ratios.[61] In summary, it appears that large monoclonal antibodies like trastuzumab are able to penetrate the CNS, but at much lower levels than that found in the serum. In the case of breast cancer, it is important to emphasize that radiation weakens the BBB and improves serum to CSF ratios of trastuzumab. Because radiation has become part of the standard therapy for GBM, its effect may decrease the role of the BBB for that disease as well.

## TUMOR-ASSOCIATED AND TUMOR-SPECIFIC ANTIGENS

One way to direct the immune system against tumors is to target it against individual antigens that are expressed by tumor cells. A possible concern with this approach is that by focusing the immune attack toward one antigen, there may be tumor cells that escape immune destruction if those cells lack or down-regulate that specific antigen. The strength of this concern depends on the importance of that specific antigen for tumorigenesis. In general, tumor antigens can be described as being either tumor-associated or tumor-specific antigens. Tumor-associated antigens are normal antigens found throughout the body but are overexpressed in tumor cells. Tumor-specific antigens are novel antigens found only on tumor cells. These specific antigens arise from gene mutations or splice variations.

Other important antigens include viral antigens that are expressed when a virus is implicated in the tumor. Examples of these antigens are the products of human papillomavirus in cervical cancer specimens,[62] antigens from Epstein-Barr virus in Burkitt's lymphoma or nasopharyngeal carcinoma specimens,[63] and possibly even antigens from *Cytomegalovirus* in GBM.[64]

Tumor-associated antigens comprise most tumor antigens targeted by immunotherapy strategies to date, and have been described in a variety of different cancers. They can be classified based on how they are presented by HLA molecules.[10] Class I-restricted tumor antigens are presented to CD8[+] T cells, and include melanoma-melanocyte differentiation antigens such as gp100,[65] MART-1,[66] and tyrosinase,[67] cancer-testes antigens such as MAGE[68-71] and NY-ESO-1,[72,73] and also MUC-1[74] and HER2/Neu.[75] Class II-restricted tumor-associated antigens, which can overlap with some Class I-restricted antigens, are recognized by CD4[+] T cells and include non-mutated protein epitopes such as gp100,[76] MAGE-3,[77] and NY-ESO-1.[78]

Although tumor-associated antigens can be used as targets for immunotherapy, it may be more difficult to provoke an immune response against a normally expressed antigen owing to preexisting immunologic tolerance to that antigen. Furthermore, any response that is generated could also have increased toxicity by the response being unintentionally directed against normal tissues. Because normal cells also express the same antigens, there may be an increased risk of autoimmune attack on normal tissue.[79,80]

Tumor-specific antigens are not expressed on normal cells and are therefore ideal targets for vaccines. The lack of expression of these antigens on normal cells allows for a focused immune response. Because this response should not be diluted by systemic antigen expression, it may be possible to achieve a stronger response across the BBB and it is hoped that systemic toxicity will be more limited. Unfortunately, many tumor-specific antigens are inconsistent and patient-specific, making them difficult to characterize and target.

One tumor-specific antigen, EGFRvIII, is consistently expressed in a wide range of malignant cancers, including approximately 40% of GBMs,[81] and it therefore has been the subject of much recent immunotherapy research. EGFRvIII is a truncated form of EGFR, resulting from an 801 base pair in-frame deletion that produces a fusion junction with a novel glycine (**Fig. 3**).[82,83]

Vaccination against EGFRvIII has shown promising results in preclinical studies. Preclinical studies performed in vitro and in vivo in a mouse tumor model demonstrated inhibition of tumor growth with passive administration of the EGFR-vIII-specific antibodies and improved long-term survival after cessation of antibody administration.[84] A DC-based vaccine derived from a peptide fragment of EGFRvIII that spans the novel glycine junction peptide fragment of EGFRvIII (PEPvIII) was subsequently developed. When injected intraperitoneally, this vaccine was efficacious against murine intracerebral tumors and greatly increased the median survival of treated mice.[85] Not only did most vaccinated mice survive without evidence of

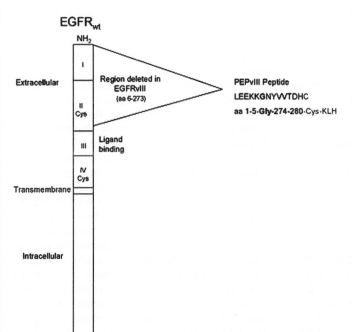

**Fig. 3.** Depiction of wild-type EGFR and the formation of EGFRvIII. Drawing illustrates the 801 base pair region that is deleted to form EGFRvIII. The inframe deletion occurs in the extracellular portion of the protein, and at the fusion site a novel glycine amino acid codon is created. The peptide used for vaccination studies, PEPvIII, is the 13 amino acid sequence that spans across this fusion region, which contains a tumor-specific epitope including the novel glycine, and is linked to a terminal cysteine, which permits conjugation of the peptide to the adjuvant KLH molecule. (*Reprinted from* Sampson JH, Archer GE, Mitchell DA, et al. Tumor-specific immunotherapy targeting the EGFRvIII mutation in patients with malignant glioma. Semin Immunol 2008;20(5):268; with permission.)

tumor recurrence, they also survived a repeat challenge of tumor inoculation, suggesting the development of long-term immune memory as well. Clinical trials with this promising vaccine are reviewed in detail in the following section.

## PEPTIDE VACCINATION TRIALS

Although few peptide vaccination studies have been performed in primary brain tumors; many more have been performed for systemic cancers, like melanoma, that often have CNS metastases. One important clinical trial involved a synthetic peptide vaccine developed from the melanoma-melanocyte differentiation antigen gp100 that was given to patients with metastatic melanoma both with and without IL-2 adminstration.[86] This trial tested vaccination of both the naturally occurring melanoma antigen gp209-217 and a synthetic peptide, called gp209-2 M, which is a modified form of this antigen that possesses a greater binding affinity to HLA-A2. Both peptides were administered subcutaneously in incomplete Freund's adjuvant (IFA) with and without intravenous IL-2 administration. Treatments before study enrollment for these patients included surgery, chemotherapy, radiation, and immunotherapy with IL-2, and 82% of study patients had received two or more of these therapies. Objective cancer regression was seen in 1 (11%) of 9 patients who received g209-217 in IFA, 0 (0%) of 11 patients who received g209-2 M in IFA, 5 (42%) of 12 patients who received g209-217 in IFA with IL-2, and 8 (42%) of 19 patients who received g209-2 M in IFA with IL-2. For comparison, previous trials of IL-2 alone in 134 melanoma patients showed a 17% response rate.[87] This study proved both that it was possible to generate an antitumor response against a self-antigen and that the combination of the cytokine IL-2 with vaccination improves clinical regression rates when compared with either vaccine or IL-2 alone. Additionally Rosenberg and colleagues state,[86] "objective regression was seen of metastases in the brain, lung, liver, lymph nodes, muscle, skin and subcutaneous tissues." This important trial showed the highest published clinical response rate of any peptide vaccination trial for melanoma to date.[88] Other peptide vaccination trials in melanoma have reported response rates ranging from 0% to 28% using multiple different peptides derived from the tumor-associated antigens gp100, MAGE-1, MAGE-3, tyrosinase, and NY-ESO-1 and administered in various adjuvants, including IFA, IL-12, and granulocyte-macrophage colony-stimulating factor (GM-CSF).[89–95]

In 2004, Rosenberg and colleagues[96] reviewed multiple cancer vaccine trials in various metastatic cancers. According to their review of National Cancer Institute (NCI) trials that involved peptide vaccines against metastatic melanoma,[94,97–99] prostate,[100,101] breast,[101] cervical,[102] and colorectal cancer[103] along with peptide vaccines against multiple cancers,[95,104,105] they calculated a total of 7 (4%) objective responses, all in melanoma trials, out of 175 patients. This can be separated into a 7.8% response rate in melanoma peptide vaccine trials (7 of 90 patients) and 0% response rate in all other peptide vaccine trials (0 of 85 patients). Rosenberg and colleagues[96] criticized the conclusions of these individual studies, stating that their results were overly optimistic, as they relied on surrogate, subjective end points rather than using standard tumor response criteria, which should involve objective measurements of lesions.[106,107] After calculating the adjusted overall numbers, that review criticized cancer vaccine strategies in general owing to their poor results in clinical trials so far, and suggested that immunosuppressive mechanisms such as regulatory T cells may be playing a significant role.[96] Although standard chemotherapy or radiation should deplete the inhibitory regulatory T cells, at the same time it would also cause systemic lymphodepletion, thereby depleting the effector cells needed to mount a tumoricidal immune response. To eliminate the immunosuppressive cells while maintaining immune cells that can mount an effective antitumor response, Rosenberg and colleagues[96] suggest that cell transfer therapies may be a more successful immunotherapy strategy. In this approach, systemic lymphodepletion can be performed before infusion of the activated cells.

Despite the difficulty with successful translation of active vaccination strategies to the clinic, the pessimism expressed by Rosenberg and colleagues[96] appears to be somewhat misleading. As previously expressed elsewhere,[108,109] many of the earlier vaccination "failures" used different response criteria that, if translated into RECIST (response evaluation criteria in solid tumors) criteria, may actually appear to have improved results. Additionally, treatment in the neo-adjuvant or adjuvant setting may show more treatment efficacy, and previous vaccine studies have used patients who were already heavily pretreated with chemotherapy, which selects for resistant and aggressive tumors and therefore biases the results toward failure. These authors who have previously responded to these criticisms suggest that future studies may be more successful if more immunogenic tumor antigens are selected, if only patients with minimal burden of disease are treated, or if the vaccines are studied on only specific subsets of patients with particular HLA haplotypes or other immunologic variables.[108,109] Furthermore, although the results of cell transfer therapy to date have been encouraging, there has yet to be a significant study that conclusively demonstrates that this form of treatment will extend survival. Additionally, the cost and effort required for this cellular therapy that is personalized to each patient will likely prevent this approach from ever becoming widespread.

The recent experience of an overwhelming immune response to a peptide vaccine against the amyloid-β protein in Alzheimer's disease demonstrates that peptide vaccination has the ability to affect the CNS environment.[14] Amyloid-β protein is known to be involved in Alzheimer's disease, although its full role in the disease process has not been completely determined.[110] When antibodies against this protein were passively administered to a mouse model of Alzheimer's disease, clearance of the protein in the CNS occurred and the mice were symptomatically improved.[111,112] Additionally, after intraperitoneal injection of the antibody, staining was able to conclusively demonstrate that it was present within the CNS.[112]

Multiple theories have been proposed to explain how an antibody could cause clearance of Aβ plaques in the CNS. These theories suggest that either antibodies cross the BBB and directly dissolve the plaques,[113] or they cross and directly bind to the plaques, which leads to phagocytosis by microglia.[111,112] A third theory suggests that the antibody actually causes clearance of Aβ plaques near the periphery of the CNS, increasing plasma concentration of Aβ, which leads to deeper clearance via diffusion of Aβ owing to the resultant concentration gradient.[114] Which of these is the predominant mechanism of action has not been conclusively determined.

When a vaccine targeting this protein was attempted in human clinical trials, antibodies were successfully induced against the Aβ protein. However, levels of antibody titers in serum were not associated with symptom severity and 6% of patients in the trial developed meningoencephalitis, so the trial was stopped early.[115,116] Analysis of these patients suggests that the Aβ removal was secondary to antibody binding, while the meningoencephalitis was likely caused by a cell-mediated immune response.[117] After death, autopsy of some vaccine trial patients revealed large areas of cortex lacking plaques and decreased average numbers of amyloid plaques when compared with age matched nonimmunized controls,

although there was no evidence of a difference in survival or time to progression (TTP) to dementia.[118] It is important to note that the small study size would have made it extremely difficult to see a difference in clinical end points. Additionally, these studies revealed that microglia was associated with Aβ antibodies, suggesting that they may be involved in clearance of these plaques.[117]

## EPIDERMAL GROWTH FACTOR RECEPTOR VARIANT III VACCINE TRIALS

Despite the largely unimpressive results of earlier peptide vaccine trials, there have been much more encouraging data coming from our ongoing vaccine studies targeting the tumor-specific antigen, EGFRvIII. As opposed to earlier peptide vaccine trials that targeted tumor-associated antigens, these ongoing studies with the EGFRvIII vaccine may be benefited by the lack of self-tolerance to this tumor-specific antigen. Clinical testing of vaccination against the tumor-specific antigen EGFRvIII began in a Phase I trial (VICTORI) conducted at Duke University Medical Center (Principal Investigator [PI]: John H. Sampson), and continued in a Phase II multicenter trial (ACTIVATE) conducted at Duke (PI: John H. Sampson) and University of Texas, M.D. Anderson Cancer Center (PI: Amy B. Heimberger).[119] The Phase I trial, VICTORI, enrolled 20 patients with World Health Organization (WHO) grade III or IV malignant gliomas, and 16 of these patients were administered vaccine. Production of this vaccine involved autologous dendritic cells pulsed with PEPvIII conjugated to the adjuvant molecule keyhole limpet cyanin (KLH). The DC-based vaccine was delivered via intradermal injection 2 weeks following the end of radiation therapy. Patients in the trial developed both B-cell and T-cell immunity against PEPvIII and EGFRvIII, and the only adverse events that occurred were NCI Common Toxicity Criteria grade I and II local reactions at the injection site. The median survival after histologic diagnosis in the 12 patients with GBM who were treated was 22.8 months, which is significantly longer than both the published median survival of 13.9 months for carmustine wafer treatment,[120] and 14.6 months for temozolomide therapy.[2]

To eliminate the prohibitive cost and variability associated with DC-based vaccine production, the subsequent Phase II trial involved vaccination directly with PEPvIII-KLH and GM-CSF without the use of DCs. This change was supported by preclinical results that showed a 26% increase in median survival in mice receiving just one vaccination of PEPvIII-KLH in incomplete Freund's adjuvant and GM-CSF.[121] This Phase II trial entitled, ACTIVATE, enrolled patients with newly diagnosed GBM (WHO grade IV) and used the same timing of initial vaccine delivery as in VICTORI. However, unlike VICTORI, patients in ACTIVATE subsequently received monthly vaccines until evidence of tumor progression. The 18 eligible patients had a median progression-free survival (PFS) of 14.2 months (n = 18) in vaccinated patients compared with median PFS of 6.3 months (n = 17) in historical matched unvaccinated patients (gross total resection without progression during radiation, EGFRvIII+). The vaccinated cohort not only compared favorably with the unvaccinated cohort, but also with concurrent temozolomide and radiation followed by adjuvant temozolomide, which reports a median TTP of 6.9 months. Additionally, 100% of the recurrent tumors in the vaccinated cohort showed loss of EGFRvIII expression, suggesting both effective immunologic activation and elimination of EGFR-vIII+ tumor cells as well as a possible mechanism of treatment failure.[122] The results of the phase II trial confirmed that with these vaccinations, patients developed powerful immune responses against the vaccinating peptide, PEPvIII, and the native protein, EGFRvIII.[123]

A follow-up phase II multicenter trial enrolled 21 patients with newly diagnosed, EGFRvIII+ GBM and treated them with monthly PEPvIII-KLH intradermal vaccinations with concurrent monthly temozolomide on either a 5-day (200 mg/m$^2$) or 21-day (100 mg/m$^2$) regimen following standard surgical resection and combined radiation and temozolomide. The results showed a median PFS of 16.6 months in the patients who received vaccine and concurrent temozolomide, which compared favorably against the median PFS of 14.3 months in a historical matched control group ($P<.0001$) and the median PFS of 15.2 months in a subgroup treated with temozolomide alone ($P = .0078$).[124] The results from these trials are very encouraging and suggest that vaccination with PEPvIII-KLH can be efficacious in those patients with newly diagnosed GBM whose tumors express the EGFRvIII antigen. These promising results are currently awaiting confirmation in an ongoing phase III study.

## SUMMARY

So far, the only immune-based treatment against tumors that has made it to standard clinical practice with FDA approval is the passive administration of monoclonal antibodies. As described previously, antibodies have been demonstrated

to cross the BBB, and antibody infusions have demonstrated efficacy in treating solid tumors (trastuzumab, cetuximab, bevacizumab); however, cellular infusions and vaccination strategies have both produced encouraging results. Previous attempts at peptide vaccination for Alzheimer's disease have shown that peptide vaccination has the ability to not only provoke an immune response across the BBB but that this response can rise to clinically significant levels.

The extent to which antibody versus cell-mediated responses are necessary to eliminate tumors has not been completely determined. As discussed previously, both responses were generated in our experience with the EGFRvIII vaccine and also with the amyloid-β peptide vaccine against Alzheimer's disease. The antibodies that are targeted to tumor-specific antigens that these vaccines produced may have been very important in combating disease. Because there are a number of monoclonal antibodies clinically approved by the FDA for passive administration that have shown efficacy against solid tumors, this suggests that T-cell mediated killing may not be absolutely necessary against tumors. Furthermore, all standard preventative vaccines to prevent infectious disease produce antibody responses. It is difficult to extrapolate from those vaccines, however, as they are prophylactic and therefore are given before disease exposure, with the sole exception of the rabies vaccine. It is likely that some component of both humoral and cell-mediated responses will be necessary to obtain sustained tumor eradication, but the evidence is mounting in support of the important role played by antibodies in this process.

Because it can be difficult to control an immune response once it has begun, one possible avenue to prevent the immunotherapy from causing overwhelming systemic toxicity is to focus it toward a tumor-specific antigen, such as EGFR-vIII, where the cross-reactivity with normal cellular antigens should be minimized. The lack of systemic cross-reactivity also may increase the fraction of antibody that penetrates the BBB. Our initial promising results with peptide vaccination against EGFRvIII are being confirmed in ongoing studies. It is hoped that this treatment will become a significant advance in the treatment of GBM patients.

GBM is a devastating disease and although standard treatment is able to prolong survival, there is an urgent need to find new, more effective therapies. Immunotherapy may provide a solution to this problem. Although passive antibody administration is certainly the most successful immune strategy against existing solid tumors to date, peptide vaccination has also been able to elicit significant antitumor responses, via both B-cell and T-cell mediated pathways. The results of ongoing clinical studies will help to clarify the predominant mechanism through which these effects are mediated, and will conclusively determine the magnitude of treatment effect that can be achieved with this treatment approach.

## REFERENCES

1. CBTRUS. CBTRUS statistical report: primary brain and central nervous system tumors diagnosed in the United States in 2000–2004. Hinsdale (IL): Central Brain Tumor Registry of the United States; 2008. Available at: http://www.cbtrus.org.
2. Stupp R, Mason WP, van den Bent MJ, et al. Radiotherapy plus concomitant and adjuvant temozolomide for glioblastoma. N Engl J Med 2005; 352(10):987–96.
3. Mocellin S, Mandruzzato S, Bronte V, et al. Part I: vaccines for solid tumours. Lancet Oncol 2004; 5(11):681–9.
4. Pejawar-Gaddy S, Finn OJ. Cancer vaccines: accomplishments and challenges. Crit Rev Oncol Hematol 2008;67(2):93–102.
5. Rosenberg SA, Lotze MT, Muul LM, et al. Observations on the systemic administration of autologous lymphokine-activated killer cells and recombinant interleukin-2 to patients with metastatic cancer. N Engl J Med 1985;313(23):1485–92.
6. Rosenberg SA, Yang JC, White DE, et al. Durability of complete responses in patients with metastatic cancer treated with high-dose interleukin-2: identification of the antigens mediating response. Ann Surg 1998;228(3):307–19.
7. Fyfe G, Fisher RI, Rosenberg SA, et al. Results of treatment of 255 patients with metastatic renal cell carcinoma who received high-dose recombinant interleukin-2 therapy. J Clin Oncol 1995;13(3):688–96.
8. Atkins MB, Lotze MT, Dutcher JP, et al. High-dose recombinant interleukin 2 therapy for patients with metastatic melanoma: analysis of 270 patients treated between 1985 and 1993. J Clin Oncol 1999;17(7):2105–16.
9. Rosenberg SA. Shedding light on immunotherapy for cancer. N Engl J Med 2004;350(14):1461–3.
10. Rosenberg SA. Progress in human tumour immunology and immunotherapy. Nature 2001; 411(6835):380–4.
11. Janeway CA, Travers P, Walport M, et al, editors. Immunobiology: the immune system in health and disease. 6th edition. New York: Garland Science Publishing; 2005. p. 169–202.
12. Sehgal A, Berger MS. Basic concepts of immunology and neuroimmunology. Neurosurg Focus 2000;9(6):e1.
13. Medawar PB. Immunity to homologous grafted skin: the fate of skin homografts transplanted to the brain, to subcutaneous tissue, and to the anterior chamber of the eye. Br J Exp Pathol 1948; 29(1):58–69.
14. Mitchell DA, Fecci PE, Sampson JH. Immunotherapy of malignant brain tumors. Immunol Rev 2008;222:70–100.
15. Gehrmann J, Matsumoto Y, Kreutzberg GW. Microglia: intrinsic immuneffector cell of the brain. Brain Res Brain Res Rev 1995;20(3):269–87.
16. Cserr HF, Harling-Berg CJ, Knopf PM. Drainage of brain extracellular fluid into blood and deep cervical lymph and its immunological significance. Brain Pathol 1992;2(4):269–76.
17. Zalutsky MR, Moseley RP, Coakham HB, et al. Pharmacokinetics and tumor localization of 131I-labeled anti-tenascin monoclonal antibody 81C6 in patients with gliomas and other intracranial malignancies. Cancer Res 1989;49(10):2807–13.
18. Scott AM, Lee FT, Tebbutt N, et al. A phase I clinical trial with monoclonal antibody ch806 targeting transitional state and mutant epidermal growth factor receptors. Proc Natl Acad Sci U S A 2007; 104(10):4071–6.
19. Perera RM, Zoncu R, Johns TG, et al. Internalization, intracellular trafficking, and biodistribution of monoclonal antibody 806: a novel anti-epidermal growth factor receptor antibody. Neoplasia 2007; 9(12):1099–110.
20. Dalmau J, Rosenfeld MR. Paraneoplastic syndromes of the CNS. Lancet Neurol 2008;7(4):327–40.
21. Sansing LH, Tuzun E, Ko MW, et al. A patient with encephalitis associated with NMDA receptor antibodies. Nat Clin Pract Neurol 2007;3(5):291–6.
22. Bataller L, Dalmau J. Paraneoplastic neurologic syndromes. Neurol Clin 2003;21(1):221–47, ix.
23. Dalmau J, Bataller L. Clinical and immunological diversity of limbic encephalitis: a model for paraneoplastic neurologic disorders. Hematol Oncol Clin North Am 2006;20(6):1319–35.
24. Rosenfeld MR, Dalmau J. The clinical spectrum and pathogenesis of paraneoplastic disorders of the central nervous system. Hematol Oncol Clin North Am 2001;15(6):1109–28, vii.
25. Dalmau J. Limbic encephalitis and variants related to neuronal cell membrane autoantigens. Rinsho Shinkeigaku 2008;48(11):871–4.
26. Tuzun E, Dalmau J. Limbic encephalitis and variants: classification, diagnosis and treatment. Neurologist 2007;13(5):261–71.
27. Rosenfeld MR, Dalmau J. Current therapies for paraneoplastic neurologic syndromes. Curr Treat Options Neurol 2003;5(1):69–77.
28. Bataller L, Dalmau J. Paraneoplastic neurologic syndromes: approaches to diagnosis and treatment. Semin Neurol 2003;23(2):215–24.

29. Engelhardt B, Ransohoff RM. The ins and outs of T-lymphocyte trafficking to the CNS: anatomical sites and molecular mechanisms. Trends Immunol 2005;26(9):485–95.

30. Wekerle H, Sun D, Oropeza-Wekerle RL, et al. Immune reactivity in the nervous system: modulation of T-lymphocyte activation by glial cells. J Exp Biol 1987;132:43–57.

31. van den Berg MP, Merkus P, Romeijn SG, et al. Uptake of melatonin into the cerebrospinal fluid after nasal and intravenous delivery: studies in rats and comparison with a human study. Pharm Res 2004;21(5):799–802.

32. Merkus P, Guchelaar HJ, Bosch DA, et al. Direct access of drugs to the human brain after intranasal drug administration? Neurology 2003;60(10): 1669–71.

33. Bobo RH, Laske DW, Akbasak A, et al. Convection-enhanced delivery of macromolecules in the brain. Proc Natl Acad Sci U S A 1994;91(6):2076–80.

34. Morrison PF, Laske DW, Bobo H, et al. High-flow microinfusion: tissue penetration and pharmacodynamics. Am J Physiol 1994;266(1 Pt 2):R292–305.

35. Sampson JH, Reardon DA, Friedman AH, et al. Sustained radiographic and clinical response in patient with bifrontal recurrent glioblastoma multiforme with intracerebral infusion of the recombinant targeted toxin TP-38: case study. Neuro Oncol 2005;7(1):90–6.

36. Vogelbaum MA, Sampson JH, Kunwar S, et al. Convection-enhanced delivery of cintredekin besudotox (interleukin-13-PE38QQR) followed by radiation therapy with and without temozolomide in newly diagnosed malignant gliomas: phase 1 study of final safety results. Neurosurgery 2007;61(5): 1031–7 [discussion: 1037–8].

37. Rand RW, Kreitman RJ, Patronas N, et al. Intratumoral administration of recombinant circularly permuted interleukin-4-Pseudomonas exotoxin in patients with high-grade glioma. Clin Cancer Res 2000;6(6):2157–65.

38. Teicher BA. Transforming growth factor-beta and the immune response to malignant disease. Clin Cancer Res 2007;13(21):6247–51.

39. Houston A, Bennett MW, O'Sullivan GC, et al. Fas ligand mediates immune privilege and not inflammation in human colon cancer, irrespective of TGF-beta expression. Br J Cancer 2003;89(7): 1345–51.

40. Finn OJ. Cancer immunology. N Engl J Med 2008; 358(25):2704–15.

41. Rabinovich GA, Gabrilovich D, Sotomayor EM. Immunosuppressive strategies that are mediated by tumor cells. Annu Rev Immunol 2007;25:267–96.

42. Shevach EM, McHugh RS, Piccirillo CA, et al. Control of T-cell activation by CD4+ CD25+ suppressor T cells. Immunol Rev 2001;182:58–67.

43. Hori S, Takahashi T, Sakaguchi S. Control of autoimmunity by naturally arising regulatory CD4+ T cells. Adv Immunol 2003;81:331–71.

44. Sakaguchi S, Sakaguchi N, Asano M, et al. Immunologic self-tolerance maintained by activated T cells expressing IL-2 receptor alpha-chains (CD25). Breakdown of a single mechanism of self-tolerance causes various autoimmune diseases. J Immunol 1995;155(3):1151–64.

45. Fecci PE, Mitchell DA, Whitesides JF, et al. Increased regulatory T-cell fraction amidst a diminished CD4 compartment explains cellular immune defects in patients with malignant glioma. Cancer Res 2006;66(6):3294–302.

46. Davila E, Kennedy R, Celis E. Generation of antitumor immunity by cytotoxic T lymphocyte epitope peptide vaccination, CpG-oligodeoxynucleotide adjuvant, and CTLA-4 blockade. Cancer Res 2003;63(12):3281–8.

47. Yang JC, Haworth L, Sherry RM, et al. A randomized trial of bevacizumab, an anti-vascular endothelial growth factor antibody, for metastatic renal cancer. N Engl J Med 2003;349(5):427–34.

48. Vredenburgh JJ, Desjardins A, Herndon JE 2nd, et al. Bevacizumab plus irinotecan in recurrent glioblastoma multiforme. J Clin Oncol 2007;25(30): 4722–9.

49. Korsisaari N, Ross J, Wu X, et al. Blocking vascular endothelial growth factor-A inhibits the growth of pituitary adenomas and lowers serum prolactin level in a mouse model of multiple endocrine neoplasia type 1. Clin Cancer Res 2008;14(1): 249–58.

50. Fuh G, Wu P, Liang WC, et al. Structure-function studies of two synthetic anti-vascular endothelial growth factor Fabs and comparison with the Avastin Fab. J Biol Chem 2006;281(10):6625–31.

51. Slamon DJ, Leyland-Jones B, Shak S, et al. Use of chemotherapy plus a monoclonal antibody against HER2 for metastatic breast cancer that overexpresses HER2. N Engl J Med 2001;344(11): 783–92.

52. Pestalozzi BC, Zahrieh D, Price KN, et al. Identifying breast cancer patients at risk for Central Nervous System (CNS) metastases in trials of the International Breast Cancer Study Group (IBCSG). Ann Oncol 2006;17(6):935–44.

53. Stemmler HJ, Heinemann V. Central nervous system metastases in HER-2-overexpressing metastatic breast cancer: a treatment challenge. Oncologist 2008;13(7):739–50.

54. Lin NU, Winer EP. Brain metastases: the HER2 paradigm. Clin Cancer Res 2007;13(6):1648–55.

55. Bartsch R, Rottenfusser A, Wenzel C, et al. Trastuzumab prolongs overall survival in patients with brain metastases from Her2 positive breast cancer. J Neurooncol 2007;85(3):311–7.

56. Gori S, Rimondini S, De Angelis V, et al. Central nervous system metastases in HER-2 positive metastatic breast cancer patients treated with trastuzumab: incidence, survival, and risk factors. Oncologist 2007;12(7):766–73.

57. Burstein HJ, Lieberman G, Slamon DJ, et al. Isolated central nervous system metastases in patients with HER2-overexpressing advanced breast cancer treated with first-line trastuzumab-based therapy. Ann Oncol 2005;16(11):1772–7.

58. Fuchs IB, Loebbecke M, Buhler H, et al. HER2 in brain metastases: issues of concordance, survival, and treatment. J Clin Oncol 2002;20(19):4130–3.

59. Stemmler HJ, Schmitt M, Willems A, et al. Ratio of trastuzumab levels in serum and cerebrospinal fluid is altered in HER2-positive breast cancer patients with brain metastases and impairment of blood-brain barrier. Anticancer Drugs 2007;18(1):23–8.

60. Pestalozzi BC, Brignoli S. Trastuzumab in CSF. J Clin Oncol 2000;18(11):2349–51.

61. Baculi RH, Suki S, Nisbett J, et al. Meningeal carcinomatosis from breast carcinoma responsive to trastuzumab. J Clin Oncol 2001;19(13):3297–8.

62. zur Hausen H. Human papillomaviruses in the pathogenesis of anogenital cancer. Virology 1991;184(1):9–13.

63. Hislop AD, Taylor GS, Sauce D, et al. Cellular responses to viral infection in humans: lessons from Epstein-Barr virus. Annu Rev Immunol 2007;25:587–617.

64. Mitchell DA, Xie W, Schmittling R, et al. Sensitive detection of human cytomegalovirus in tumors and peripheral blood of patients diagnosed with glioblastoma. Neuro Oncol 2008;10(1):10–8.

65. Kawakami Y, Eliyahu S, Delgado CH, et al. Identification of a human melanoma antigen recognized by tumor-infiltrating lymphocytes associated with in vivo tumor rejection. Proc Natl Acad Sci U S A 1994;91(14):6458–62.

66. Kawakami Y, Eliyahu S, Delgado CH, et al. Cloning of the gene coding for a shared human melanoma antigen recognized by autologous T cells infiltrating into tumor. Proc Natl Acad Sci U S A 1994;91(9):3515–9.

67. Brichard V, Van Pel A, Wolfel T, et al. The tyrosinase gene codes for an antigen recognized by autologous cytolytic T lymphocytes on HLA-A2 melanomas. J Exp Med 1993;178(2):489–95.

68. van der Bruggen P, Traversari C, Chomez P, et al. A gene encoding an antigen recognized by cytolytic T lymphocytes on a human melanoma. Science 1991;254(5038):1643–7.

69. Visseren MJ, van der Burg SH, van der Voort EI, et al. Identification of HLA-A*0201-restricted CTL epitopes encoded by the tumor-specific MAGE-2 gene product. Int J Cancer 1997;73(1):125–30.

70. Gaugler B, Van den Eynde B, van der Bruggen P, et al. Human gene MAGE-3 codes for an antigen recognized on a melanoma by autologous cytolytic T lymphocytes. J Exp Med 1994;179(3):921–30.

71. Panelli MC, Bettinotti MP, Lally K, et al. A tumor-infiltrating lymphocyte from a melanoma metastasis with decreased expression of melanoma differentiation antigens recognizes MAGE-12. J Immunol 2000;164(8):4382–92.

72. Jager E, Chen YT, Drijfhout JW, et al. Simultaneous humoral and cellular immune response against cancer-testis antigen NY-ESO-1: definition of human histocompatibility leukocyte antigen (HLA)-A2-binding peptide epitopes. J Exp Med 1998;187(2):265–70.

73. Wang RF, Johnston SL, Zeng G, et al. A breast and melanoma-shared tumor antigen: T cell responses to antigenic peptides translated from different open reading frames. J Immunol 1998;161(7):3598–606.

74. Jerome KR, Barnd DL, Bendt KM, et al. Cytotoxic T-lymphocytes derived from patients with breast adenocarcinoma recognize an epitope present on the protein core of a mucin molecule preferentially expressed by malignant cells. Cancer Res 1991;51(11):2908–16.

75. Ioannides CG, Fisk B, Fan D, et al. Cytotoxic T cells isolated from ovarian malignant ascites recognize a peptide derived from the HER-2/neu proto-oncogene. Cell Immunol 1993;151(1):225–34.

76. Li K, Adibzadeh M, Halder T, et al. Tumour-specific MHC-class-II-restricted responses after in vitro sensitization to synthetic peptides corresponding to gp100 and Annexin II eluted from melanoma cells. Cancer Immunol Immunother 1998;47(1):32–8.

77. Chaux P, Vantomme V, Stroobant V, et al. Identification of MAGE-3 epitopes presented by HLA-DR molecules to CD4(+) T lymphocytes. J Exp Med 1999;189(5):767–78.

78. Zeng G, Touloukian CE, Wang X, et al. Identification of CD4+ T cell epitopes from NY-ESO-1 presented by HLA-DR molecules. J Immunol 2000;165(2):1153–9.

79. Gilboa E. The promise of cancer vaccines. Nat Rev Cancer 2004;4(5):401–11.

80. Gilboa E. The makings of a tumor rejection antigen. Immunity 1999;11(3):263–70.

81. Moscatello DK, Holgado-Madruga M, Godwin AK, et al. Frequent expression of a mutant epidermal growth factor receptor in multiple human tumors. Cancer Res 1995;55(23):5536–9.

82. Libermann TA, Nusbaum HR, Razon N, et al. Amplification, enhanced expression and possible rearrangement of EGF receptor gene in primary human brain tumours of glial origin. Nature 1985;313(5998):144–7.

83. Bigner SH, Humphrey PA, Wong AJ, et al. Characterization of the epidermal growth factor receptor in

human glioma cell lines and xenografts. Cancer Res 1990;50(24):8017–22.

84. Sampson JH, Crotty LE, Lee S, et al. Unarmed, tumor-specific monoclonal antibody effectively treats brain tumors. Proc Natl Acad Sci U S A 2000;97(13):7503–8.

85. Heimberger AB, Archer GE, Crotty LE, et al. Dendritic cells pulsed with a tumor-specific peptide induce long-lasting immunity and are effective against murine intracerebral melanoma. Neurosurgery 2002;50(1):158–64 [discussion: 164].

86. Rosenberg SA, Yang JC, Schwartzentruber DJ, et al. Immunologic and therapeutic evaluation of a synthetic peptide vaccine for the treatment of patients with metastatic melanoma. Nat Med 1998;4(3):321–7.

87. Rosenberg SA, Yang JC, Topalian SL, et al. Treatment of 283 consecutive patients with metastatic melanoma or renal cell cancer using high-dose bolus interleukin 2. JAMA 1994;271(12):907–13.

88. Parmiani G, Castelli C, Dalerba P, et al. Cancer immunotherapy with peptide-based vaccines: what have we achieved? Where are we going? J Natl Cancer Inst 2002;94(11):805–18.

89. Cormier JN, Salgaller ML, Prevette T, et al. Enhancement of cellular immunity in melanoma patients immunized with a peptide from MART-1/Melan A. Cancer J Sci Am 1997;3(1):37–44.

90. Rosenberg SA, Yang JC, Schwartzentruber DJ, et al. Impact of cytokine administration on the generation of antitumor reactivity in patients with metastatic melanoma receiving a peptide vaccine. J Immunol 1999;163(3):1690–5.

91. Wang F, Bade E, Kuniyoshi C, et al. Phase I trial of a MART-1 peptide vaccine with incomplete Freund's adjuvant for resected high-risk melanoma. Clin Cancer Res 1999;5(10):2756–65.

92. Lee P, Wang F, Kuniyoshi J, et al. Effects of interleukin-12 on the immune response to a multipeptide vaccine for resected metastatic melanoma. J Clin Oncol 2001;19(18):3836–47.

93. Marchand M, van Baren N, Weynants P, et al. Tumor regressions observed in patients with metastatic melanoma treated with an antigenic peptide encoded by gene MAGE-3 and presented by HLA-A1. Int J Cancer 1999;80(2):219–30.

94. Scheibenbogen C, Schmittel A, Keilholz U, et al. Phase 2 trial of vaccination with tyrosinase peptides and granulocyte-macrophage colony-stimulating factor in patients with metastatic melanoma. J Immunother 2000;23(2):275–81.

95. Jager E, Gnjatic S, Nagata Y, et al. Induction of primary NY-ESO-1 immunity: CD8+ T lymphocyte and antibody responses in peptide-vaccinated patients with NY-ESO-1+ cancers. Proc Natl Acad Sci U S A 2000;97(22):12198–203.

96. Rosenberg SA, Yang JC, Restifo NP. Cancer immunotherapy: moving beyond current vaccines. Nat Med 2004;10(9):909–15.

97. Slingluff CL Jr, Petroni GR, Yamshchikov GV, et al. Clinical and immunologic results of a randomized phase II trial of vaccination using four melanoma peptides either administered in granulocyte-macrophage colony-stimulating factor in adjuvant or pulsed on dendritic cells. J Clin Oncol 2003;21(21):4016–26.

98. Cebon J, Jager E, Shackleton MJ, et al. Two phase I studies of low dose recombinant human IL-12 with Melan-A and influenza peptides in subjects with advanced malignant melanoma. Cancer Immun 2003;3:7.

99. Peterson AC, Harlin H, Gajewski TF. Immunization with Melan-A peptide-pulsed peripheral blood mononuclear cells plus recombinant human interleukin-12 induces clinical activity and T-cell responses in advanced melanoma. J Clin Oncol 2003;21(12):2342–8.

100. Noguchi M, Kobayashi K, Suetsugu N, et al. Induction of cellular and humoral immune responses to tumor cells and peptides in HLA-A24 positive hormone-refractory prostate cancer patients by peptide vaccination. Prostate 2003;57(1):80–92.

101. Vonderheide RH, Domchek SM, Schultze JL, et al. Vaccination of cancer patients against telomerase induces functional antitumor CD8+ T lymphocytes. Clin Cancer Res 2004;10(3):828–39.

102. van Driel WJ, Ressing ME, Kenter GG, et al. Vaccination with HPV16 peptides of patients with advanced cervical carcinoma: clinical evaluation of a phase I-II trial. Eur J Cancer 1999;35(6):946–52.

103. Sato Y, Maeda Y, Shomura H, et al. A phase I trial of cytotoxic T-lymphocyte precursor-oriented peptide vaccines for colorectal carcinoma patients. Br J Cancer 2004;90(7):1334–42.

104. Khleif SN, Abrams SI, Hamilton JM, et al. A phase I vaccine trial with peptides reflecting ras oncogene mutations of solid tumors. J Immunother 1999;22(2):155–65.

105. Tanaka S, Harada M, Mine T, et al. Peptide vaccination for patients with melanoma and other types of cancer based on pre-existing peptide-specific cytotoxic T-lymphocyte precursors in the periphery. J Immunother 2003;26(4):357–66.

106. Therasse P, Arbuck SG, Eisenhauer EA, et al. New guidelines to evaluate the response to treatment in solid tumors. European Organization for Research and Treatment of Cancer, National Cancer Institute of the United States, National Cancer Institute of Canada. J Natl Cancer Inst 2000;92(3):205–16.

107. James K, Eisenhauer E, Christian M, et al. Measuring response in solid tumors: unidimensional versus bidimensional measurement. J Natl Cancer Inst 1999;91(6):523–8.

108. Mocellin S, Mandruzzato S, Bronte V, et al. Cancer vaccines: pessimism in check. Nat Med 2004; 10(12):1278–9 [author reply: 1279–80].

109. Timmerman JM, Levy R. Cancer vaccines: pessimism in check. Nat Med 2004;10(12):1279 [author reply: 1279–80].

110. Wisniewski T, Konietzko U. Amyloid-beta immunisation for Alzheimer's disease. Lancet Neurol 2008;7(9):805–11.

111. Bacskai BJ, Kajdasz ST, Christie RH, et al. Imaging of amyloid-beta deposits in brains of living mice permits direct observation of clearance of plaques with immunotherapy. Nat Med 2001;7(3):369–72.

112. Bard F, Cannon C, Barbour R, et al. Peripherally administered antibodies against amyloid beta-peptide enter the central nervous system and reduce pathology in a mouse model of Alzheimer disease. Nat Med 2000;6(8):916–9.

113. Solomon B, Koppel R, Frankel D, et al. Disaggregation of Alzheimer beta-amyloid by site-directed mAb. Proc Natl Acad Sci U S A 1997;94(8): 4109–12.

114. DeMattos RB, Bales KR, Cummins DJ, et al. Peripheral anti-A beta antibody alters CNS and plasma A beta clearance and decreases brain A beta burden in a mouse model of Alzheimer's disease. Proc Natl Acad Sci U S A 2001;98(15):8850–5.

115. Gilman S, Koller M, Black RS, et al. Clinical effects of Abeta immunization (AN1792) in patients with AD in an interrupted trial. Neurology 2005;64(9):1553–62.

116. Orgogozo JM, Gilman S, Dartigues JF, et al. Subacute meningoencephalitis in a subset of patients with AD after Abeta42 immunization. Neurology 2003;61(1):46–54.

117. Nicoll JA, Wilkinson D, Holmes C, et al. Neuropathology of human Alzheimer disease after immunization with amyloid-beta peptide: a case report. Nat Med 2003;9(4):448–52.

118. Holmes C, Boche D, Wilkinson D, et al. Long-term effects of Abeta42 immunisation in Alzheimer's disease: follow-up of a randomised, placebo-controlled phase I trial. Lancet 2008;372(9634): 216–23.

119. Sampson JH, Archer GE, Mitchell DA, et al. Tumor-specific immunotherapy targeting the EGFRvIII mutation in patients with malignant glioma. Semin Immunol 2008;20(5):267–75.

120. Westphal M, Hilt DC, Bortey E, et al. A phase 3 trial of local chemotherapy with biodegradable carmustine (BCNU) wafers (Gliadel wafers) in patients with primary malignant glioma. Neuro Oncol 2003;5(2):79–88.

121. Heimberger AB, Crotty LE, Archer GE, et al. Epidermal growth factor receptor VIII peptide vaccination is efficacious against established intracerebral tumors. Clin Cancer Res 2003;9(11): 4247–54.

122. Heimberger A, Hussain SF, Aldape K, et al. Tumor-specific peptide vaccination in newly-diagnosed patients with GBM. 2006 ASCO Annual Meeting Proceedings Part I. J Clin Oncol 2006;24(18S Suppl):2529.

123. Schmittling RJ, Archer GE, Mitchell DA, et al. Detection of humoral response in patients with glioblastoma receiving EGFRvIII-KLH vaccines. J Immunol Methods 2008;339(1):74–81.

124. Sampson JH, Archer GE, Bigner DD, et al. Effect of EGFRvIII-targeted vaccine (CDX-110) on immune response and TTP when given with simultaneous standard and continuous temozolomide in patients with GBM [abstract]. J Clin Oncol 2008;26(Suppl): 2011.

# Heat Shock Proteins in Glioblastomas

Isaac Yang, MD*, Shanna Fang, BS,
Andrew T. Parsa, MD, PhD

## KEYWORDS

- Immunotherapy • Major histocompatibility complex
- Antigens • T cell

Glioblastoma multiforme (GBM) is the most common primary central nervous system tumor, affecting as many as 17,000 patients every year just in the United States.[1] The prognosis for these malignant brain tumors is poor, with a median survival of 14 months and a 5-year survival rate below 2%. Development of novel treatments such as immunotherapy is essential to improving survival and quality of life for these patients.

## VACCINES AND IMMUNOTHERAPY

Advances in cancer immunology have led to the development of various therapies using tumor-specific T cells to generate antitumor activity. Current approaches to immunotherapy are based on the principle that tumor-specific antigens are capable of inducing cytotoxic T lymphocytes (CTLs) to specifically target the antigen-presenting cells (APCs).[2,3] Internalization of the antigens by APCs, such as dendritic cells or macrophages, results in their presentation by major histocompatibility complex (MHC) class I molecules, eliciting antigen-specific CTL responses.[4–6] Much attention has been given to enhancing APC activation, manipulating processing of tumor-specific antigens, and ultimately improving the specific killing of tumor cells while sparing normal tissue, an aspect especially important to preservation of normal brain tissue in treatment of gliomas.[7–9] To exploit the ability of the immune system to generate antitumor responses, vaccinations against cancer that have been developed to date, which range from use of purified peptides and antigens to whole tumor lysates or cells.

Active immunotherapy may also address some of the most challenging obstacles in cancer immunotherapy: the tumor's ability to escape immune detection or exertion of immunosuppressive mechanisms.[10] Endogenous heat shock proteins (HSPs) have been implicated in mediation of both adaptive and innate immunity, and there is a rising interest in the use of this safe and multifaceted HSP vaccine therapy as a promising treatment for human cancers, including GBM (**Fig. 1**).[11]

### Discovery of HSP

First discovered in flies, it was observed that environmental temperature increases led to the transient expression of specific proteins.[12] Other studies showed that these "heat shock proteins (HSPs)" were also stimulated by any environmental or pathologic insults or trauma that resulted in protein misfolding, including such conditions as hyperthermia, anoxia, glucose deprivation, oxidative damage, irradiation, infection, and inflammation.[13] Highly conserved, these abundant proteins are best known for their functions as molecular chaperones, playing important roles in the proper folding, assembly, transport of nascent peptides, and degradation of misfolded proteins. Under normal conditions, HSPs account for approximately 10% of proteins in the cell,[14] but exhibit as much as a threefold increase in expression levels in response to stressful cellular conditions to counteract abnormal protein folding and dysfunction.[14–16] There are five major classes of HSPs: Hsp60, Hsp70, Hsp90, Hsp100, and small HSPs.[17] In addition to these main HSPs that reside

Department of Neurological Surgery, University of California at San Francisco, 505 Parnassus Avenue, Room M779, Campus 0112, San Francisco, CA 94143, USA
* Corresponding author.
*E-mail address:* yangi@neurosurg.ucsf.edu (I. Yang).

Neurosurg Clin N Am 21 (2010) 111–123
doi:10.1016/j.nec.2009.09.002

neurosurgery.theclinics.com

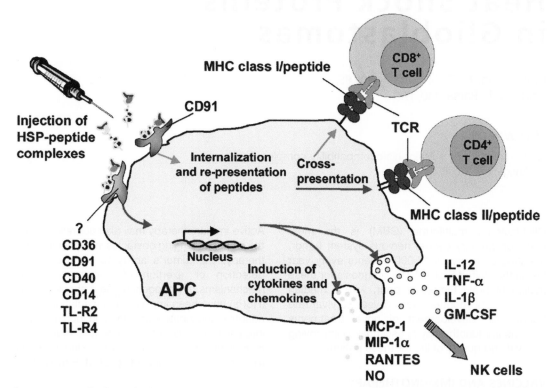

**Fig. 1.** Diagram for heat shock protein vaccine injection and postulated induced immune response and interactions with immune cells.

in the nucleus and cytosol, stress proteins include glucose[18–21] regulated proteins (Grp) that are found in the endoplasmic reticulum (ER).[22] This stress-inducible family of proteins (Grp78/BiP, grp94/96, and grp170) is induced by conditions effecting ER function, such as hyopoglycemia, hypoxia, heavy metals, and glycosylation and calcium homeostasis interference[23,24] and function to exert similar functions as HSPs. Although intracellular HSPs function to protect cells from death, extracellular and membrane-bound HSPs play important immunomodulatory functions.[17] Not all HSPs though have the ability to stimulate antigen-specific CTL immunity. Among stress proteins, Gp96, hsp90, hsp70, calreticulin, hsp110, and hsp170 appear to be among the most immunogenic stress proteins.[25,26]

### Role of HSP in GBM

The increasing interest in the use of immunogenic chaperone proteins in cancer has led to use of this vaccine for various cancers in immunotherapeutic clinical trials; however, the application of this therapy has not yet been widely explored for the treatment of brain tumors.

Some aspects of HSPs though have been characterized in human brain tumors.[11] Considering the stressful conditions of the glioma environment, such as hypoxia, high proliferation, increased levels of metabolism, and genetic instability, chaperone proteins have been found to be highly upregulated in brain tumor cells.[18–21] Tumor cell overexpression of HSPs may exploit the advantage of protection and homeostasis that is normally conferred by HSPs, and may permit cancer progression and therapeutic resistance of the cancerous tumor.[19] This abundance and overexpression of HSP and its functions in brain tumor cells may provide a possible therapeutic intervention to enhance targeted attacks against these tumor cells.

GBM is associated with a multitude of genetic mutations, the most frequent of which includes epidermal growth factor receptor (EGFR) amplification, PTEN deletion, inactivation of TP53, mdm2 overexpression, and loss of chromosomes 1p and 19q.[27–29] Many of these genes and proteins that play a role in glioma genesis have been found to interact with HSPs. HSPs are involved in the cellular proliferation, evasion of apoptosis, metastatic motility, invasion of normal issue, and angiogenesis associated with gliomas.[14,29] Although predominantly intracellular studies have begun to reveal that there are also cell surface expression and extracellular functions of HSPs in cancerous tumors.[18,30–33] Under stressful conditions, glial cells have been shown to release chaperone proteins, such as Hsp70, Hsp110, and Grp78.[18,31,34–36]

### Hsp90 interactions in GBM

Expression of Hsp90 protein seems to play an important role in mediating mechanisms that promote tumor survival and growth.[14,37,38] It has been identified to be an important chaperone protein associating with key oncogenic proteins, growth factor receptors, and cell cycle regulators in known brain tumor signaling pathways. Hsp90 has been found to form complexes with many chaperone clients known to play important roles in glioma formation, such as EGFR (vIII), PDGFR, FAK, AKT, hTERT, p53, cdk4, MAPK, PI3K, EF-2 kinase, HIF-1α, Akt, c-Src, Raf-1, Brc-Abl, and MMP 2.[14,29,31]

The main functions of Hsp90 are the binding of unstable tertiary protein structures, prevention of protein degradation, and antiapoptosis properties.[37–40] Normally functioning to stabilize proteins and transcription factors for cell growth, Hsp90 acts in cancer as a buffer to tolerate the effects and altered signals of malignant genetic alterations.[14,41,42] Hsp90 has two isoforms: the minor Hsp90β is expressed constitutively, whereas the expression of major Hsp90α is inducible.[38,43] Hsp90α protein and mRNA have been shown to be highly expressed in both glioma cells and in cancer tissue samples.[38]

### HSP interaction with EGFR mutations

The EGFR growth factor pathway is a strongly implicated molecular pathway in brain tumor pathogenesis; its mutations alter many factors that contribute to formation, maintenance, and progression of cancer. The most common genetic mutation found in GBM is the epidermal growth factor receptor (EGFRvIII), which results in the truncated form because of deletion mutations of exon 2-7.[44,45] The mutant form of EGFR is found in 40% to 50% of GBMs and has been associated with poorer prognosis of patients.[21,45–48] This mutation of EGFR receptor deletes the ligand binding region and subsequently results in constitutive expression of tyrosine kinase, leading to signaling alterations that promote malignant growth and survival.[49,50] Hsp90 associates with EGFRvIII by forming a complex along with proteins Cdc37 and p60/Hop to maintain elevated levels of EGFRvIII expression.[21] Hsp90 also directly interacts with c-Myc, a proto-oncogene highly expressed in high-grade gliomas, at its binding site on the Hsp90 promoter.[21,51] Like in other cancers, the Hsp90–c-Myc interaction is essential in mediating proliferation and promotion of malignant glioma cells survival, with a special role in the regulation of glioma stem cells.[51,52]

### HSP interactions with AKT

Another brain tumor relevant client protein of Hsp90α is Akt, a frequently hyperactivated downstream effector of phosphatidylinositol 3-kinase (PI3K) in the PTEN/PI3K/AKT pathway known to be aberrently upregulated in malignant gliomas.[29,53–55] In GBM, the common mutation of the AKT inhibitor, phosphatase, and tensin homolog deleted on chromosome 10 (PTEN) results in dysregulation of Akt and allows for downstream promotion of cell survival.[56–58] In addition to protection against apoptosis, activation of Akt is also known to be involved in immunoresistance of gliomas by upregulation of B7 homolog 1 (B7-H1) protein expression establishing Akt as a useful point for intervention.[59] Stabilization of the AKT protein kinase relies on interactions with Hsp90α to prevent protein degradation and to maintain its functions in tumor progression and cell survival.[37,53,60–63] Consistent with the essential stabilization of AKT by Hsp90α, the suppression of Hsp90α using SiRNA results in decreased expression of phosphorylated AKT in glioma cells.[37] Inhibition of Hsp90α disrupts its complex with AKT and results in proteosome-dependent degradation of Akt protein.[62] Suppression of the PI3K-AKT-mammalian target of rapamycin pathway not only downregulates antiapoptotic FLIP, it also decreases expression of the immunosuppressive B7-H1 protein making tumor cells more amenable to immunotherapeutic treatments.[59,64]

Recent studies may explain the antiapoptotic effects of Hsp90α in glioma cells that are especially resistant to apoptosis. Tumor necrosis factor-α related apoptosis inducing ligand (TRAIL) is a key apoptotic factor in gliomas and is shown to interact with the α form of Hsp90. In a recent study, Hsp90α was found to bind FLIP and subsequently regulate the sensitivity of TRAIL-induced apoptosis in gliomas through recruitment and localization of antiapoptotic protein, FLIP, rather than through alteration of FLIP stability.[37] The recruitment and stabilization of FLIP and other antiapoptotic molecules to the death-inducing signaling complex allows Hsp90α to regulate TRAIL resistance through an ATP-dependent N-terminal domain interaction.[37] Using SiRNA targeting Hsp90α, sensitization of previously resistant glioma cells rendered glioma cells vulnerable to apoptosis by TRAIL-dependent mechanisms.[37] The roles in cell cycle regulation and its ability to stabilize malignant characteristics suggest Hsp90 α may be a potential therapeutic target for brain tumors.[37,38]

### HSP role in glioma angiogenesis

Another tumor promoting function of Hsp90 is its involvement in cancer angiogenesis and malignant migration. Angiogenesis is important in cancer to sustain the growth of tumors because the highly proliferating tumors cells demand increased metabolism because of high proliferation states of tumor cells. Hsp90 binds and stabilizes hypoxia-inducible factor-1α (H1F1α), the major sensor of hypoxic conditions present in cancer cells.[14,39,65] In GBM, transcription factor H1F1α is highly overexpressed especially in the most invasive regions of the tumor, and also correlates with glioma tumor grades.[66–68] The hypoxic environment of GBM induces H1F1α to increase vascular endothelial growth factor stimulating nitric oxide synthase expression, resulting in proper signaling required for angiogenesis.[39,69] The treatment of glioma cells with an Hsp90 inhibitor in vitro results in the rapid proteolytic degradation of H1F1α and prevention of vascular endothelial growth factor induction.[69,70] The Hsp90 client protein, H1F1α, is also thought to contribute to malignant invasion and metastatic migration of gliomas. Interference of the Hsp90 and H1F1α interaction decreases the cellular migration of human glioma cells in culture by inhibition of focal adhesion kinase (FAK) phosphorylation.[67] These findings suggest the importance of Hsp90 in tumor angiogenesis and its therapeutic potential in mediating antiangiogenic mechanisms of GBM.

### Hsp90 inhibition

The instability of cancer signaling molecules resulting from disruption of HSP complexes using HSP inhibitors suggest that HSP-specific inhibitors could be used as therapeutic treatments or adjuvants.[31,62,71] Experiments using geldanamycin, an antibiotic inhibitor of Hsp90, demonstrated the widespread involvement of the HSP in many important tumor signaling pathways.[72] The anamycin antibiotics geldanamycin and 17-allyl-17-dimethoxygeldanamycin inhibit Hsp90 by binding to its ATP-binding domain so the treatment of cancer with Hsp90 inhibitors destabilize client proteins and causes their degradation.[55,73,74] In addition to decreasing stability of essential proteins, another mechanism of action of Hsp90 inhibitor may be the enhancement of complement-dependent cell lysis of cancer cells.[75]

17-Allyl-17-dimethoxygeldanamycin is the less hepatoxic geldanamycin analog that has recently been tested in phase I and II trials for metastatic melanoma, prostate, and breast cancer, renal cell carcinoma, leukemia, and other solid advanced cancers.[73,76–83] Combination treatments of 17-allyl-17-dimethoxygeldanamycin have been combined with chemotherapeutic agents, such as irinotecan, paclitaxel, and angiogenesis inhibitors, and have been shown to be promising in treating some cancers. Hsp90 inhibitors continue to be investigated as a potential therapeutic adjuvant.[14,79,83–85] Because Hsp90 interacts with client proteins that are highly dysregulated in the pathogenesis of GBM, such as EGFR, p53, AKT, HIF1α, and MMP2, Hsp90 inhibitors may provide a novel method for simultaneously targeting multiple aspects contributing to the rapid progression of GBM.

### Hsp70 interactions in GBM

Hsp70 is an important target for anticancer therapies because of its expression on the tumor cell surface, acting as a target for natural killer (NK) cells.[86] The CD94 lectin receptor on NK cell recognizes a specific 14 amino acid peptide of Hsp70 that is presented on the plasma membrane of tumor cells and initiates cell lysis.[87–89] Detection of the peptide causes NK cells to release cytotoxic lymphocyte product, granzyme B, which is subsequently taken up by tumor cells and rendering these Hsp70-positive tumor cells more vulnerable to cytolytic killing.[90] In addition to soluble chaperone Hsp70 that are known to be released by glial cells,[34] some tumor cells are also known to release detergent-soluble exosomes containing the membrane-bound Hsp70, which can stimulate the cytotoxic activities of NK cells.[17,90,91] These exosomes derived from Hsp70-positive tumor cells can also induce the specific migration of CD94-positive NK cells to target tumor cells.[90] The ability of these secreted exosomes to stimulate immune reactions of macrophages and dendritic cells is functionally effective in causing tumor reduction of autologous and allogeneic animal models bearing cancerous tumors.[92]

P53 is a crucial tumor suppressor protein normally functioning to regulate genomic damage and defects, abnormal oncogene activation, and hypoxic and metabolic stresses.[29,93,94] TP53 is a frequent genetic mutation in gliomas and is deleted or absent in approximately 40% of GBM.[95,96] Inactivated in almost all cancers, p53 deletion leads to the dysregulation of normal cellular growth cycle, angiogenesis, apoptosis, and oncogenic regulation, all of which are important processes that contribute to tumorigenesis.[94,97]

Interestingly, a major regulator of HSP is p53 and the loss of HSP promoter repression by p53 in cancer may contribute to the increased rates of HSP transcription in cancers.[39,98,99] Human

Hsp70 is normally transcriptionally repressed by p53 binding of transcription factors including NF-Y and (CCAATT binding factor) CBF.[39,98,100] Absence of p53 caused by TP53 mutations results in the lack of normal defenses against tumorigenesis, and studies have demonstrated that Hsp70 binds mutant p53 and accumulates abnormally in tumor cells of various cancers.[39,101–103]

One of the mechanisms by which Hsp70 may be exerting its antiapoptotic protection of cancer cells is stabilization of lysosomes. In human cancers, Hsp70 localizes to the plasma membrane of lysosomes and prevents permealization ultimately halting tumor necrosis factor–induced apoptosis.[104] Indeed, depletion of Hsp70 using antisense Hsp70 cDNA decreases survival of glioblastoma cells in vitro and induces caspase independent cell death. In vivo, its depletion results in tumor reduction and promotes survival of glioblastoma xenograft mice compared with control mice.[105] The variety of immunostimulatory and antiapoptotic capabilities of Hsp70 makes this chaperone protein a potent activator of the immune system and a potentially effective therapeutic target.

### Hsp27

A prognostic role has been suggested for antiapoptotic chaperone protein Hsp27, both in murine models and in human cancers.[106,107] Hsp27 is characterized as an apoptotic HSP that is associated with improved prognosis in esophageal squamous cell carcinoma and malignant fibrous histiocytomas, but decreased survival in prostate and gastric cancer for patients with high expression of Hsp27.[108–110] A recent study revealed that constitutional expression of Hsp27 in tumor cells did not correlate significantly with clinical outcome of patients with medulloblastoma.[107] In a large study of 198 human brain tumors, all glioblastomas were found to be intensely immunopositive for Hsp27.[20] Although increased expression levels of Hsp27 has been associated with higher-grade gliomas compared with their lower-grade counterpart, it is not shown to be prognostic and the Hsp27 expression level has not been found to be significantly increased in GBM patients undergoing radiation treatment.[19,20,111] The lack of prognostic correlation may be in part attributed to the high baseline overexpression of Hsp27 in GBM, in which further elevation may not contribute to the already present chemotherapy- and radiation-resistant phenotype of GBM.[30,101] In vitro experiments using GBM cell culture also did not reveal any protective effects of induced Hsp27.[19]

## HSP CANCER VACCINES
### Immunogenic Properties of HSP

Realization that cancer cells extracted from tumor provided immune protection in host mice on subsequent challenge prompted studies that revealed the importance of HSPs in the immune response. That mice were immunized against the specific cancers used for rechallenge, but not against other types of cancers they harbored, established the unique and individual-tumor specificity of cancer immunity.[112–114] To isolate the immunogenic component of tumors, cancer homogenates were fractionated by chromatographic techniques and represented to host animals testing for cancer rejection potential.[115] Molecules capable of immunizing animals were then purified by repeated fractionation until homogenous, and further identified to be proteins belonging to the heat shock family, such as Hsp90, Hsp70, Hsp110, Hsp170, calreticulin, and Gp96.[25,114–116] This surprising discovery revealed the immunogenic properties of these HSPs; however, the HSPs isolated from adjacent normal tissue or other tumors were unable to elicit the immune protection seen by its tumor-derived counterpart.[114]

### Origin of Immunogenicity

Attempts to explain the tumor specificity of cancer-derived HSP were not revealed by differences in DNA sequencing, structural variation, or somatic polymorphisms when compared with nontumor HSPs.[22] It was a series of experiments showing large groups of peptides to be associated with homogenous Gp96-HSP preparations that suggested peptide groups to be the immunogenic origins. The ability of HSP-protein complex to induce cellular immunity was later confirmed by loss of immune protection under peptide deprivation conditions.[114] Furthermore, the replenishment of peptide to HSP proteins reconstituted effective antitumor protection in host animals.[117] Interestingly, these peptides carried by other types of proteins, such as serum albumin, did not elicit CTL induction and failed to provide immunogenicity.[117] These studies confirmed that neither peptide nor HSP were immunogenic individually, but antigenic peptides chaperoned by HSPs could induce antigen-specific CD8+ T cell[117,118] in immunized animals.[119–121]

### HSP vaccine

Based on the properties of chaperone proteins to generate the desired specialized targeting of malignant cells, the idea of harnessing HSP immunogenicity led to the development of HSP-peptide complex cancer vaccines. Although HSP vaccines have been successfully developed for clinical trials of melanoma, sarcoma, colorectal, renal, and pancreatic cancer, and non-Hodgkin's lymphoma, there is currently a single clinical trial studying the use of HSP in malignant brain tumors.[122–125] This promising vaccine therapy uses heat shock peptide-complex to generate a combination of tumor-specific adaptive immunity but also induces the activation of innate immune mechanisms, maximizing antitumor activity. Oncophage (HSP-peptide complex-96; vitespen) vaccines are composed of Hsp96 (Gp96) complexed with the autologous tumor antigenic peptides.[126] The specificity of the vaccine against the tumor of origin is caused by the ability of chaperone proteins to form strong noncovalent bonds with the unique antigens of the individual tumor. An ongoing clinical trial is currently investigating the HSP-peptide complex-96 in the treatment of patients with recurrent or progressive high-grade gliomas, such as GBM, gliosarcoma, anaplastic gliomas, anaplastic astrocytoma, anaplastic oligo-dendroglioma, anaplastic infiltrating glioma, and mixed malignant glioma (http://clinicaltrials.gov/ct2/show/NCT00293423). The vaccine is derived from autologous tumor cells obtained from individual patients during standard intracranial surgical resection, generating immune responses only against the specific tumor from which it was derived.

### HSP polyvalent antigen interaction

By representing the broad range of tumor-associated antigen peptides characterizing individual cancers, the HSP vaccine provides a polyvalent method to improve targeting of tumors. The ability for the HSP-peptide complex vaccine to represent the wide antigenic fingerprint of gliomas makes this vaccine an individualized cancer therapy, conveniently circumventing the need to characterize specific antigens for a certain cancer type, especially in such cancers as GBM, in which these antigenic epitopes have not yet been sufficiently identified.[25,117,127,128] In addition, HSP peptide complexes encompass the entire antigenic repertoire, which can also overcome the common issue of immunoresistance and immune escape mechanisms by cancerous tumors.[14,127]

### Presentation on APCs

The Gp96-peptide complexes isolated and purified from patients' glioma samples are complexed with the specific variety of tumor-specific peptides making up the antigenic profile of the tumor. The ability of HSPs to chaperone these antigenic peptides confers the ability to elicit specific immunity against the origin of the peptides, within tumors and other malignancies. The specific mechanism by which HSP-peptide complexes accomplish immune induction is beginning to be understood through investigation of its interaction with APCs. To generate a successful immune response against tumor tissue, antigens must be processed and displayed by APCs on MHC class I molecules for induction and expansion of antigen-specific CD8+ T cells. The ability of tumor-derived HSP vaccination to elicit specific immunity against the origin of the antigenic peptides indicates that HSP-peptide complexes are involved in the antigen processing pathway. Depletion of both macrophages and APCs from host animals confirmed the dependence of HSP-peptide complex to induce immune protection on phagocytic mechanisms.[114,128] These studies also suggested the essential role of macrophages in transfer of antigenic material from chaperone proteins to APCs for MHC class I presentation, rather than a direct exchange of peptides between chaperone and APCs, to exert immune induction.[112]

## MORE EFFICIENT ANTIGEN PRESENTATION ON MHC

The high sensitivity of APCs to HSP-peptide complexes led to early suspicion of HSP-specific receptors on APCs that account for the efficient uptake of small quantities of HSP complexes.[129] Further evidence supporting indirect antigen is the finding that HSP-chaperoned peptides are significantly more efficient at loading antigens onto MHC class I molecules than that of free peptides and inducing recognition by CTLs.[112,130,131] There is now evidence that HSP-peptide complexes undergo internalization by macrophages through clathrin-coated receptor-mediated endocytic mechanisms, and some HSP-specific receptors have been identified on the surface of APCs.[132]

On injection of Oncophage into the host, the HSP-peptide complex is internalized by HSP-specific receptors, such as CD91 on APCs. The exogenous peptides complexed with chaperone proteins then undergo antigen processing through intracellular compartments of MHC class I and II molecules to be presented or re-expressed on the surface of APCs.[120,129,133] Activated APCs carrying antigenic peptides, including dendritic cells, macrophages, or Langerhans cells, exert their immunostimulatory effects by circulating systemically to be recognized by naive T cells in the lymph node of the host.[112,113,129] Naive T cells stimulated by recognition of these tumor-specific peptides expand into CD8+ and CD4+ T cells that exert specific immunity against the range of antigens present in the tumor. Both glioma relevant HSPs (Hsp70 and Hsp90) have been shown to play essential roles in the activation of CD8+ T cells by this process of representing tumor-specific antigens on surfaces of MHC class I molecules.[40]

## HSP Activation of Innate Immunity

In addition to eliciting adaptive immunity, this HSP vaccine also has the advantage of generating activation of innate immunity. Apart from its involvement in the antigen presentation pathway, the internalization of chaperone-peptide complexes results in the maturation and subsequent functional activation of APCs, defined by the expression of costimulatory molecules and cytokine activity.[134,135] Exposure to various HSPs causes differential expression of MHC class II and costimulatory molecules, such as CD80 (B7-1), CD86 (B7-2), and CD40, to be upregulated on the surface of APCs.[39,131] Interaction with Gp96 induces the surface expression MHC class II and B7-2, but not B7-1 on dendritic cells, whereas another HSP, Hsp70, induces upregulation of B7-1, but not MHC II and B7-2.[23,136,137]

The other consequence of the interaction between isolated HSP and APCs is the natural stimulation of cytokine release by macrophages and dendritic cells.[136] Important cytokines released by APCs on exposure to gp96, Hsp70, and Hsp 90 include interleukin-1b, -12, and -6; tumor necrosis factor-$\alpha$; granulocyte-macrophage colony–stimulating factor; chemokines, such as MCP-1, MIP-1, and RANTES; and nitric oxide.[23,25,138] In particular, it is thought that the cytokine interleukin-12 released from exposure to HSP may be responsible for expansion of NK cells[26] in vaccine-treated cancer patients. The presence of HSP itself, regardless of bound peptides, can stimulate release of these potent proinflammatory agents known to be important in antigen-specific immunity, serving as a convenient adjuvant for enhancing protective immunity.[23]

Specific interaction between HSP-peptide complex and APCs leads to induction of dendritic cell maturation, release of cytokines by both macrophages and DCs, and the stimulation of NK cells to enhance antitumor activity of T cells. NK cells are essential for innate immunity and the activation of these cells has been observed following immunization by tumor derived HSP-peptide complexes.[26,113] The multiple effects on APCs may be caused by the observation that exposure to Gp96 and Hsp70 causes translocation of NFkB into the nucleus of APC, a well conserved pathway for immunologic signal transduction.[26,39,135] Activation of NFkB through HSP influence mediates important downstream proteins that regulate the growth, progression, and antiapoptotic capabilities of cancer cells to enhance malignancy.[119,136] Acting in conjunction with the activation of antigen-specific CD8 T cell and CD4 T cells, important players in innate immunity are stimulated by the HSP-peptide complex vaccine.

## Limitations of an HSP Vaccine for GBM

The HSP-peptide complex vaccine requires the isolation of significant amounts of HSP-peptide complexes from the patient's tumor, which can be limited by the size of tumors extracted during standard surgical resection, even though the vaccine itself is relatively easy to produce.[23] Although this may not be an issue for cancers characterized by larger tumors, the significantly smaller tumor able to be resected from GBM patients sometimes limits the availability of HSP vaccine treatment as an option.[23,121,139] In addition to the quantity of HSPs and tumor sample, another level of challenge for patients to receive the potent immune vaccines is the purity criteria during processing necessary to generate the vaccine for patients to proceed with the treatment. Although the sample is processed as soon as possible after surgery, the time required to generate the vaccine may sometimes create difficulty especially in aggressive tumors that can progress rapidly and prevent use of this treatment modality.[139,140]

The polyvalent chaperoning capabilities of the HSP-peptide vaccine are advantageous and effective in treatment of cancers not yet sufficiently characterized antigenically, as in the case of GBM. The lack of characterization also results in less efficient immunomonitoring, however, which may assist in the further understanding and development of other targeted cancer strategies.[121] Concern for adverse autoimmune responses is countered by excellent safety profiles have been observed for all autologous HSP clinical trials. Patients report good quality of life and only occasional patients experience transient side effects, such as low-grade fever and mild local responses.[139,140] The ongoing clinical trial of the vaccine for patients with recurrent high-grade gliomas is rigorously assessing the safety, dosage, and efficacy of this vaccine for the treatment of these fatal brain tumors (http://clinicaltrials.gov/ct2/show/NCT00293423).

### Advantages of an HSP vaccine for GBM

The multifactorial effects of HSP vaccines seem to be a promising immunotherapeutic approach for treating malignant gliomas, which tend to have very high rates of recurrence even after standard modern treatment. The potential to efficiently chaperone potent antigenic peptides, activate APCs, and exert proinflammatory stimulation of NK cells are important properties of HSPs that allow the use of tumor-derived HSP-peptide complexes to maximize specific immunity against cancer cells. The unique ability to chaperone the wide range of a tumor's antigenic fingerprint is not only capable of stimulating potent specific immunity against this tumor but also activates innate immunity to aid targeting of the malignancy.

Although tumor-associated antigens are now being investigated and characterized in human cancers, most current immunotherapeutic treatments require identification of characteristic tumor antigens for respective cancers. Although tumor-associated antigens are continuing to be investigated in human gliomas, most specific glioma antigens remain to be sufficiently characterized. By representing the antigenic repertoire of glioma antigens from the particular tumor extracted from the patient, the HSP vaccine provides a strictly individualized treatment vaccine and also bypasses the usual difficulty of identifying a set of immunogenic antigens that characterize a certain cancer, such as GBM. In addition, the chaperoning of the entire antigenic fingerprint precludes the immune evasion and escape capabilities from single antigen therapies, issues faced especially by aggressive cancers like GBM. Because the variety of antigens chaperoned by the isolated HSPs include some self-antigens expected to be chaperoned in addition to the desired tumor antigens, the risk of autoimmunity from administration of the vaccine might be expected.[23] The occurrence of autoimmune reactions or serious side effects has not been observed, however, in any HSP-peptide vaccine patients to date.[139,141,142] The ability of these potent immunogenic properties of the HSP vaccine to efficiently elicit protective immunity against cancers, combined with the safety and success of clinical trials against other cancers, has established a promising and novel avenue of investigation for neuro-oncologists against malignant gliomas.

## REFERENCES

1. Greenlee RT, Murray T, Bolden S, et al. Cancer statistics, 2000. CA Cancer J Clin 2000;50(1):7–33.

2. Boudreau CR, Yang I, Liau LM. Gliomas: advances in molecular analysis and characterization. Surg Neurol 2005;64(4):286–94 [discussion: 294].

3. Yang I, Kremen TJ, Giovannone AJ, et al. Modulation of major histocompatibility complex class I molecules and major histocompatibility complex-bound immunogenic peptides induced by interferon-alpha and interferon-gamma treatment of human glioblastoma multiforme. J Neurosurg 2004;100(2):310–9.

4. Disis ML, Bernhard H, Jaffee EM. Use of tumour-responsive t cells as cancer treatment. Lancet 2009;373(9664):673–83.

5. Gajewski TF, Chesney J, Curriel TJ. Emerging strategies in regulatory t-cell immunotherapies. Clin Adv Hematol Oncol 2009;7(1):1–10 [quiz: 11–12].

6. Yamanaka R. Cell- and peptide-based immunotherapeutic approaches for glioma. Trends Mol Med 2008;14(5):228–35.

7. Das S, Raizer JJ, Muro K. Immunotherapeutic treatment strategies for primary brain tumors. Curr Treat Options Oncol 2008;9(1):32–40.

8. Luptrawan A, Liu G, Yu JS. Dendritic cell immunotherapy for malignant gliomas. Rev Recent Clin Trials 2008;3(1):10–21.

9. Mitchell DA, Fecci PE, Sampson JH. Immunotherapy of malignant brain tumors. Immunol Rev 2008;222:70–100.

10. Vega EA, Graner MW, Sampson JH. Combating immunosuppression in glioma. Future Oncol 2008;4(3):433–42.

11. Graner MW, Bigner DD. Therapeutic aspects of chaperones/heat-shock proteins in neuro-oncology. Expert Rev Anticancer Ther 2006;6(5):679–95.

12. Park HG, Han SI, Oh SY, et al. Cellular responses to mild heat stress. Cell Mol Life Sci 2005;62(1):10–23.

13. Young JC, Agashe VR, Siegers K, et al. Pathways of chaperone-mediated protein folding in the cytosol. Nat Rev Mol Cell Biol 2004;5(10):781–91.

14. Soo ET, Yip GW, Lwin ZM, et al. Heat shock proteins as novel therapeutic targets in cancer. In Vivo 2008;22(3):311–5.

15. Pockley AG. Heat shock proteins as regulators of the immune response. Lancet 2003;362(9382):469–76.

16. Voellmy R. Feedback regulation of the heat shock response. Handb Exp Pharmacol 2006;172:43–68.

17. Schmitt E, Gehrmann M, Brunet M, et al. Intracellular and extracellular functions of heat shock proteins: repercussions in cancer therapy. J Leukoc Biol 2007;81(1):15–27.

18. Graner MW, Cumming RI, Bigner DD. The heat shock response and chaperones/heat shock proteins in brain tumors: surface expression, release, and possible immune consequences. J Neurosci 2007;27(42):11214–27.

19. Hermisson M, Strik H, Rieger J, et al. Expression and functional activity of heat shock proteins in human glioblastoma multiforme. Neurology 2000; 54(6):1357–65.

20. Hitotsumatsu T, Iwaki T, Fukui M, et al. Distinctive immunohistochemical profiles of small heat shock proteins (heat shock protein 27 and alpha b-crystallin) in human brain tumors. Cancer 1996;77(2): 352–61.

21. Shervington A, Cruickshanks N, Wright H, et al. Glioma: what is the role of c-myc, hsp90 and telomerase? Mol Cell Biochem 2006;283(1–2):1–9.

22. Srivastava PK. Peptide-binding heat shock proteins in the endoplasmic reticulum: role in immune response to cancer and in antigen presentation. Adv Cancer Res 1993;62:153–77.

23. Manjili MH, Wang XY, Park J, et al. Immunotherapy of cancer using heat shock proteins. Front Biosci 2002;7:d43–52.

24. Subjeck JR, Shyy TT. Stress protein systems of mammalian cells. Am J Physiol 1986;250(1 Pt 1): C1–17.

25. Binder RJ. Heat shock protein vaccines: from bench to bedside. Int Rev Immunol 2006;25(5–6): 353–75.

26. Srivastava PK, Amato RJ. Heat shock proteins: the Swiss Army Knife vaccines against cancers and infectious agents. Vaccine 2001;19(17–19):2590–7.

27. Burton EC, Lamborn KR, Forsyth P, et al. Aberrant p53, mdm2, and proliferation differ in glioblastomas from long-term compared with typical survivors. Clin Cancer Res 2002;8(1):180–7.

28. Hill C, Hunter SB, Brat DJ. Genetic markers in glioblastoma: prognostic significance and future therapeutic implications. Adv Anat Pathol 2003;10(4): 212–7.

29. Rich JN, Bigner DD. Development of novel targeted therapies in the treatment of malignant glioma. Nat Rev Drug Discov 2004;3(5):430–46.

30. Calderwood SK, Theriault JR, Gong J. Message in a bottle: role of the 70-kda heat shock protein family in anti-tumor immunity. Eur J Immunol 2005;35(9):2518–27.

31. Graner MW, Bigner DD. Chaperone proteins and brain tumors: potential targets and possible therapeutics. Neuro Oncol 2005;7(3):260–78.

32. Multhoff G, Hightower LE. Cell surface expression of heat shock proteins and the immune response. Cell Stress Chaperones 1996;1(3):167–76.

33. Shin BK, Wang H, Yim AM, et al. Global profiling of the cell surface proteome of cancer cells uncovers an abundance of proteins with chaperone function. J Biol Chem 2003;278(9):7607–16.

34. Guzhova I, Kislyakova K, Moskaliova O, et al. In vitro studies show that hsp70 can be released by glia and that exogenous hsp70 can enhance neuronal stress tolerance. Brain Res 2001;914(1–2):66–73.

35. Hightower LE, Guidon PT Jr. Selective release from cultured mammalian cells of heat-shock (stress) proteins that resemble glia-axon transfer proteins. J Cell Physiol 1989;138(2):257–66.

36. Tytell M, Greenberg SG, Lasek RJ. Heat shock-like protein is transferred from glia to axon. Brain Res 1986;363(1):161–4.

37. Panner A, Murray JC, Berger MS, et al. Heat shock protein 90alpha recruits flips to the death-inducing signaling complex and contributes to trail resistance in human glioma. Cancer Res 2007;67(19): 9482–9.

38. Shervington A, Cruickshanks N, Lea R, et al. Can the lack of hsp90alpha protein in brain normal tissue and cell lines, rationalise it as a possible therapeutic target for gliomas? Cancer Invest 2008;26(9):900–4.

39. Calderwood SK, Khaleque MA, Sawyer DB, et al. Heat shock proteins in cancer: chaperones of tumorigenesis. Trends Biochem Sci 2006;31(3): 164–72.

40. Tesniere A, Panaretakis T, Kepp O, et al. Molecular characteristics of immunogenic cancer cell death. Cell Death Differ 2008;15(1):3–12.

41. Rahmani M, Reese E, Dai Y, et al. Cotreatment with suberanoylanilide hydroxamic acid and 17-allylamino 17-demethoxygeldanamycin synergistically induces apoptosis in Bcr-Abl+ Cells sensitive and resistant to STI571 (imatinib mesylate) in association with down-regulation of Bcr-Abl, abrogation of signal transducer and activator of transcription 5 activity, and Bax conformational change. Mol Pharmacol 2005;67(4):1166–76.

42. Whitesell L, Lindquist SL. Hsp90 and the chaperoning of cancer. Nat Rev Cancer 2005;5(10): 761–72.

43. Hightower LE. Heat shock, stress proteins, chaperones, and proteotoxicity. Cell 1991;66(2):191–7.

44. Sugawa N, Ekstrand AJ, James CD, et al. Identical splicing of aberrant epidermal growth factor receptor transcripts from amplified rearranged genes in human glioblastomas. Proc Natl Acad Sci U S A 1990;87(21):8602–6.

45. Wong AJ, Ruppert JM, Bigner SH, et al. Structural alterations of the epidermal growth factor receptor gene in human gliomas. Proc Natl Acad Sci U S A 1992;89(7):2965–9.

46. Lavictoire SJ, Parolin DA, Klimowicz AC, et al. Interaction of hsp90 with the nascent form of the mutant epidermal growth factor receptor egfrviii. J Biol Chem 2003;278(7):5292–9.

47. Mischel PS, Shai R, Shi T, et al. Identification of molecular subtypes of glioblastoma by gene expression profiling. Oncogene 2003;22(15): 2361–73.

48. Wikstrand CJ, Hale LP, Batra SK, et al. Monoclonal antibodies against egfrviii are tumor specific and

react with breast and lung carcinomas and malignant gliomas. Cancer Res 1995;55(14):3140–8.

49. Frederick L, Wang XY, Eley G, et al. Diversity and frequency of epidermal growth factor receptor mutations in human glioblastomas. Cancer Res 2000;60(5):1383–7.

50. Gan HK, Kaye AH, Luwor RB. The egfrviii variant in glioblastoma multiforme. J Clin Neurosci 2009;16: 748–54.

51. Wang J, Wang H, Li Z, et al. C-myc is required for maintenance of glioma cancer stem cells. PLoS One 2008;3(11):e3769.

52. Soucek L, Whitfield J, Martins CP, et al. Modelling Myc inhibition as a cancer therapy. Nature 2008; 455(7213):679–83.

53. Basso AD, Solit DB, Chiosis G, et al. Akt forms an intracellular complex with heat shock protein 90 (Hsp90) and Cdc37 and is destabilized by inhibitors of Hsp90 function. J Biol Chem 2002;277(42): 39858–66.

54. Choe G, Horvath S, Cloughesy TF, et al. Analysis of the phosphatidylinositol 3'-kinase signaling pathway in glioblastoma patients in vivo. Cancer Res 2003;63(11):2742–6.

55. Georgakis GV, Li Y, Younes A. The heat shock protein 90 inhibitor 17-AAG induces cell cycle arrest and apoptosis in mantle cell lymphoma cell lines by depleting cyclin D1, Akt, Bid and activating caspase 9. Br J Haematol 2006; 135(1):68–71.

56. Maehama T, Dixon JE. PTEN: a tumour suppressor that functions as a phospholipid phosphatase. Trends Cell Biol 1999;9(4):125–8.

57. Muise-Helmericks RC, Grimes HL, Bellacosa A, et al. Cyclin D expression is controlled post-transcriptionally via a phosphatidylinositol 3-kinase/ akt-dependent pathway. J Biol Chem 1998; 273(45):29864–72.

58. Yu C, Rahmani M, Almenara J, et al. Induction of apoptosis in human leukemia cells by the tyrosine kinase inhibitor adaphostin proceeds through a raf-1/mek/erk- and akt-dependent process. Oncogene 2004;23(7):1364–76.

59. Parsa AT, Waldron JS, Panner A, et al. Loss of tumor suppressor PTEN function increases b7-h1 expression and immunoresistance in glioma. Nat Med 2007;13(1):84–8.

60. Fujita N, Sato S, Ishida A, et al. Involvement of hsp90 in signaling and stability of 3-phosphoinositide-dependent kinase-1. J Biol Chem 2002; 277(12):10346–53.

61. Neckers L. Heat shock protein 90: the cancer chaperone. J Biosci 2007;32(3):517–30.

62. Premkumar DR, Arnold B, Jane EP, et al. Synergistic interaction between 17-aag and phosphatidylinositol 3-kinase inhibition in human malignant glioma cells. Mol Carcinog 2006;45(1):47–59.

63. Sato S, Fujita N, Tsuruo T. Modulation of Akt kinase activity by binding to Hsp90. Proc Natl Acad Sci U S A 2000;97(20):10832–7.

64. Panner A, James CD, Berger MS, et al. Mtor controls flips translation and trail sensitivity in glioblastoma multiforme cells. Mol Cell Biol 2005; 25(20):8809–23.

65. Zhou J, Schmid T, Frank R, et al. Pi3k/akt is required for heat shock proteins to protect hypoxia-inducible factor 1alpha from pvhl-independent degradation. J Biol Chem 2004;279(14): 13506–13.

66. Semenza GL. Involvement of hypoxia-inducible factor 1 in human cancer. Intern Med 2002;41(2): 79–83.

67. Zagzag D, Nomura M, Friedlander DR, et al. Geldanamycin inhibits migration of glioma cells in vitro: a potential role for hypoxia-inducible factor (hif-1alpha) in glioma cell invasion. J Cell Physiol 2003;196(2):394–402.

68. Zagzag D, Zhong H, Scalzitti JM, et al. Expression of hypoxia-inducible factor 1alpha in brain tumors: association with angiogenesis, invasion, and progression. Cancer 2000;88(11):2606–18.

69. Sun J, Liao JK. Induction of angiogenesis by heat shock protein 90 mediated by protein kinase Akt and endothelial nitric oxide synthase. Arterioscler Thromb Vasc Biol 2004;24(12):2238–44.

70. Mabjeesh NJ, Post DE, Willard MT, et al. Geldanamycin induces degradation of hypoxia-inducible factor 1alpha protein via the proteosome pathway in prostate cancer cells. Cancer Res 2002;62(9): 2478–82.

71. Prodromou C, Roe SM, O'brien R, et al. Identification and structural characterization of the ATP/ ADP-binding site in the hsp90 molecular chaperone. Cell 1997;90(1):65–75.

72. Neckers L, Neckers K. Heat-shock protein 90 inhibitors as novel cancer chemotherapeutic agents. Expert Opin Emerg Drugs 2002;7(2):277–88.

73. Sausville EA, Tomaszewski JE, Ivy P. Clinical development of 17-allylamino, 17-demethoxygeldanamycin. Curr Cancer Drug Targets 2003;3(5): 377–83.

74. Solit DB, Rosen N. Hsp90: a novel target for cancer therapy. Curr Top Med Chem 2006;6(11):1205–14.

75. Sreedhar AS, Nardai G, Csermely P. Enhancement of complement-induced cell lysis: a novel mechanism for the anticancer effects of hsp90 inhibitors. Immunol Lett 2004;92(1–2):157–61.

76. Blagosklonny MV, Fojo T, Bhalla KN, et al. The Hsp90 inhibitor geldanamycin selectively sensitizes Bcr-Abl-expressing leukemia cells to cytotoxic chemotherapy. Leukemia 2001;15(10):1537–43.

77. Heath EI, Hillman DW, Vaishampayan U, et al. A phase II trial of 17-allylamino-17-demethoxygeldanamycin in patients with hormone-refractory

metastatic prostate cancer. Clin Cancer Res 2008; 14(23):7940–6.

78. Neckers L. Heat shock protein 90 inhibition by 17-allylamino-17- demethoxygeldanamycin: a novel therapeutic approach for treating hormone-refractory prostate cancer. Clin Cancer Res 2002;8(5): 962–6.

79. Ramalingam SS, Egorin MJ, Ramanathan RK, et al. A phase I study of 17-allylamino-17-demethoxygeldanamycin combined with paclitaxel in patients with advanced solid malignancies. Clin Cancer Res 2008;14(11):3456–61.

80. Ramanathan RK, Trump DL, Eiseman JL, et al. Phase I pharmacokinetic-pharmacodynamic study of 17-(allylamino)-17-demethoxygeldanamycin (17AAG, NSC 330507), a novel inhibitor of heat shock protein 90, in patients with refractory advanced cancers. Clin Cancer Res 2005;11(9): 3385–91.

81. Ronnen EA, Kondagunta GV, Ishill N, et al. A phase II trial of 17-(allylamino)-17-demethoxygeldanamycin in patients with papillary and clear cell renal cell carcinoma. Invest New Drugs 2006;24(6):543–6.

82. Solit DB, Osman I, Polsky D, et al. Phase II trial of 17-allylamino-17-demethoxygeldanamycin in patients with metastatic melanoma. Clin Cancer Res 2008;14(24):8302–7.

83. Tse AN, Klimstra DS, Gonen M, et al. A phase 1 dose-escalation study of irinotecan in combination with 17-allylamino-17-demethoxygeldanamycin in patients with solid tumors. Clin Cancer Res 2008; 14(20):6704–11.

84. De Candia P, Solit DB, Giri D, et al. Angiogenesis impairment in id-deficient mice cooperates with an hsp90 inhibitor to completely suppress HER2/ neu-dependent breast tumors. Proc Natl Acad Sci U S A 2003;100(21):12337–42.

85. Modi S, Stopeck AT, Gordon MS, et al. Combination of trastuzumab and tanespimycin (17-aag, kos-953) is safe and active in trastuzumab-refractory her-2 overexpressing breast cancer: a phase I dose-escalation study. J Clin Oncol 2007;25(34):5410–7.

86. Multhoff G. Activation of natural killer cells by heat shock protein 70. Int J Hyperthermia 2002;18(6): 576–85.

87. Botzler C, Li G, Issels RD, et al. Definition of extracellular localized epitopes of hsp70 involved in an NK immune response. Cell Stress Chaperones 1998;3(1):6–11.

88. Gross C, Schmidt-Wolf IG, Nagaraj S, et al. Heat shock protein 70-reactivity is associated with increased cell surface density of CD94/CD56 on primary natural killer cells. Cell Stress Chaperones 2003;8(4):348–60.

89. Multhoff G, Pfister K, Gehrmann M, et al. A 14-mer hsp70 peptide stimulates natural killer (NK) cell activity. Cell Stress Chaperones 2001;6(4):337–44.

90. Gastpar R, Gehrmann M, Bausero MA, et al. Heat shock protein 70 surface-positive tumor exosomes stimulate migratory and cytolytic activity of natural killer cells. Cancer Res 2005;65(12):5238–47.

91. Lancaster GI, Febbraio MA. Exosome-dependent trafficking of hsp70: a novel secretory pathway for cellular stress proteins. J Biol Chem 2005; 280(24):23349–55.

92. Cho JA, Lee YS, Kim SH, et al. Mhc independent anti-tumor immune responses induced by hsp70-enriched exosomes generate tumor regression in murine models. Cancer Lett 2009;275(2):256–65.

93. Vogelstein B, Lane D, Levine AJ. Surfing the p53 network. Nature 2000;408(6810):307–10.

94. Whibley C, Pharoah PD, Hollstein M. P53 polymorphisms: cancer implications. Nat Rev Cancer 2009; 9(2):95–107.

95. Rasheed BK, Mclendon RE, Herndon JE, et al. Alterations of the tp53 gene in human gliomas. Cancer Res 1994;54(5):1324–30.

96. Watanabe K, Sato K, Biernat W, et al. Incidence and timing of p53 mutations during astrocytoma progression in patients with multiple biopsies. Clin Cancer Res 1997;3(4):523–30.

97. Vousden KH, Lane DP. P53 in health and disease. Nat Rev Mol Cell Biol 2007;8(4):275–83.

98. Agoff SN, Hou J, Linzer DI, et al. Regulation of the human hsp70 promoter by p53. Science 1993; 259(5091):84–7.

99. Wu G, Osada M, Guo Z, et al. Deltanp63alpha up-regulates the hsp70 gene in human cancer. Cancer Res 2005;65(3):758–66.

100. Taira T, Sawai M, Ikeda M, et al. Cell cycle-dependent switch of up-and down-regulation of human hsp70 gene expression by interaction between c-myc and CBF/NF-Y. J Biol Chem 1999;274(34): 24270–9.

101. Ciocca DR, Calderwood SK. Heat shock proteins in cancer: diagnostic, prognostic, predictive, and treatment implications. Cell Stress Chaperones 2005;10(2):86–103.

102. Lane DP, Midgley C, Hupp T. Tumour suppressor genes and molecular chaperones. Philos Trans R Soc Lond B Biol Sci 1993;339(1289):369–72 [discussion: 372–3].

103. Pinhasi-Kimhi O, Michalovitz D, Ben-Zeev A, et al. Specific interaction between the p53 cellular tumour antigen and major heat shock proteins. Nature 1986;320(6058):182–4.

104. Gyrd-Hansen M, Nylandsted J, Jaattela M. Heat shock protein 70 promotes cancer cell viability by safeguarding lysosomal integrity. Cell Cycle 2004; 3(12):1484–5.

105. Nylandsted J, Wick W, Hirt UA, et al. Eradication of glioblastoma, and breast and colon carcinoma xenografts by HSP70 depletion. Cancer Res 2002;62(24):7139–42.

106. Bausero MA, Page DT, Osinaga E, et al. Surface expression of HSP25 and HSP72 differentially regulates tumor growth and metastasis. Tumour Biol 2004;25(5–6):243–51.

107. Hauser P, Hanzely Z, Jakab Z, et al. Expression and prognostic examination of heat shock proteins (HSP 27, HSP 70, and HSP 90) in medulloblastoma. J Pediatr Hematol Oncol 2006;28(7):461–6.

108. Cornford PA, Dodson AR, Parsons KF, et al. Heat shock protein expression independently predicts clinical outcome in prostate cancer. Cancer Res 2000;60(24):7099–105.

109. Lo Muzio L, Leonardi R, Mariggio MA, et al. HSP 27 as possible prognostic factor in patients with oral squamous cell carcinoma. Histol Histopathol 2004;19(1):119–28.

110. Tetu B, Lacasse B, Bouchard HL, et al. Prognostic influence of HSP-27 expression in malignant fibrous histiocytoma: a clinicopathological and immunohistochemical study. Cancer Res 1992;52(8):2325–8.

111. Khalid H, Tsutsumi K, Yamashita H, et al. Expression of the small heat shock protein (HSP) 27 in human astrocytomas correlates with histologic grades and tumor growth fractions. Cell Mol Neurobiol 1995;15(2):257–68.

112. Suto R, Srivastava PK. A mechanism for the specific immunogenicity of heat shock protein-chaperoned peptides. Science 1995;269(5230):1585–8.

113. Tamura Y, Peng P, Liu K, et al. Immunotherapy of tumors with autologous tumor-derived heat shock protein preparations. Science 1997;278(5335):117–20.

114. Udono H, Srivastava PK. Comparison of tumor-specific immunogenicities of stress-induced proteins gp96, hsp90, and hsp70. J Immunol 1994;152(11):5398–403.

115. Srivastava PK, Deleo AB, Old LJ. Tumor rejection antigens of chemically induced sarcomas of inbred mice. Proc Natl Acad Sci U S A 1986;83(10):3407–11.

116. Srivastava PK, Menoret A, Basu S, et al. Heat shock proteins come of age: primitive functions acquire new roles in an adaptive world. Immunity 1998;8(6):657–65.

117. Blachere NE, Li Z, Chandawarkar RY, et al. Heat shock protein-peptide complexes, reconstituted in vitro, elicit peptide-specific cytotoxic T lymphocyte response and tumor immunity. J Exp Med 1997;186(8):1315–22.

118. Przepiorka D, Srivastava PK. Heat shock protein–peptide complexes as immunotherapy for human cancer. Mol Med Today 1998;4(11):478–84.

119. Castelli C, Rivoltini L, Rini F, et al. Heat shock proteins: biological functions and clinical application as personalized vaccines for human cancer. Cancer Immunol Immunother 2004;53(3):227–33.

120. Nicchitta CV, Carrick DM, Baker-Lepain JC. The messenger and the message: Gp96 (grp94)-peptide interactions in cellular immunity. Cell Stress Chaperones 2004;9(4):325–31.

121. Wang XY, Li Y, Yang G, et al. Current ideas about applications of heat shock proteins in vaccine design and immunotherapy. Int J Hyperthermia 2005;21(8):717–22.

122. Belli F, Testori A, Rivoltini L, et al. Vaccination of metastatic melanoma patients with autologous tumor-derived heat shock protein gp96-peptide complexes: clinical and immunologic findings. J Clin Oncol 2002;20(20):4169–80.

123. Li Z, Qiao Y, Liu B, et al. Combination of imatinib mesylate with autologous leukocyte-derived heat shock protein and chronic myelogenous leukemia. Clin Cancer Res 2005;11(12):4460–8.

124. Mazzaferro V, Coppa J, Carrabba MG, et al. Vaccination with autologous tumor-derived heat-shock protein gp96 after liver resection for metastatic colorectal cancer. Clin Cancer Res 2003;9(9):3235–45.

125. Younes A. A phase II study of heat shock protein-peptide complex-96 vaccine therapy in patients with indolent non-Hodgkin's lymphoma. Clin Lymphoma 2003;4(3):183–5.

126. Cancer vaccine–antigenics. BioDrugs 2002;16(1):72–4.

127. Srivastava P. Interaction of heat shock proteins with peptides and antigen presenting cells: chaperoning of the innate and adaptive immune responses. Annu Rev Immunol 2002;20:395–425.

128. Wang XY, Kaneko Y, Repasky E, et al. Heat shock proteins and cancer immunotherapy. Immunol Invest 2000;29(2):131–7.

129. Srivastava PK, Udono H, Blachere NE, et al. Heat shock proteins transfer peptides during antigen processing and CTL priming. Immunogenetics 1994;39(2):93–8.

130. Roigas J, Wallen ES, Loening SA, et al. Heat shock protein (HSP72) surface expression enhances the lysis of a human renal cell carcinoma by IL-2 stimulated NK cells. Adv Exp Med Biol 1998;451:225–9.

131. Binder RJ, Blachere NE, Srivastava PK. Heat shock protein-chaperoned peptides but not free peptides introduced into the cytosol are presented efficiently by major histocompatibility complex I molecules. J Biol Chem 2001;276(20):17163–71.

132. Arnold-Schild D, Hanau D, Spehner D, et al. Cutting edge: receptor-mediated endocytosis of heat shock proteins by professional antigen-presenting cells. J Immunol 1999;162(7):3757–60.

133. Nishikawa M, Takemoto S, Takakura Y. Heat shock protein derivatives for delivery of antigens to

antigen presenting cells. Int J Pharm 2008; 354(1–2):23–7.

134. Scheibel T, Weikl T, Buchner J. Two chaperone sites in hsp90 differing in substrate specificity and ATP dependence. Proc Natl Acad Sci U S A 1998;95(4):1495–9.

135. Strbo N, Podack ER. Secreted heat shock protein gp96-ig: an innovative vaccine approach. Am J Reprod Immunol 2008;59(5):407–16.

136. Basu S, Binder RJ, Suto R, et al. Necrotic but not apoptotic cell death releases heat shock proteins, which deliver a partial maturation signal to dendritic cells and activate the NF-kappa B pathway. Int Immunol 2000;12(11):1539–46.

137. Manjili MH, Wang XY, Park J, et al. Cancer immunotherapy: stress proteins and hyperthermia. Int J Hyperthermia 2002;18(6):506–20.

138. Wang HH, Mao CY, Teng LS, et al. Recent advances in heat shock protein-based cancer vaccines. Hepatobiliary Pancreat Dis Int 2006; 5(1):22–7.

139. Parmiani G, Testori A, Maio M, et al. Heat shock proteins and their use as anticancer vaccines. Clin Cancer Res 2004;10(24):8142–6.

140. Wood C, Srivastava P, Bukowski R, et al. An adjuvant autologous therapeutic vaccine (hsppc-96; vitespen) versus observation alone for patients at high risk of recurrence after nephrectomy for renal cell carcinoma: a multicentre, open-label, randomised phase III trial. Lancet 2008;372(9633): 145–54.

141. Janetzki S, Blachere NE, Srivastava PK. Generation of tumor-specific cytotoxic T lymphocytes and memory T cells by immunization with tumor-derived heat shock protein gp96. J Immunother 1998;21(4): 269–76.

142. Testori A, Richards J, Whitman E, et al. Phase III comparison of vitespen, an autologous tumor-derived heat shock protein gp96 peptide complex vaccine, with physician's choice of treatment for stage IV melanoma: the c-100-21 study group. J Clin Oncol 2008;26(6):955–62.

# The Role of Tregs in Glioma-Mediated Immunosuppression: Potential Target for Intervention

William Humphries, MD[a], Jun Wei, PhD[a],
John H. Sampson, MD, PhD, MHSc[b], Amy B. Heimberger, MD[a],*

**KEYWORDS**

- Regulatory T cells • Glioblastoma multiforme
- Central nervous system • Immunotherapy
- Vaccine • Prognosis

The function of the immune system is to recognize foreign materials in the body and distinguish them from normal body tissues and cells. Immune responses consist of cell-mediated (T cells, natural killer cells, and phagocytes) or humoral (B cells, antibodies, and complement) responses modified and regulated by cytokines. Antigen-presenting cells (APCs) such as dendritic cells (DCs) and macrophages take up antigens, partially degrade them, and present them to T cells in the context of major histocompatibility complex (MHC) molecules. To activate fully the adaptive immune response, the T cells must receive two signals: one through the T cell receptor and the other through the costimulatory receptor CD28, which recognizes the costimulatory molecules CD80 and CD86 expressed on the surface of APCs. Failure to do so will result in T cell anergy.[1] T cells have a number of functions, including potentiating cytotoxic T cell responses (CD4+ helper T cells [Th1 cells]), assisting B cells in the production of antibodies (CD4+ helper T cells [Th2 cells]), recognizing and destroying virally infected or tumor cells (CD8+ effector T cells), and limiting the level of reactivity in the immune system (CD4+ CD25+ [forkhead box P3+] Foxp3+ regulatory T cells [Tregs]).

Tregs are a physiologic subset of CD4+ T cells that curtail the function of T cells, B cells,[2,3] DCs,[4–6] monocytes or macrophages,[6] natural killer T cells,[7] and natural killer cells.[8,9] Tregs potently inhibit T cell cytokine secretion and proliferation by down-regulating interleukin (IL-2) and interferon-γ (IFN-γ) production[10–14]; increase Th2 cytokine skewing[15]; directly curtail the generation and expansion of endogenous or induced immune responses by suppressing proinflammatory cytokine production[16–24]; and, apparently, play a significant role in hindering immunity to tumor-associated antigens.[25,26] Furthermore, studies of murine models of immunogenic tumors have shown that adoptively transferred Tregs inhibit tumor-reactive effector T cells and that elimination of Tregs in vivo enhances antitumor immunity.[15]

---

This work was supported by The Dr Marnie Rose Foundation, the Anthony D. Bullock III Foundation, an institutional research grant from The University of Texas M. D. Anderson Cancer Center, and National Institutes of Health grants CA120813-01 and A177225-01 (to A.B.H.).
[a] Department of Neurosurgery, The University of Texas M. D. Anderson Cancer Center, 1515 Holcombe Boulevard, Houston, TX 77030, USA
[b] Division of Neurosurgery, Duke University Medical Center, 220 Sands Building, Box 3050, Durham, NC 27710, USA
* Corresponding author.
*E-mail address:* aheimber@mdanderson.org (A.B. Heimberger).

Neurosurg Clin N Am 21 (2010) 125–137
doi:10.1016/j.nec.2009.08.012
1042-3680/09/$ – see front matter © 2010 Elsevier Inc. All rights reserved.

More specifically, in murine tumor challenge models of established gliomas, in vivo depletion of Tregs has resulted in enhanced tumor rejection and increased median survival durations.[27–29]

Since the discovery of Tregs,[30] understanding of the types and functions of these cells has increased greatly. Tregs are classified into three subtypes based on their induction site, cytokine profile, and respective cell surface markers: natural Tregs (nTregs), Th3 cells, and Tr1 cells (**Fig. 1**).[31–34] nTregs (CD4+ CD25+ Foxp3+) are thymically derived, bind with intermediate affinity to the MHC/peptide complex, and are capable of recognizing both self-generated and foreign antigens. Upon their exportation to the periphery from the thymus, nTregs exert their effect on peripheral effector T cells primarily via cell-to-cell contact. Although the mechanism by which nTregs exert their effects on the effector T cells has yet to be fully elucidated,[31–34] it likely results from down-regulation of IL-2 cytokine production and may involve membrane-bound cytotoxic T lymphocyte antigen-4 (CTLA-4), a negative regulator of T cell activation, a member of the CD28 immunoglobulin superfamily that is constitutively expressed on Tregs,[35] and whose expression is up-regulated in activated T cells.[36,37] The development of nTregs is regulated by the Foxp3 gene in CD4+ CD25+ T cells.[38] The primary role of nTregs is suspected to be maintenance of a constant homeostatic balance by curtailing the effects of autoreactive T cells in noninflammatory settings.[32]

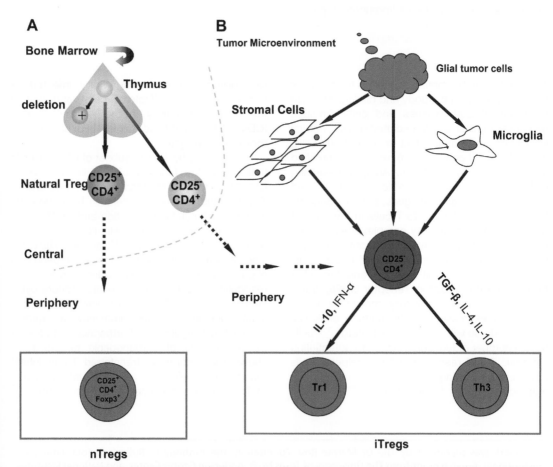

**Fig. 1.** Treg development. (*A*) The development of nTregs. nTregs are selected with an intermediate affinity for the MHC II/self-peptide complex in the thymus. They then enter the peripheral circulation as CD4+ CD25+ Foxp3+ cells. The nTregs exert their effect on immune effector cells primarily via cell-to-cell contact both peripherally and within the tumor microenvironment. (*B*) The development of iTregs. Tr1 and Th3 cells fall under the rubric of iTregs and are also derived from the thymus. However, they enter the peripheral circulation as naïve (CD4+ CD25− Foxp3−) T cells. They are then induced in the periphery to differentiate into regulatory T cells via a myriad of redundant pathways emanating from the tumor microenvironment. Differentiation of naïve CD4+ cells into Tr1 and Th3 cells is cytokine-dependent, as is the mechanism by which the iTregs exert their effects on immune effector cells.

Tregs in circulating peripheral blood include not only nTregs differentiated in the thymus but also Foxp3$^+$ Tregs generated extrathymically by the conversion of naïve T cells via chronic encounters with antigens present in suboptimal doses[39] or by the suppressive cytokine milieu secreted by the glioma. In vitro experiments have demonstrated that peripheral T cells retain the ability to induce Foxp3 expression upon T cell receptor cross-linking in the presence of TGF-β[40] or by the CD28/B7 interaction.[41] However, the overall contribution of the peripheral conversion of Tregs to immune suppression and its functional significance are not clear. Investigators have described two populations of peripherally induced CD4$^+$ Tregs: Tr1 and Th3 cells. Tr1 cells require IL-10 for induction, predominantly secrete IL-10, and to a lesser degree TGF-β and INF-γ. Tr1 cells inhibit naïve, memory, and helper T cells and the ability of DCs to induce T cell proliferation.[42] In contrast, Th3 cells[43] are induced by IL-10 and TGF-β[44] and predominantly secrete TGF-β and IL-10 at levels lower than Tr1 cells do. It is suspected that these induced Tregs (iTregs) play a primary role in mitigating pathologic immune responses such as those seen in cases of infection and autoimmune-mediated inflammation.[32]

## BIOLOGIC ROLE OF TREGS IN PATIENTS WITH GLIOMA

Studies have indicated that Tregs mediate immunosuppression in patients with a number of different malignancies, including ovarian, pancreatic, breast, colorectal, lung, and esophageal cancer.[25,45,46] For example, Curiel and colleagues[25] showed that the Treg fraction was higher in ascites of patients with ovarian cancer compared with that of patients with nonmalignant ascites. The investigators showed that Tregs preferentially migrated to the tumor microenvironment induced by CCL22 secreted by the tumor cells and macrophages. Furthermore, Tregs inhibited the function of tumor-infiltrating T cells by inhibiting production of IL-12 and INF-γ.

Patients with malignant gliomas have severe defects in host humoral and cellular immune responses.[47] These defects are characterized by dramatic reductions in CD4$^+$ T cell number[27] and function,[48,49] and a disproportionate presence of immunosuppressive Tregs.[27] This increase in Treg fractions corresponds with a decrease in effector T cell functions. Furthermore, the removal of the Treg fraction from T cells obtained from patients with glioblastoma multiforme (GBM) restores T cell proliferation and cytokine responses to normal levels.[27] Moreover, in vitro depletion of

Tregs from peripheral blood results in the successful reversal of effector T cell function, including increased T cell proliferation and a switch from Th2 to a Th1 (IL-2$^+$, tumor necrosis factor-α [TNF-α)$^+$, IFN-γ$^+$] cytokine profile. These findings demonstrate the important role of Tregs in glioma-mediated immunosuppression.

In the glioma microenvironment, the anti-tumor effector T cells can be critically suppressed or overwhelmed by Tregs. Researchers have obtained human glioma tissue during surgery, dissociated the tumors into single-cell suspensions, and stained them for the CD8$^+$ and CD4$^+$ subsets of T cells.[50] They found that tumor-infiltrating CD8$^+$ T cells were phenotypically CD8$^+$ and CD25$^-$, indicating that these effector cells were not activated or proliferating. The CD4$^+$ T cells were more numerous than CD8$^+$ T cells within the gliomas, and the majority of CD4$^+$ T cells were Tregs as evidenced by positive intracellular staining for Foxp3. In another study, the CD4$^+$ CD25$^+$ Foxp3$^+$ T cells were found only in gliomas, whereas Tregs were absent from control brain tissue specimens.[51] The presence of Tregs within the glioma microenvironment is secondary to the elaboration of the chemokine CCL2 by gliomas which induces the migration of Tregs.[52] Finally, in murine models of syngeneic murine glioma, investigators have observed a time-dependent accumulation of Foxp3$^+$ Tregs in brain tumors.[53] These data indicate that Tregs can not only inhibit the initial systemic anti-tumor immune activation but also prevent effector T cell responses in the tumor microenvironment and thus are a potential therapeutic target for inhibition.

## PROGNOSTIC SIGNIFICANCE OF TREGS IN PATIENTS WITH GLIOMA

T cells in the central nervous system (CNS) of healthy humans are a rare finding. However, during inflammatory responses, T cells are evident within the CNS. T cells require activation before entry into the CNS,[54] but antigen specificity is not necessary for this entry. T cell infiltrates are commonly identified in human gliomas,[55] and multiple studies have attempted to correlate the intensity of T cell infiltration with survival.[55–57] However, this prognostic significance has not been seen consistently.[58] These types of immunohistochemical assays used in the aforementioned studies do not take into account the functional activity of these T cells or the influence of the immune inhibitory Tregs. Thus, although these T cells are activated in the systemic circulation, their functional activity likely becomes impaired upon entry into the glioma microenvironment.[60] Thus, the fact that the T cells presence in a glioma is not a definitive prognostic marker is not surprising.

Researchers showed that CD8[+] T cells were present in the majority of glioma specimens regardless of tumor grade. However, the number of patients with CD4[+] T cell populations (including Tregs) increased as the tumor grade increased (39% for World Health Organization [WHO] grade II tumors to 73% for WHO grade III tumors to 98% for grade WHO grade IV tumors).[59] Foxp3[+] Tregs are not usually seen in normal brain tissue specimens and are very rare in patients with oligodendroglioma (WHO grade II), mixed oligoastrocytoma (WHO grade II), or anaplastic oligodendroglioma (WHO grade III) (**Fig. 2**). In contrast, 39% of the anaplastic mixed oligoastrocytoma specimens (WHO grade III), 53% of the anaplastic astrocytoma specimens (WHO grade III), 48% of the GBM specimens (WHO grade IV), and 83% of the gliosarcoma specimens (WHO grade IV) had Foxp3[+] Tregs.[60] Thus, Tregs were more common in high-grade astrocytic gliomas than in low-grade oligodendroglioma-type tumors.

Because the presence of Foxp3[+] Tregs correlates with the overall malignant behavior of astrocytic tumors, the expectation that the presence of Tregs in the tumor microenvironment will act as a negative prognostic indicator is reasonable. Univariate analysis demonstrated that, similar to other established parameters such as the Karnofsky performance score, patient age, and tumor grade, the presence or absence of Foxp3[+] Tregs and absolute number of Foxp3[+] Tregs per tumor sample were prognostic factors. However, a multivariate analysis performed to account for confounding factors, such as patient age and Karnofsky performance score, found that the presence of Foxp3 Tregs did not have a prognostic impact.[60] Although some cancers may mediate immunosuppression predominantly via Tregs, high-grade gliomas have multiple mechanisms mediating immunosuppression. Thus, the lack of a prognostic impact of one mechanism in this setting, such as the presence or absence of Foxp3[+] Tregs, is not entirely surprising and emphasizes the redundancy of immunosuppressive pathways. Furthermore, this type of study does not account for the prognostic influence of Tregs in the systemic, peripheral blood compartment.

## MECHANISMS OF MODULATING TREG RESPONSES

It is widely recognized that tumors evade the host immune response through a number of mechanisms, including elaboration of immunosuppressive cytokines, alteration of signal transduction, and the induction of Tregs. Thus, at the core of the development of more effective immunotherapeutic strategies for brain tumors is simultaneous stimulation of more potent immune responses against these tumors while overcoming immunosuppressive mechanisms induced by the tumors themselves. Overcoming Treg-induced immunosuppression can be achieved using a variety of approaches, including administration of denileukin diftitox (Ontak; a recombinant protein of diphtheria toxin and IL-2),[61] cyclophosphamide (CTX),[62] an anti-CD25 antibody (targeting the IL-2 receptor),[29] CTLA-4 blockade (inhibits co-stimulation),[28] and signal transcription and activator of translation (STAT)-3–blocking agents that also block transcriptional activation of Foxp3[63,64]; inhibition of intratumoral Treg trafficking (ie, inhibition of CCL2) with temozolomide[65]; and, nonspecifically, lymphodepletion to augment immunologic responses, which investigators have described in both murine models[62,66] and human patients with cancer.[67,68] Antitumor responses enhanced by lymphodepletion may be secondary to the removal of competition at the surface of APCs,[69] enhanced availability of cytokines that augment T cell activity (such as IL-7 and IL-15),[70] or the depletion of immune inhibitory Tregs.[71]

Developing an optimal approach to modulating or suppressing the Treg population for therapeutic purposes in cancer patients is controversial. CTX, an alkylating agent with therapeutic effects against tumors at high doses, preferentially inhibits Tregs at lower doses. CTX can abolish the function of CD4[+] CD25[+] Foxp3[+] T cells and enhance cytotoxic T cell responses.[72] Treatment with CTX before antitumor vaccination results in activation of tumor-specific CD8[+] T cells.[73] When CTX is administered at subtumoricidal doses in combination with IL-12 in mice, it improves immune response and eradicates large established sarcomas.[74] This combination enhances CD4[+] T cells, CD8[+] T cells, and macrophage infiltration in tumors and skews the immune responses to the Th1 phenotype.[74] In addition to its induction of immunity to new antigens, CTX can overcome immune tolerance. For example, administration of CTX in mice bearing established plasmacytomas resulted in a cure in 92% of the mice, and further studies demonstrated that the cured mice rejected a subsequent tumor challenge.[75,76] The mechanisms of efficacy appeared to include both generation of CD8[+] cytotoxic T cells and upregulation of expression of B7-1 (a co-stimulatory molecule).

Multiple clinical trials have demonstrated enhanced immune responses and improved

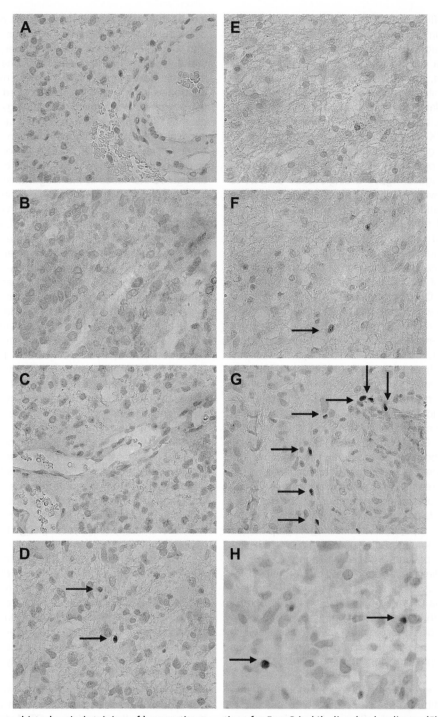

**Fig. 2.** Immunohistochemical staining of human tissue sections for Foxp3 in (*A*) oligodendroglioma, (*B*) mixed oligoastrocytoma, (*C*) anaplastic oligodendroglioma, (*D*) anaplastic mixed oligodendroglioma, (*E*) low-grade astrocytoma, (*F*) anaplastic astrocytoma, (*G*) glioblastoma, and (*H*) gliosarcoma. Tissue sections for Foxp3 show faint staining with few nonclustering Tregs (*D, F*). The Treg number increased as the tumor grade increased (*E–G*), although they were nearly absent from tumors with oligo-based histologies (*A* and *C*). All of the images were taken at a magnification of 400x.

clinical efficacy when CTX was administered before immunotherapy.[77,78] For example, when CTX was administered to augment an autologous melanoma vaccine in patients with metastatic melanoma, there were enhanced delayed-type hypersensitivity responses.[79] Researchers have seen similar potentiation of immune responses in metastatic breast cancer and renal cell carcinoma cases. CTX has also been used in a phase I clinical trial of glioma patients that demonstrated evidence of clinical efficacy. In this trial, Plautz and colleagues[80] gave a single dose of CTX to patients with newly diagnosed glioma before administration of adoptively transferred T cells harvested from the patients' lymph nodes. They conducted this study without the benefit of the current understanding of the influence of CTX on Tregs; thus, the contribution of CTX to the clinical efficacy of this immune therapeutic strategy is unknown. Despite the use of CTX in clinical trials, the timing and dosing of CTX for optimal Treg inhibition[81,82] relative to each type of vaccination or immunotherapy strategy still needs further refinement.

Researchers have also studied temozolomide, which is capable of suppressing Tregs, in clinical trials of immunotherapy for GBM. Temozolomide is the standard of care for GBM and an alkylating agent that causes cell death by inducing cell-cycle arrest at G2/M phase and, likely, autophagy without apoptosis.[83] In addition to inhibiting the proliferation of lymphocytes, temozolomide can deplete Tregs[84] and inhibit trafficking of Tregs into the glioma microenvironment.[65] The use of temozolomide has proven to be beneficial in combination with a peptide vaccine targeting epidermal growth factor receptor variant III in a phase II clinical trial in patients with newly diagnosed GBM.[85] Another clinical trial, sponsored by Northwest Biotherapeutics (Bethesda, MD), is using GBM patient autologous DCs for an immunotherapy in combination with temozolomide in a similar manner. The use of temozolomide as a possible Treg modulator has particular appeal in the glioma patient population since it is the current standard of care.

Inactivation of Tregs by treatment with an anti-CD25 antibody[29,53,86] or CTLA-4 blockade[28,53] have demonstrated efficacy in murine glioma models. Various studies support the notion that CTLA-4 blockade can enhance antitumor immune responses by limiting suppression of effector T cell responses[87] either by directly activating effector T cells or indirectly inactivating Tregs. Although some studies have shown that CTLA-4 blockade fails to suppress Tregs,[87] others have indicated that Tregs and CTLA-4 blockade act independently and that the effects of CTLA-4 blockade are not focused on Tregs,[88,89] such that CTLA-4 blockade may be synergistic with strategies that inhibit Tregs.[89] In one study of systemic delivery of CTLA-4 blocking monoclonal antibodies in mice with well-established malignant astrocytomas recapitulating the biology of human gliomas,[90] the treatment produced a long-term survival rate of 80% without induction of autoimmune encephalomyelitis.[28] CTLA-4 blockade also re-established normal CD4$^+$ T cell counts and abrogated increases in the Treg fractions elicited by the tumors. Significant increases in total and CD4$^+$ T cell counts were also observed in individual mice treated with anti-CTLA-4 when compared with mean counts in the untreated group, suggesting a mechanism independent of tumor destruction. Furthermore, CTLA-4 blockade restored CD4$^+$ T cell proliferative capacity and enhanced antitumor immune responses. Interestingly, the benefits of CTLA-4 blockade appear to be bestowed exclusively upon activated CD4$^+$ CD25$^-$ T cells but not the Tregs. In the study described above, the CD4$^+$ CD25$^-$ T cells obtained from treated mice demonstrated both improved proliferative responses and Treg resistance, whereas Tregs obtained from the same mice remained anergic in vitro and exhibited no restriction of their suppressive effect on effector T cells not treated with CTLA-4 monoclonal antibodies. This absence of a direct effect of anti-CTLA-4 antibodies on Tregs strengthens the notion that CTLA-4 blockade may be synergistic with strategies designed to remove Tregs.[89] Although eliminating suppression of endogenous antitumor immune responses through the removal of Tregs may enhance tumor immune clearance, it is accompanied by a potential risk of inducing autoimmunity, although investigators did not find this in murine models. Strategies that induce Th17 responses but not necessarily Treg inhibition likely are the primary mechanisms of inducing CNS autoimmunity.[91] Nevertheless, CTLA-4 blockade has demonstrated safety and significant efficacy as an antitumor strategy in a variety of animal models.[92–95]

The greatest overall clinical experience of Treg modulation in cancer patients is with antibodies that abrogate the function of CTLA-4, including some clinical studies that have included patients with metastatic brain tumors.[96,97] These fully human antibodies (Pfizer and Bristol-Meyers Squibb, New York, NY, USA; and Medarex, Princeton, NJ, USA) were created using strains of mice with engineered human immune systems. Their use in clinical trials, mostly for melanoma and prostate cancer,[98,99] has been associated with a spectrum of autoimmune-associated side effects, such as dermatitis, enterocolitis, hepatitis, uveitis, and hypophysitis.[100] In some cases they are associated with clinical response and sustainable progression-free survival.[97,101] Specifically, in one study in which an anti-CTLA-4 antibody was administered with gp100 melanoma-associated antigens to patients with melanoma, 36% of patients with at least grade 3 autoimmune toxic effects had a clinical response, whereas only 5% of those with no autoimmune toxic effects had a clinical response (overall response was 13% regardless of autoimmune toxicity).[102] This CTLA-4 blockade has been shown to enhance both tumor-specific humoral and cytotoxic responses in patients.[103] Another study found that anti-CTLA-4 immunotherapy with IL-2 in a phase I-II clinical trial in patients with melanoma had an objective response rate of 22%.[104] Anti-CTLA-4 therapy has generated clinically meaningful antitumor immunity without autoimmune toxic effects in patients with melanoma or ovarian cancer who were previously vaccinated with irradiated autologous tumor cells engineered to secrete granulocyte-macrophage colony-stimulating factor (GM-CSF),[105] suggesting that anti-CTLA-4 therapy may be beneficial in previously vaccinated patients. Unfortunately, anti-CTLA-4 therapy has yet to be studied in patients with malignant glioma, but given the aforementioned data, it may be appropriate for use in those glioma patients who have previously received vaccination or immune therapeutics who may be in early stages of progression to provide an immunologic boost. Furthermore, the authors propose that the therapeutic efficacy of epidermal growth factor receptor variant III-targeted vaccination[106,107] may be enhanced in combination with CTLA-4 blockade in patients with GBM who have residual disease through reversal of Treg-mediated immunosuppression and may enhance vaccine-induced and endogenous antitumor immune responses.

In the case of anti-CD25, two different immunotoxins have been created that could be exploited for inhibiting Tregs. One is linked to ricin A (RFT5.SMPT-DGA),[108,109] whereas the other is linked to *Pseudomonas* exotoxin (LMB-2).[110] Investigators have administered these two immunotoxins in patients with heavily pretreated refractory Hodgkin disease and hairy cell leukemia, respectively, and observed clinical responses. The toxic effects of RFT5.SMPT-DGA included weakness, edema, dyspnea, and myalgia,[111] whereas those of LMB-2 consisted primarily of transaminase-level elevations and fever.[112] As with the anti-CTLA-4 approaches, neither of these agents or the other anti-CD25 preclinical approaches that have been investigated in murine models[29,53,86] have been attempted in glioma patients but these agents could also be used in combination with other immune therapeutics or in the setting of residual disease.

In a study of patients with metastatic renal carcinoma, treatment with Ontak (anti-IL-2) specifically depleted Tregs without inducing toxic effects and significantly improved stimulation of tumor-specific T cell responses when those patients were stimulated with tumor RNA-transfected DCs.[113] Without tumor vaccination, researchers have shown that Ontak is efficacious as a single agent against relapsed or refractory B-cell non-Hodgkin lymphoma and cutaneous T cell lymphoma.[114] However, Ontak has not been particularly effective in depleting Tregs in patients with melanoma,[60] a tumor of similar neuroectodermal derivation as glioma. Furthermore, Ontak targets IL-2, which is expressed in effector T cells. Because the effector T cell immune population is already compromised in patients with GBM,[115–117] further suppression of the antitumor effector T cell population may be deleterious in these patients.

Investigators have reported that targeting of the Toll-like receptor (TLR) elicits effective antitumor responses against various neoplasms, including experimental brain tumors,[118] which may partially neutralize the effects of Tregs. For instance, one study has shown that the stimulation with synthetic or natural ligands for human TLR8, and the subsequent transfer of TLR-8 ligand-stimulated Tregs into tumor-bearing mice led to the enhancement of anti-tumor immunity.[119] Furthermore, a study showed that TLR stimulation by CpG-oligodeoxynucleotides in murine GL261 gliomas enhanced CD8$^+$ T cell mediated immune responses and demonstrated a marked increase in the ratio of CD4$^+$ effector T cells to Foxp3$^+$ Tregs.[120] However, TLR agonists may not be able to reverse the other mechanisms of immunosuppression in patients with glioma, including immune inhibitory microglia or macrophages present in the tumor microenvironment.[50]

## FUTURE DIRECTIONS

An emerging approach to modulating Tregs is administration of agents that block or disrupt Notch signaling and STAT-3 inhibitors. Notch plays a role in regulating the responses of T cells and can induce the differentiation of CD4$^+$ T cells into Tregs.[121] However, which members of the Notch family that must be blocked is unclear. As described previously,[63,64] the STAT-3 inhibitors are a new class of compounds that are potent inhibitors of Tregs that will soon be tested in clinical trials. Researchers have shown that STAT-3 activation is required for both TGF-β and IL-10 production by CD4[+] T cells[122]; both of these factors are necessary for the generation of tumor-associated Tregs. In addition, a study has shown that IL-2 regulates Foxp3 expression in human CD4[+] CD25[+] Tregs via STAT-3 binding of the first intron of the *Foxp3* gene.[123] Previous studies in mice showed that ablation of *Stat3* in the hematopoietic system using the *Mx1-Cre-loxP* system was accompanied by a reduction in the number of tumor-infiltrating Tregs.[124] We have reported that a small molecular inhibitor of the STAT-3 pathway, WP1066, inhibited the induction of Foxp3 expression in peripheral T cells and down-regulated Foxp3 expression in nTregs[63,64] and that this likely accounted for the marked in vivo antitumor effects and enhancement of cytotoxic T cell responses. Additionally, we reported that STAT-3 blockade had negligible inhibitory effects on effector T cell cytotoxicity (which is mediated by the STAT-5 activation pathway), which may compromise immunologic tumor clearance. In comparison, many of the other types of anti-Treg agents (Ontak, anti-CD25 antibodies, CTLA-4–blocking agents, etc) are cross-reactive with other T cell populations that exert effector responses.

Despite recent advancements in immunotherapies for malignant gliomas, the overall prognosis for individuals with these tumors remains very poor. Given the cellular complexity of this very aggressive tumor, any single treatment modality alone is unlikely to be effective against it. Ultimately, improving outcomes in patients with malignant gliomas will require a multifaceted treatment approach combining various treatment modalities. Given the multiplicity of immunosuppressive mechanisms, anti-Treg agents may be most beneficial in patients whose immunosuppression is dependent on this mechanism (ie, elevated number or fraction of CD4[+] Foxp3[+] Tregs in the peripheral blood or marked intratumoral infiltration with Tregs). Future studies of Treg inhibition or modulation in combination with other immunotherapeutics, such as IFN-α, IL-2, GM-CSF, monoclonal antibodies against tumor antigens, peptides, DCs, and anticancer vaccines, would present an opportunity to further potentiate these agents' therapeutic efficacy, and not just for malignant gliomas. The recent success of several clinical trials of immunotherapy for glioma patients further stresses the need for development of promising adjunct treatments, especially combination treatments, of malignant gliomas. However, these and other future developments must be integrated into a comprehensive treatment program incorporating current treatment modalities.

## REFERENCES

1. Yi-qun Z, Lorre K, de Boer M, et al. B7-blocking agents, alone or in combination with cyclosporin A, induce antigen-specific anergy of human memory T cells. J Immunol 1997;158:4734–40.
2. Lim HW, Hillsamer P, Banham AH, et al. Cutting edge: direct suppression of B cells by CD4+ CD25+ regulatory T cells. J Immunol 2005;175:4180–3.
3. Zhao DM, Thornton AM, DiPaolo RJ, et al. Activated CD4+CD25+ T cells selectively kill B lymphocytes. Blood 2006;107:3925–32.
4. Fallarino F, Grohmann U, Hwang KW, et al. Modulation of tryptophan catabolism by regulatory T cells. Nat Immunol 2003;4:1206–12.
5. Misra N, Bayry J, Lacroix-Desmazes S, et al. Cutting edge: human CD4+CD25+ T cells restrain the maturation and antigen-presenting function of dendritic cells. J Immunol 2004;172:4676–80.
6. Taams LS, van Amelsfort JM, Tiemessen MM, et al. Modulation of monocyte/macrophage function by human CD4+CD25+ regulatory T cells. Hum Immunol 2005;66:222–30.
7. Azuma T, Takahashi T, Kunisato A, et al. Human CD4+ CD25+ regulatory T cells suppress NKT cell functions. Cancer Res 2003;63:4516–20.
8. Ralainirina N, Poli A, Michel T, et al. Control of NK cell functions by CD4+CD25+ regulatory T cells. J Leukoc Biol 2007;81:144–53.
9. Smyth MJ, Teng MW, Swann J, et al. CD4+CD25+ T regulatory cells suppress NK cell-mediated immunotherapy of cancer. J Immunol 2006;176:1582–7.
10. Dieckmann D, Plottner H, Berchtold S, et al. Ex vivo isolation and characterization of CD4(+)CD25(+) T cells with regulatory properties from human blood. J Exp Med 2001;193:1303–10.
11. Fontenot JD, Gavin MA, Rudensky AY. Foxp3 programs the development and function of CD4+CD25+ regulatory T cells. Nat Immunol 2003;4:330–6.
12. Jonuleit H, Schmitt E, Stassen M, et al. Identification and functional characterization of human CD4(+)CD25(+) T cells with regulatory properties isolated from peripheral blood. J Exp Med 2001;193:1285–94.
13. Khattri R, Cox T, Yasayko SA, et al. An essential role for Scurfin in CD4+CD25+ T regulatory cells. Nat Immunol 2003;4:337–42.
14. Thornton AM, Shevach EM. CD4+CD25+ immunoregulatory T cells suppress polyclonal T cell

activation in vitro by inhibiting interleukin 2 production. J Exp Med 1998;188:287–96.

15. Sakaguchi S. Naturally arising CD4+ regulatory T cells for immunologic self-tolerance and negative control of immune responses. Annu Rev Immunol 2004;22:531–62.

16. Asano M, Toda M, Sakaguchi N, et al. Autoimmune disease as a consequence of developmental abnormality of a T cell subpopulation. J Exp Med 1996;184:387–96.

17. Bagavant H, Thompson C, Ohno K, et al. Differential effect of neonatal thymectomy on systemic and organ-specific autoimmune disease. Int Immunol 2002;14:1397–406.

18. Miyara M, Sakaguchi S. Natural regulatory T cells: mechanisms of suppression. Trends Mol Med 2007;13:108–16.

19. Sakaguchi S, Sakaguchi N, Asano M, et al. Immunologic self-tolerance maintained by activated T cells expressing IL-2 receptor alpha-chains (CD25). Breakdown of a single mechanism of self-tolerance causes various autoimmune diseases. J Immunol 1995;155:1151–64.

20. Salomon B, Lenschow DJ, Rhee L, et al. B7/CD28 costimulation is essential for the homeostasis of the CD4+CD25+ immunoregulatory T cells that control autoimmune diabetes. Immunity 2000;12: 431–40.

21. Seddon B, Mason D. Regulatory T cells in the control of autoimmunity: the essential role of transforming growth factor beta and interleukin 4 in the prevention of autoimmune thyroiditis in rats by peripheral CD4(+)CD45RC- cells and CD4(+)CD8(-) thymocytes. J Exp Med 1999;189: 279–88.

22. Stephens LA, Mason D. CD25 is a marker for CD4+ thymocytes that prevent autoimmune diabetes in rats, but peripheral T cells with this function are found in both CD25+ and CD25- subpopulations. J Immunol 2000;165:3105–10.

23. Taguchi O, Kontani K, Ikeda H, et al. Tissue-specific suppressor T cells involved in self-tolerance are activated extrathymically by self-antigens. Immunology 1994;82:365–9.

24. Taguchi O, Nishizuka Y. Self tolerance and localized autoimmunity. Mouse models of autoimmune disease that suggest tissue-specific suppressor T cells are involved in self tolerance. J Exp Med 1987;165:146–56.

25. Curiel TJ, Coukos G, Zou L, et al. Specific recruitment of regulatory T cells in ovarian carcinoma fosters immune privilege and predicts reduced survival. Nat Med 2004;10:942–9.

26. Somasundaram R, Jacob L, Swoboda R, et al. Inhibition of cytolytic T lymphocyte proliferation by autologous CD4+/CD25+ regulatory T cells in a colorectal carcinoma patient is mediated by transforming growth factor-beta. Cancer Res 2002;62:5267–72.

27. Fecci PE, Mitchell DA, Whitesides JF, et al. Increased regulatory T-cell fraction amidst a diminished CD4 compartment explains cellular immune defects in patients with malignant glioma. Cancer Res 2006;66:3294–302.

28. Fecci PE, Ochiai H, Mitchell DA, et al. Systemic CTLA-4 blockade ameliorates glioma-induced changes to the CD4+ T cell compartment without affecting regulatory T-cell function. Clin Cancer Res 2007;13:2158–67.

29. Fecci PE, Sweeney AE, Grossi PM, et al. Systemic anti-CD25 monoclonal antibody administration safely enhances immunity in murine glioma without eliminating regulatory T cells. Clin Cancer Res 2006;12:4294–305.

30. Gershon RK, Kondo K. Infectious immunological tolerance. Immunology 1971;21:903–14.

31. Knutson KL, Disis ML, Salazar LG. CD4 regulatory T cells in human cancer pathogenesis. Cancer Immunol Immunother 2007;56:271–85.

32. Bluestone JA, Abbas AK. Natural versus adaptive regulatory T cells. Nat Rev Immunol 2003;3:253–7.

33. Mitchell DA, Fecci PE, Sampson JH. Immunotherapy of malignant brain tumors. Immunol Rev 2008;222:70–100.

34. Jonuleit H, Schmitt E. The regulatory T cell family: distinct subsets and their interrelations. J Immunol 2003;171:6323–7.

35. Takahashi T, Tagami T, Yamazaki S, et al. Immunologic self-tolerance maintained by CD25(+)CD4(+) regulatory T cells constitutively expressing cytotoxic T lymphocyte-associated antigen 4. J Exp Med 2000;192:303–10.

36. Brunet JF, Denizot F, Luciani MF, et al. A new member of the immunoglobulin superfamily—CTLA-4. Nature 1987;328:267–70.

37. Walunas TL, Lenschow DJ, Bakker CY, et al. CTLA-4 can function as a negative regulator of T cell activation. Immunity 1994;1:405–13.

38. Hori S, Sakaguchi S. Foxp3: a critical regulator of the development and function of regulatory T cells. Microbes Infect 2004;6:745–51.

39. Kretschmer K, Apostolou I, Hawiger D, et al. Inducing and expanding regulatory T cell populations by foreign antigen. Nat Immunol 2005;6: 1219–27.

40. Chen W, Jin W, Hardegen N, et al. Conversion of peripheral CD4+CD25- naive T cells to CD4+CD25+ regulatory T cells by TGF-beta induction of transcription factor Foxp3. J Exp Med 2003;198:1875–86.

41. Scotta C, Soligo M, Camperio C, et al. FOXP3 induced by CD28/B7 interaction regulates CD25 and anergic phenotype in human CD4+CD25- T lymphocytes. J Immunol 2008;181:1025–33.

42. Groux H. Type 1 T-regulatory cells: their role in the control of immune responses. Transplantation 2003;75:8S–12S.

43. Chen Y, Kuchroo VK, Inobe J, et al. Regulatory T cell clones induced by oral tolerance: suppression of autoimmune encephalomyelitis. Science 1994; 265:1237–40.

44. Weiner HL. Induction and mechanism of action of transforming growth factor-beta-secreting Th3 regulatory cells. Immunol Rev 2001;182:207–14.

45. Liyanage UK, Moore TT, Joo HG, et al. Prevalence of regulatory T cells is increased in peripheral blood and tumor microenvironment of patients with pancreas or breast adenocarcinoma. J Immunol 2002;169:2756–61.

46. Wolf AM, Wolf D, Steurer M, et al. Increase of regulatory T cells in the peripheral blood of cancer patients. Clin Cancer Res 2003;9:606–12.

47. Dix AR, Brooks WH, Roszman TL, et al. Immune defects observed in patients with primary malignant brain tumors. J Neuroimmunol 1999;100: 216–32.

48. Morford LA, Elliott LH, Carlson SL, et al. T cell receptor-mediated signaling is defective in T cells obtained from patients with primary intracranial tumors. J Immunol 1997;159:4415–25.

49. Roszman TL, Brooks WH. Immunobiology of primary intracranial tumours. III. Demonstration of a qualitative lymphocyte abnormality in patients with primary brain tumours. Clin Exp Immunol 1980;39:395–402.

50. Hussain SF, Yang D, Suki D, et al. The role of human glioma-infiltrating microglia/macrophages in mediating antitumor immune responses. Neuro Oncol 2006;8:261–79.

51. El Andaloussi A, Lesniak MS. An increase in CD4+CD25+FOXP3+ regulatory T cells in tumor-infiltrating lymphocytes of human glioblastoma multiforme. Neuro Oncol 2006;8:234–43.

52. Jordan JT, Sun WH, Hussain SF, et al. Preferential migration of regulatory T cells mediated by glioma-secreted chemokines can be blocked with chemotherapy. Cancer Immunol Immunother 2008;57:123–31.

53. Grauer OM, Nierkens S, Bennink E, et al. CD4+FoxP3+ regulatory T cells gradually accumulate in gliomas during tumor growth and efficiently suppress antiglioma immune responses in vivo. Int J Cancer 2007;121:95–105.

54. Hickey WF, Hsu BL, Kimura H. T-lymphocyte entry into the central nervous system. J Neurosci Res 1991;28:254–60.

55. von Hanwehr RI, Hofman FM, Taylor CR, et al. Mononuclear lymphoid populations infiltrating the microenvironment of primary CNS tumors. Characterization of cell subsets with monoclonal antibodies. J Neurosurg 1984;60:1138–47.

56. Brooks WH, Markesbery WR, Gupta GD, et al. Relationship of lymphocyte invasion and survival of brain tumor patients. Ann Neurol 1978;4:219–24.

57. Strik HM, Stoll M, Meyermann R. Immune cell infiltration of intrinsic and metastatic intracranial tumours. Anticancer Res 2004;24:37–42.

58. Safdari H, Hochberg FH, Richardson EP Jr. Prognostic value of round cell (lymphocyte) infiltration in malignant gliomas. Surg Neurol 1985;23:221–6.

59. Heimberger AB, Reina-Ortiz C, Yang DS, et al. Incidence and prognostic impact of FoxP3+ regulatory T cells in human gliomas. Clin Cancer Res 2008;14: 5166–72.

60. Attia P, Maker AV, Haworth LR, et al. Inability of a fusion protein of IL-2 and diphtheria toxin (Denileukin Diftitox, DAB389IL-2, ONTAK) to eliminate regulatory T lymphocytes in patients with melanoma. J Immunother 2005;28:582–92.

61. Foss F. Clinical Experience With Denileukin Diftitox (ONTAK). Semin Oncol 2006;33:11–6.

62. North RJ. Cyclophosphamide-facilitated adoptive immunotherapy of an established tumor depends on elimination of tumor-induced suppressor T cells. J Exp Med 1982;155:1063–74.

63. Kong L-K, Wei J, Sharma AK, et al. A novel phosphorylated STAT3 inhibitor enhances T cell cytotoxicity against melanoma through inhibition of regulatory T cells. Cancer Immunol Immunother 2008;58:1023–32.

64. Kong LY, Abou-Ghazal MK, Wei J, et al. A novel inhibitor of STAT3 activation is efficacious against established central nervous system melanoma and inhibits regulatory T cells. Clin Cancer Res 2008;14:5759–68.

65. Jordan JT, Sun WH, Hussain SF, et al. Preferential migration of regulatory T cells mediated by glioma-secreted chemokines can be blocked with chemotherapy. Cancer Immunol Immunother 2008;57:123–31.

66. Cheever MA, Greenberg PD, Fefer A. Specificity of adoptive chemoimmunotherapy of established syngeneic tumors. J Immunol 1980;125:711–4.

67. Dudley ME, Wunderlich JR, Robbins PF, et al. Cancer regression and autoimmunity in patients after clonal repopulation with antitumor lymphocytes. Science 2002;298:850–4.

68. Dudley ME, Wunderlich JR, Yang JC, et al. Adoptive cell transfer therapy following non-myeloablative but lymphodepleting chemotherapy for the treatment of patients with refractory metastatic melanoma. J Clin Oncol 2005;23:2346–57.

69. Kedl RM, Rees WA, Hildeman DA, et al. T cells compete for access to antigen-bearing antigen-presenting cells. J Exp Med 2000;192:1105–13.

70. Gattinoni L, Finkelstein SE, Klebanoff CA, et al. Removal of homeostatic cytokine sinks by lymphodepletion enhances the efficacy of adoptively

transferred tumor-specific CD8+ T cells. J Exp Med 2005;202:907–12.

71. Klebanoff CA, Khong HT, Antony PA, et al. Sinks, supressors and antigen presenters: how lympho-depletion enhances T cell-mediated tumor immuno-therapy [Erratum appears in Trends Immunol 2005;26:298]. Trends Immunol 2005;26:111–7.

72. Taieb J, Chaput N, Schartz N, et al. Chemoimmuno-therapy of tumors: cyclophosphamide synergizes with exosome based vaccines. J Immunol 2006; 176:2722–9.

73. Ercolini AM, Ladle BH, Manning EA, et al. Recruit-ment of latent pools of high-avidity CD8+ T cells to the antitumor immune response. J Exp Med 2005;201:1591–602.

74. Tsung K, Meko JB, Tsung YL, et al. Immune response against large tumors eradicated by treat-ment with cyclophosphamide and IL-12. J Immunol 1998;160:1369–77.

75. Hengst JCD, Mokyr MB, Dray S. Importance of timing in cyclophosphamide therapy in MOPC-315 tumor-bearing mice. Cancer Res 1980;40: 2135–41.

76. Hengst JCD, Mokyr MB, Dray S. Cooperation between cyclophosphamide tumoricidal activity and host antitumor immunity in the cure of mice bearing large MOPC-315 tumors. Cancer Res 1981;41:2163–7.

77. Holtl L, Ramoner R, Zelle-Rieser C, et al. Alloge-neic dendritic cell vaccination against metastatic renal cell carcinoma with or without cyclophos-phamide. Cancer Immunol Immunother 2005;54: 663–70.

78. MacLean GD, Miles DW, Rubens RD, et al. Enhancing the effect of THERATOPE STn-KLH cancer vaccine in patients with metastatic breast cancer by pretreatment with low-dose intravenous cyclophosphamide. J Immunother Emphasis Tumor Immunol 1996;19:309–16.

79. Berd D, Maguire HC, McCue P, et al. Treatment of metastatic melanoma with an autologous tumor-cell vaccine: clinical and immunological results in 64 patients. J Clin Oncol 1990;8:1858–67.

80. Plautz GE, Miller DW, Barnett GH, et al. T cell adop-tive immunotherapy of newly diagnosed gliomas. Clin Cancer Res 2000;6:2209–18.

81. Hermans IF, Chong TW, Palmowski MJ, et al. Synergistic effect of metronomic dosing of cyclo-phosphamide combined with specific antitumor immunotherapy in a murine melanoma model. Cancer Res 2003;63:8408–13.

82. Ghiringhelli F, Menard C, Puig PE, et al. Metronomic cyclophosphamide regimen selectively depletes CD4+CD25+ regulatory T cells and restores T and NK effector functions in end stage cancer patients. Cancer Immunol Immunother 2007;56: 641–8.

83. Kanzawa T, Germano IM, Komata T, et al. Role of autophagy in temozolomide-induced cytotoxicity for malignant glioma cells. Cell Death Differ 2004; 11:448–57.

84. Su YB, Sohn S, Krown SE, et al. Selective CD4+ lymphopenia in melanoma patients treated with temozolomide: a toxicity with therapeutic implica-tions. J Clin Oncol 2004;22:610–6.

85. Sampson JH, Archer GE, Bigner DD, et al. Effect of EGFRvIII-targeted vaccine (CDX-110) induces immune responses and prolongs TTP when given with simultaneous standard and continuous temo-zolomide in patients with GBM. J Clin Oncol 2008;26(Suppl):92s.

86. El Andaloussi A, Han Y, Lesniak MS. Prolongation of survival following depletion of CD4+CD25+ regulatory T cells in mice with experimental brain tumors. J Neurosurg 2006;105:430–7.

87. Read S, Malmstrom V, Powrie F. Cytotoxic T lymphocyte-associated antigen 4 plays an essen-tial role in the function of CD25(+)CD4(+) regula-tory cells that control intestinal inflammation. J Exp Med 2000;192:295–302.

88. Eggena MP, Walker LS, Nagabhushanam V, et al. Cooperative roles of CTLA-4 and regulatory T cells in tolerance to an islet cell antigen. J Exp Med 2004;199:1725–30.

89. Sutmuller RP, van Duivenvoorde LM, van Elsas A, et al. Synergism of cytotoxic T lymphocyte-associ-ated antigen 4 blockade and depletion of CD25(+) regulatory T cells in antitumor therapy reveals alternative pathways for suppression of au-toreactive cytotoxic T lymphocyte responses. J Exp Med 2001;194:823–32.

90. Sampson JH, Ashley DM, Archer GE, et al. Charac-terization of a spontaneous murine astrocytoma and abrogation of its tumorigenicity by cytokine secretion. Neurosurgery 1997;41:1365–72 [discus-sion: 72–3].

91. Oukka M. Interplay between pathogenic Th17 and regulatory T cells. Ann Rheum Dis 2007;66 (Suppl 3):iii87–90.

92. Leach DR, Krummel MF, Allison JP. Enhancement of antitumor immunity by CTLA-4 blockade. Science 1996;271:1734–6.

93. Shrikant P, Khoruts A, Mescher MF. CTLA-4 blockade reverses CD8+ T cell tolerance to tumor by a CD4+ T cell- and IL-2-dependent mechanism. Immunity 1999;11:483–93.

94. Sotomayor EM, Borrello I, Tubb E, et al. In vivo blockade of CTLA-4 enhances the priming of responsive T cells but fails to prevent the induction of tumor antigen-specific tolerance. Proc Natl Acad Sci U S A 1999;96:11476–81.

95. Yang YF, Zou JP, Mu J, et al. Enhanced induction of antitumor T-cell responses by cytotoxic T lympho-cyte-associated molecule-4 blockade: the effect

is manifested only at the restricted tumor-bearing stages. Cancer Res 1997;57:4036–41.

96. Hodi FS, Mihm MC, Soiffer RJ, et al. Biologic activity of cytotoxic T lymphocyte-associated antigen 4 antibody blockade in previously vaccinated metastatic melanoma and ovarian carcinoma patients. Proc Natl Acad Sci U S A 2003;100:4712–7.

97. Phan GQ, Yang JC, Sherry RM, et al. Cancer regression and autoimmunity induced by cytotoxic T lymphocyte-associated antigen 4 blockade in patients with metastatic melanoma. Proc Natl Acad Sci U S A 2003;100:8372–7.

98. Small EJ, Tchekmedyian NS, Rini BI, et al. A pilot trial of CTLA-4 blockade with human anti-CTLA-4 in patients with hormone-refractory prostate cancer. Clin Cancer Res 2007;13:1810–5.

99. Theoret MR, Arlen PM, Pazdur M, et al. Phase I trial of an enhanced prostate-specific antigen-based vaccine and anti-CTLA-4 antibody in patients with metastatic androgen-independent prostate cancer. Clin Genitourin Cancer 2007;5:347–50.

100. Blansfield JA, Beck KE, Tran K, et al. Cytotoxic T-lymphocyte–associated antigen-4 blockage can induce autoimmune hypophysitis in patients with metastatic melanoma and renal cancer. J Immunother 2005;28:593–8.

101. Reuben JM, Lee BN, Shen DY, et al. Therapy with human monoclonal anti-CTLA-4 antibody, CP-675,206, reduces regulatory T cells and IL-10 production in patients with advanced malignant melanoma [abstract 7505]. In: 2005 American Society of Clinical Oncology Annual Meeting. Orlando (FL), May 13–17, 2005.

102. Attia P, Phan GQ, Maker AV, et al. Autoimmunity correlates with tumor regression in patients with metastatic melanoma treated with anti-cytotoxic T-lymphocyte antigen-4. J Clin Oncol 2005;23:6043–53.

103. Yuan J, Gnjatic S, Li H, et al. CTLA-4 blockade enhances polyfunctional NY-ESO-1 specific T cell responses in metastatic melanoma patients with clinical benefit. Proc Natl Acad Sci U S A 2008;105:20410–5.

104. Maker AV, Phan GQ, Attia P, et al. Tumor regression and autoimmunity in patients treated with cytotoxic T lymphocyte-associated antigen 4 blockade and interleukin 2: a phase I/II study. Ann Surg Oncol 2005;12:1005–16.

105. Hodi FS, Butler M, Oble DA, et al. Immunologic and clinical effects of antibody blockade of cytotoxic T lymphocyte-associated antigen 4 in previously vaccinated cancer patients. Proc Natl Acad Sci U S A 2008;105:3005–10.

106. Heimberger AB, Hussain SF, Aldape K, et al. Tumor-specific peptide vaccination in newly-diagnosed patients with GBM. J Clin Oncol 2006;24. Part 1.

107. Sampson JH, Aldape KD, Gilbert MR, et al. Temozolomide as a vaccine adjuvant in GBM. J Clin Oncol 2007;25(Suppl):18S.

108. Engert A, Diehl V, Schnell R, et al. A phase-I study of an anti-CD25 ricin A-chain immunotoxin (RFT5-SMPT-dgA) in patients with refractory Hodgkin's lymphoma. Blood 1997;89:403–10.

109. Schnell R, Vitetta E, Schindler J, et al. Clinical trials with an anti-CD25 ricin A-chain experimental and immunotoxin (RFT5-SMPT-dgA) in Hodgkin's lymphoma. Leuk Lymphoma 1998;30:525–37.

110. Kreitman RJ, Wilson WH, Robbins D, et al. Responses in refractory hairy cell leukemia to a recombinant immunotoxin. Blood 1999;94:3340–8.

111. Schnell R, Vitetta E, Schindler J, et al. Treatment of refractory Hodgkin's lymphoma patients with an anti-CD25 ricin A-chain immunotoxin. Leukemia 2000;14:129–35.

112. Kreitman RJ, Wilson WH, White JD, et al. Phase I trial of recombinant immunotoxin anti-Tac(Fv)-PE38 (LMB-2) in patients with hematologic malignancies. J Clin Oncol 2000;18:1622–36.

113. Dannull J, Su Z, Rizzieri D, et al. Enhancement of vaccine-mediated antitumor immunity in cancer patients after depletion of regulatory T cells. J Clin Invest 2005;115:3623–33.

114. Dang NH, Hagemeister FB, Pro B, et al. Phase II study of denileukin diftitox for relapsed/refractory B-Cell non-Hodgkin's lymphoma. J Clin Oncol 2004;22:4095–102.

115. Miescher S, Whiteside TL, de Tribolet N, et al. In situ characterization, clonogenic potential, and antitumor cytolytic activity of T lymphocytes infiltrating human brain cancers. J Neurosurg 1988;68:438–48.

116. Fontana A, Hengartner H, de Tribolet N, et al. Glioblastoma cells release interleukin 1 and factors inhibiting interleukin 2-mediated effects. J Immunol 1984;132:1837–44.

117. Roszman TL, Brooks WH, Elliott LH. Inhibition of lymphocyte responsiveness by a glial tumor cell-derived suppressive factor. J Neurosurg 1987;67:874–9.

118. Meng Y, Carpentier AF, Chen L, et al. Successful combination of local CpG-ODN and radiotherapy in malignant glioma. Int J Cancer 2005;116:992–7.

119. Peng G, Guo Z, Kiniwa Y, et al. Toll-like receptor 8-mediated reversal of CD4+ regulatory T cell function. Science 2005;309:1380–4.

120. Grauer OM, Molling JW, Bennink E, et al. TLR ligands in the local treatment of established intracerebral murine gliomas. J Immunol 2008;181:6720–9.

121. Hoyne GF, Le Roux I, Corsin-Jimenez M, et al. Serrate1-induced notch signalling regulates the decision between immunity and tolerance made by peripheral CD4(+) T cells. Int Immunol 2000;12:177–85.

122. Kinjyo I, Inoue H, Hamano S, et al. Loss of SOCS3 in T helper cells resulted in reduced immune responses and hyperproduction of interleukin 10 and transforming growth factor-beta 1. J Exp Med 2006;203:1021–31.

123. Zorn E, Nelson EA, Mohseni M, et al. IL-2 regulates FOXP3 expression in human CD4+CD25+ regulatory T cells through a STAT-dependent mechanism and induces the expansion of these cells in vivo. Blood 2006;108:1571–9.

124. Kortylewski M, Kujawski M, Wang T, et al. Inhibiting Stat3 signaling in the hematopoietic system elicits multicomponent antitumor immunity. Nat Med 2005;11:1314–21.

# Dendritic Cell Vaccines for Brain Tumors

Won Kim, MD, Linda M. Liau, MD, PhD*

**KEYWORDS**

- Brain tumor • Immunotherapy • Dendritic cells
- Cancer vaccines

Dendritic cells (DC) have long been regarded as the most potent antigen-presenting cells within the immune system. Their ability to sample environmental antigens and stimulate T-cell activity in a major histocompatibility complex (MHC)–restricted manner has attracted much attention given the poor antigen-presenting ability and immunogenicity of tumor cells.[1,2] Although DCs constitute approximately 0.3% of all circulating blood leukocytes, they serve as the sentinels of the immune system and are found nearly ubiquitously throughout the body.[3] In their immature state, DCs are highly specialized antigen samplers capable of surveying their microenvironment through several mechanisms including engulfment, macropinocytosis, and receptor-mediated endocytosis.[3] On encountering an antigen the DC processes it through MHC pathways and directs it to the cell surface to form an MHC-peptide complex (**Fig. 1**). In line with traditional antigen presentation following uptake from the environment, many antigens are channeled through MHC-class II pathways with resultant MHC-peptide complexes being capable of stimulating CD4+ T cells. In addition, DC possesses the unique ability to "cross-present" acquired antigens. In this process, DC endosomes release captured antigenic material into the cytosol where it is broken down by proteasomes.[4] The degraded peptides are then transported to the endoplasmic reticulum by a transporter-associated protein and bound to MHC-class I molecules for presentation to CD8+ T cells.[5,6] These distinct mechanisms allow DCs to stimulate T cells in an MHC-class I and II manner, overcoming classical restrictions in antigen processing and presentation[7] and diversifying the resultant immune response.

DCs are capable of handling a vast range of antigenic mediums. The sources of antigen that have been used in DC immunotherapy include exogenous MHC-restricted peptides, acid-eluted tumor peptides, tumor RNA and cDNA, viral vectors, apoptotic tumor cells, tumor cell lysate, and whole tumor cells. Many of these methods have been used with varying degrees of success. A growing sentiment has emerged, however, which argues for the use of a diverse range of antigens that cover both MHC classes rather than constructing specific MHC-matched peptides. The reasoning for this is multifold. First, stimulating T cells with a broad range of antigens reduces the likelihood of an escape phenomenon in which tumor cells lacking the specific antigens of interest avoid immune detection and continue to grow unhindered. Second, it is now well established that the stimulation of both CD4+ and CD8+ T cells is crucial in the activation and maintenance of antitumor immunity.[7–10] By allowing DCs to present and cross-present antigens on MHC-class II and I molecules, respectively, one avoids having to laboriously engineer peptides for each MHC class.[9,11] Finally, the methods used to load the spectrum of antigens for a particular tumor obviate the need of characterizing each individual antigen used. Although the use of unfractionated tumor material containing unknown antigens has long raised the concern of inducing autoimmunity, particularly in the form of experimental allergic encephalomyelitis, no reports of this complication have been seen following DC vaccination in humans to date.[3]

DC vaccine is defined as DCs loaded with antigens (eg, those found on glioma), which are

UCLA Department of Neurosurgery, David Geffen School of Medicine at UCLA, 10833 Le Conte Avenue, CHS 74-145, Los Angeles, CA 90095–6901, USA
* Corresponding author.
*E-mail address:* lliau@mednet.ucla.edu (L.M. Liau).

Neurosurg Clin N Am 21 (2010) 139–157
doi:10.1016/j.nec.2009.09.005

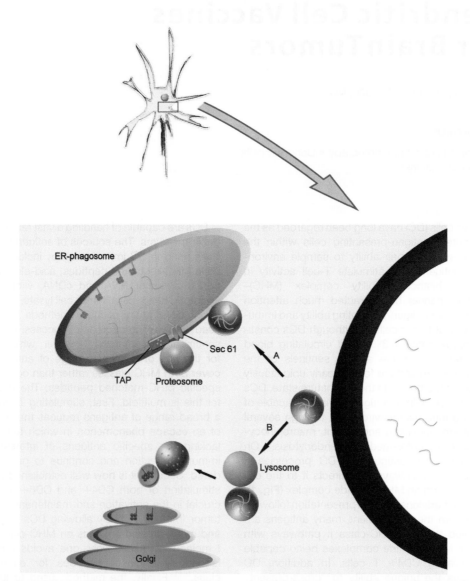

**Fig. 1.** Schematic of DC antigen processing and presentation by distinct MHC-I and MHC-II targeted pathways. Foreign antigens are sampled from the environment by dendritic cell phagocytosis or pinocytosis. Once vacuolized, antigen-containing vesicles are directed down one of two MHC pathways that result in cell surface presentation. (*A*) Antigen-containing vesicle encounters endoplasmic reticulum (ER)-phagosome. Antigen is retro-translocated into the cytoplasm by Sec 61 where proteosome complexes mediate peptide degradation. The resultant epitopes are translocated back into the ER-phagosome by the transporter-associated protein (TAP), where they are loaded onto MHC-I complexes and extruded for membrane integration and antigen presentation on the cell surface. (*B*) Antigen-containing vesicle encounters lysosome, which cleaves peptides using acid proteases. MHC-II complexes formed within the ER and subsequently processed and extruded from the Golgi apparatus are transported to peptide-containing endosomes for antigen loading.

administered to patients to induce an antigen-specific T-cell mediated antitumor response.[12] Although immature DC are not functionally ideal for the loading of antigens, they are unable to activate lymphocytes until an inflammatory signal or pathogen induces their maturation.[3,9,11] Some groups argue that ex vivo maturation of DCs through CD40L or interferon (IFN)-$\gamma$[13] is necessary

before vaccine administration to ensure proper antigen presentation and T-cell activation.[14–17] Others maintain that maturation occurs naturally, and that no prior stimulus is required.[18] In the process of maturation, DCs lose their ability to uptake and process antigens. Moreover, they exchange their immature molecular signature for a mature (CD83+) phenotype, increasing expression of MHC-antigen complexes, lymphocyte costimulatory molecules (eg, CD80/B7-1 and CD86/B7-2), tumor necrosis factor and tumor necrosis factor receptor molecules (eg, CD40), and many chemokines and chemokine receptors (eg, interleukin [IL]-12, -15, -18) to aid in T-cell recruitment and DC navigation to lymphoid tissues (as reviewed by Steinman and Dhodapkar[11] and Soling and Rainov[9]).

On localization to lymph organs rich in naive T cells, mature DCs present their processed antigens in a MHC-restricted manner. Through various interactions they are able to mobilize many different arms of the immune system, including CD8+ cytotoxic T cells (CTLs), CD4+ helper T cells, natural killer (NK) cells, and NK-like

T cells.[11] Each of these cell types plays an essential role in the antitumor response (**Fig. 2**). T cells expressing CD8 coreceptors recognize and lyse tumor cells in an MHC-class I restricted fashion, and have received much of the credit as the primary effector cell in immunotherapy. CD4+ T cells have traditionally been known for their part in the expansion and maintenance of CD8+ CTLs, secretion of stimulatory cytokines, and the induction of lasting immunity. Their critical role in immunotherapy has become increasingly appreciated over the past few years, as studies have demonstrated that their absence may result in deficient DC maturation and CTL tolerance.[7,8] Finally, NK and NK-like T cells have a unique niche in the leukocyte armament, being able to

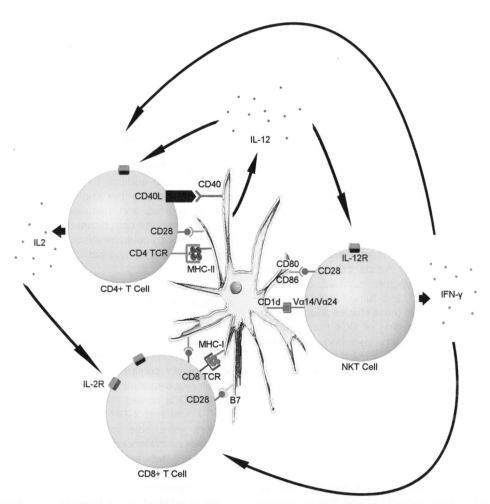

**Fig. 2.** Diagram depicting the multiple DC-lymphocyte interactions that take place in the immune cascade following antigen processing and presentation by DCs. DC activation of NK T cells through self ligands (not shown) and IL-12 results in IFN-γ release and subsequent activation of CD4+ and CD8+ T cells. CD4 and CD8 T cell receptors (TCR) interact with peptide-MHC II and I complexes, respectively. CD40L-CD40 interactions between CD4+ T cells and a DC and CD28-B7 interactions between CD8+ T cells and a DC are critical costimulatory interactions that must occur for appropriate T-cell signaling and immune responsiveness.

recognize and kill tumor cells that do not express surface markers, such as MHC-class I. Although the exact mechanism of recognition and elimination of tumor cells in the absence of MHC-restriction is yet to be elucidated, they serve as an important complement in the killing of tumor cells that may possess diminished surface marker presentation and avoid CTL detection.[3,11]

## ANIMAL MODELS

Preclinical animal models explored many of the methodologies and safety concerns regarding DC vaccines. In the late 1990s, Liau and colleagues were among the first to describe the effectiveness of DC vaccines in the antitumor immunity of gliomas using a rat model.[19] Over the past decade, many groups have published similar studies with varying permutations in the choice of antigen, timing of vaccinations, and measures of therapeutic efficacy. The dissimilarities between study designs make it difficult to compare methodologies and their associated outcomes. Their value, however, lies within their ability to demonstrate the effectiveness of multiple different DC vaccine techniques in inducing antigen-specific cytotoxicity in vitro and in vivo. These studies have shown improved survival outcomes and the safety of the strategy.

Many of the initial animal studies were key in evaluating the effectiveness of DC vaccination techniques for tumors located in the "immunologically privileged" central nervous system (CNS). Antigen sources used included synthetic peptides[20,21]; acid-eluted tumor peptides[19]; tumor lysate[21–26]; DC-tumor fusion cells (FCs)[27]; and antigen-containing vectors, such as cDNA-RNA carrying viruses[28,29] and tumor extract carrying liposomes.[30] Many of these studies adopted strategies for antigen loading of DCs from previous experiments in peripheral neoplasms and initial treatment schedules were similarly based on regimens that showed promise in non-CNS immunotherapy.[19] Nevertheless, the timing of DC administration variedly widely, with vaccinations being given before tumor inoculation,[22,24,26–28] simultaneously with,[21,23,25] or some time following tumor implantation.[19,24,27,28,30] The number of vaccinations ranged from two to five times across the various studies.

Overall, most groups concluded that vaccination with antigen-pulsed DC was able to produce a significant antitumor immune response. This was evidenced by increased overall survival in rats and mice; greater degrees of T-cell infiltration (primarily CD8+) on histologic analysis of tumors; and more robust antitumor cytotoxicity assays

when splenocytes were incubated with mouse glioma in vitro in immune responders. Although the studies conceded that pretumor vaccination resulted in greater survival in animal models, there are conflicting reports regarding the efficacy of DC vaccines when administered simultaneously or following tumor implantation.[21–25] Groups reporting no improvement in survival with DC vaccination after an established tumor suggest that it may be caused by the immune system failing to generate an appropriate response quickly enough to counteract a rapidly growing tumor within a confined cranium.[21,24] Studies in which T cell–mediated tumor killing was achieved showed, however, that the animals that did respond to DC vaccination obtained lasting antitumor memory, with significantly improved survival following tumor rechallenge compared with unvaccinated controls.[21,22,26]

These animal studies played an important role in alleviating some of the concerns regarding DC immunotherapy for CNS tumors. Experimental allergic encephalomyelitis in particular was perhaps one of the most feared side effects, because previous studies have shown this lethal form of autoimmunity to occur following the injection of glioblastoma tissue into animals.[31] Such signs of autoimmunity were not reported, however, in the more recent studies conducted to date.[21,22] In addition to the information they provided regarding the applicability of different antigen sources and treatment schedules, the preclinical reports corroborated the idea that DC immunotherapy could be effectively used for intracranial neoplasms, and set the stage for further clinical studies.

## CLINICAL TRIALS

In 2000, Liau and colleagues published a case report on the first brain tumor patient to be treated with DC-based immunotherapy.[32] A patient with histologically confirmed glioblastoma multiforme (GBM) received three biweekly intradermal injections of DCs pulsed with acid-eluted, allogeneic MHC-I matched GBM peptides. Although the authors were able to appreciate an immune response as evidenced by an increased infiltration of CD3+ T cells in postvaccination tumor, there was no objective clinical response from the treatment. The patient's poor Karnofsky performance score in addition to the possible lack of antigen homology between the allogeneic GBM and the patient's tumor may have contributed to the lack of clinical response or prolonged survival.

In a phase I dose-escalation clinical trial, 12 GBM patients were treated using DCs pulsed with autologous acid-eluted MHC tumor peptides in a dose-escalation study.[33] Patients were separated into three cohorts, each receiving 1, 5, or $10 \times 10^6$ DCs per injection. Subjects tolerated the procedure well with no signs of autoimmunity. There were only minimal grade I toxicities related to the study vaccine, which were distributed similarly across all three dose groups. Although this study was not powered to measure efficacy, patients undergoing DC-based immunotherapy seemed to have an increased median time to progression (TTP) (15.5 months) and overall survival (23.4 months) compared with historical controls. Of note, tumor burden and disease progression at the time of vaccination was a critical determinant of systemic CTL activity, tumor infiltration by T cells, and overall survival. All patients who generated a systemic CTL response showed no MRI evidence of progressive disease at the time of vaccination. Conversely, no patient with actively progressive disease developed statistically significant cytotoxicity. Moreover, only patients possessing minimal tumor burden at the time of vaccination were found to have tumor-infiltrating lymphocytes (TILs) on postvaccination tissue examination. These findings suggest that active tumor progression or bulky residual burden can debilitate the initiation and propagation of an antitumor response. Interestingly, expression of the inhibitory cytokine transforming growth factor-β2 (TGF-β2) was found to be inversely proportional to the number of TILs found in tumor tissue following vaccination (IL-10 was not), implicating TGF-β2 as a possible mediator of immune evasion following vaccination. This study argues for the need for maximal resection or minimal residual disease to improve the efficacy of DC-mediated immunotherapy for glioma. Importantly, this clinical trial established the feasibility, safety, and immunologic potential of DC vaccines for brain tumor patients.

Yu and colleagues[34] reported another phase I clinical trial using DC pulsed with autologous, acid-eluted peptides for glioma patients. In this study, nine patients with newly diagnosed malignant glioma received three biweekly subcutaneous injections of DCs loaded with acid-eluted tumor peptide. Systemic antitumor cytotoxicty was detected in four of the seven patients assessed; intratumoral CD8+ CTL and CD45RO+ memory T-cell infiltration was found in two of the four patients who underwent a second resection because of tumor progression. Patients receiving DC vaccination were found to have an increased median survival (455 days) compared with that of those in the control group (257 days).

Kikuchi and colleagues[35] used DC-glioma FCs to vaccinate glioma patients in their phase I clinical trial. Eight patients with malignant gliomas received FCs intradermally every 3 weeks, with the total number of injections ranging from one to nine. An increased percentage of NK cells were found on FACS analysis in the peripheral blood of patients. In addition, an increase in IFN-γ release in peripheral blood mononuclear cells (PBMC) tumor coincubation with both autologous and allogeneic glioma was seen following DC vaccination. Two patients experienced a minor response and no serious side effects were observed. These findings suggested that nonspecific antitumor cytotoxicity may play a role in the DC-based immunotherapy of glioma.

Kobayashi and colleagues[36] vaccinated five patients with autologous glioma RNA-pulsed DCs. They were able to demonstrate the presence of a strong CD8+ CTL response against autologous glioma accompanied by a weaker NK cell–mediated cytotoxicity in their patients. This finding was significant in three of the five patients treated. Notably, in the two patients with minimal immune responses, a constitutively increased expression of the inhibitory cytokine IL-10 and decreased expression of IFN-γ by CD8+ T cells was found in vitro.

Yamanaka and colleagues[37,38] compared different routes of DC injection in their phase I-II clinical trial of 10 patients. DCs were pulsed with autologous tumor lysate and administered to patients intradermally (N = 5) or both intradermally and intratumorally by an Ommaya (N = 5) reservoir every 3 weeks for a total number of injections ranging from 1 to 10. Immunologically, they observed an increased percentage of NK cells and increased T cell–mediated antitumor activity. In addition, there was an increased intratumoral infiltration of CD4+ and CD8+ T cells in the two patients who underwent reoperation following vaccination. Radiographically, the two minor responses seen were in patients included in the combined intradermal-intratumoral administration group, suggesting that the additional intratumorally injected DCs may stimulate a more efficient antitumor immune response.

Wheeler and colleagues[39] published a report examining the correlation between thymic function, as manifest through CD8+ recent thymic emigrant production, age, and patient outcome in 17 GBM patients undergoing DC immunotherapy. They found that thymic function, as reflected by its ability to produce CD8+ T cells, was directly proportional to good clinical outcomes in mice and human GBM patients and inversely proportional to age. Although patient age has long been a predictor of mortality and prognosis, their findings suggest that it is actually thymic function, which is inversely correlated with age, which may be the more telling factor. This nonspecific immune parameter may later serve as an important prognosticator in glioma immunotherapy.

Caruso and colleagues[40] conducted a phase I study of nine pediatric brain tumor patients undergoing immunotherapy by autologous tumor RNA pulsed DCs. The cohort was comprised of a wide range of different tumor histologies (**Table 1**). Although they detected a modest increase in antitumor antibodies in some patients, they did not appreciate any increase in T cell–mediated antitumor immunity. This may be explained by their findings that their patients had impaired immunocompetency before the start of the trial. Despite this, they reported clinical responses in three patients during the course of their study.

De Vleeschouwer and colleagues[17] explored the possibility of assessing immunotherapeutic progress through the use of MRI and methionine positron emission tomography. By monitoring contrast-enhancement changes in relation to metabolic uptake ratios they could postulate at which point an immune response had occurred. This group published the findings from their phase I clinical trial of 12 recurrent malignant glioma patients who were vaccinated with tumor lysate-pulsed DC.[16] Interestingly, they were the first to induce DC maturation ex vivo for glioma immunotherapy based on recent evidence arguing that the injection of mature DCs may mediate a more potent antitumor response.[45,46] The extent of resection stressed in this study as prolonged disease-free survival was only achieved in two patients who underwent gross total resection (GTR) before vaccination. Moreover, one patient who received only partial tumor resection suffered grade IV neurotoxicity (National Cancer Institute common toxicity criteria) secondary to vaccination-induced peritumoral edema. As such, they argue that maximal resection may help avoid such dangerous complications during CNS immunotherapy. Akin to the authors' conclusions,[33] this study further champions the need for maximal resection to improve the potential efficacy of vaccination strategies for malignant gliomas.

In a phase I-II study of tumor lysate-loaded DC vaccination for malignant glioma, subcutaneous injections of DCs loaded with tumor lysate were administered biweekly for a total of three injections.[41] Elevated IFN-$\gamma$ mRNA levels in PBMCs, positive cytotoxicity assays, increased peripheral CD8+ CTLs, and increased infiltration of CD45RO+ memory and CD8+ T cells in progressive tumor corroborated a positive immune response. Additionally, this study reported an increased median survival in patients receiving vaccinations (133 weeks) compared with historical controls (30 weeks), further substantiating the viability of DC immunotherapy for glioma.

After their initial phase I clinical trial, Kikuchi and colleagues[42] continued their work with human patients through a phase I-II series modeled after their animal studies involving DC-glioma FC injection with perivaccination IL-12.[27] Fifteen patients were vaccinated intradermally with FCs on a biweekly basis for a total of three injects per course, with IL-12 administration on days 2 and 5 following each injection. IL-12 was given because it had been shown to enhance the antitumor effects of FCs in mouse models. Similarly, they found that treatment efficacy using FC–IL-12 vaccination in human patients was better than FCs alone. Although, they were able to demonstrate cellular antitumor immunity in only a few of their patients, they observed much improved clinical outcomes, including four partial responses and one mixed response as determined by imaging. Patients tolerated the treatment regimen well and there were no reported signs of autoimmunity despite the use of systemic IL-12.

Walker and colleagues[43] investigated the interaction between chemotherapy and DC vaccines in their phase I clinical trial. Thirteen patients with malignant glioma were treated with six biweekly injections (and every 6 weeks thereafter) of DCs pulsed with autologous irradiated tumor cells. Immunologically, they were able to appreciate an antitumor response by the presence of increased cytotoxic and memory T cells on postvaccination resected tumor. Of the eight patients who received adjuvant chemotherapy in addition to immunotherapy, five were reported to show objective radiologic response to treatment, including one patient who had a complete response. This mirrors findings by Wheeler and colleagues,[47] who through retrospective analysis determined that patients who received chemotherapy following DC immunotherapy did better in terms of overall survival and time to recurrence than patients who received either one alone. Although it was previously believed that chemotherapy and immunotherapy were antagonistic forms of treatment,[48] this and other studies have added to the accumulating evidence that these two therapies may be synergistic in nature.

In a recent paper, De Vleeschouwer and colleagues[14] published an update of their work on DC immunotherapy for brain tumors, including 56 patients with recurrent glioblastoma. Patients received intradermal injections of mature DCs pulsed with autologous tumor lysate according to three vaccination schedules that varied in regards to frequency of injections and the presence or absence of tumor lysate boosts (see **Table 1**). In addition, delayed-type hypersensitivity (DTH) was assessed in 21 patients from whom enough tumor material could be removed for appropriate testing. The treatment regimens were well-tolerated with the exception of one patient who developed vaccination-induced grade IV neurotoxicity as was mentioned in their previous study[16] and two patients who experienced grade II transient hematotoxicity. Analysis of patient survival and TTP revealed that GTR before vaccination was the only independent predictor of progression-free survival. Younger age (<35) and GTR were predictive of better overall survival, however, only in univariable analyses. Although it did not reach statistical significance, the regimen that included frequent vaccinations with tumor lysate boosting seemed to have improved progression-free survival. Interestingly, DTH reactivity was not shown to have any correlation with clinical outcome.

Recently, Wheeler and colleagues[44] reported on their phase II trial in which they treated 34 patients with new or recurrent glioblastoma. Patients received a total of four subcutaneous injections of autologous tumor lysate-pulsed DCs on weeks 0, 2, 4, and 10. Primary outcomes of interest were TTP and time to survival. Immunologic responses were quantified through measuring the differential expression of IFN-$\gamma$ mRNA in lysate pulsed DCs expanded from PBMCs collected before and after vaccination. Using normalized IFN-$\gamma$ production values as previously reported,[49] 17 of the 31 patients tested showed a positive vaccine response ($\geq$1.5-fold expression) after three vaccinations (responders). The magnitude of increased IFN-$\gamma$ expression correlated logarithmically with time to survival, however, only in vaccine responders. This finding was striking in that it was the first immunologic predictor of immunotherapy outcome to achieve statistical significance, likely because of the large number of vaccine responders in this trial. Clinically, vaccine responders had significantly longer time to survival (642 $\pm$ 61 days) compared with nonresponders (430 $\pm$ 50 days). Moreover, disease-free progression in vaccine responders was improved by 4.5 months, with responders and nonresponders having TTPs of 308 $\pm$ 55 days and 167 $\pm$ 22 days, respectively. It should be noted that these trends were not significant in patients with recurrent glioblastoma, only in those with newly diagnosed tumors. Finally, it was found that patients in this study experienced a 186- to 190-day increase in TTP when the course of DC injections was followed by adjuvant chemotherapy, compared with DC therapy alone. This treatment effect was observed indiscriminately between responders and nonresponders, with differences only appreciable when comparing patients with fivefold IFN-$\gamma$ increase with all others. These findings supported recent data suggesting that chemotherapy may possibly potentiate the clinical effects of DC-based immunotherapy.[47,48]

## CURRENT STATUS OF DC VACCINES FOR BRAIN TUMORS
### Safety

DC immunotherapy for brain tumors, throughout the 16 different clinical trials and over 200 patients treated to date, seems to be well tolerated across all variations in treatment protocols. A notable exception was one patient who experienced a grade IV neurotoxicity following DC administration, which was believed to be caused by peritumoral edema from the gross residual tumor.[14] Another patient, interestingly, developed a subcutaneous glioblastoma with single lymph node involvement following DTH testing.[41] Despite these outliers, most groups have predominantly reported grade I and II toxicities in response to DC vaccine administration, with no treatment-associated deaths or permanent neurologic defects. The most common reason for discontinuing DC-immunotherapy was tumor recurrence or progression, as is the case with any other treatment modality for glioblastoma. Overall, the relative lack of serious adverse effects supports the safety of DC-based immunotherapies when used in the management of brain tumor patients.

### Measures of Outcome

One of the major criticisms of immunotherapy has been the lack of evidence supporting its objective clinical benefit (by MRI response criteria) despite the numerous studies that have validated its immunologic antitumor response.[50] This assertion was posed while evaluating clinical outcomes of immunotherapy using antiquated imaging criteria, however, which many now argue may not be an appropriate means of assessment in the presence of improved imaging technologies and greater emphasis on disease control and stability, quality of life, and overall survival.[43,51,52] Moreover, although systemic evidence of antitumor responses following DC immunotherapy has been demonstrated on many occasions both in vitro and in vivo, its correlation with actual tumor lysis in human patients is inconsistent at best.

Several groups have tried to determine an immunologic correlate of clinical efficacy in their

**Table 1**
Summary of phase I and II clinical trials of DC vaccination for CNS tumors

| Series | Number of Patients (Type of Trial) | Tumor Characteristics | Antigen Source | Dendritic Cell Characteristics | Immunologic Response | Clinical Response | Toxicity |
|---|---|---|---|---|---|---|---|
| Liau et al (2000)[32] | 1 (case report) | Recurrent GBM (N = 1) | Acid-eluted allogeneic MHC-I matched GBM | PBMCs differentiated with GM-CSF and IL-4; three biweekly i.d. injections | In vitro T-cell proliferative response against allogenic tumor peptides | None | None |
| Yu et al (2001)[34] | 9 (phase I) | AA (N = 2) and GBM (N = 7) | Autologous acid-eluted tumor peptides | PBMCs differentiated with GM-CSF and IL-4; three biweekly s.c. injections | JAM assay: systemic T-cell mediated cytotoxicity against tumor (N = 4 of 7 tested) IHC: increased infiltration of CD8+ and CD45RO+ T cells in tumor following vaccination (N = 2 of 4) | Increased median survival time compared with controls (455 d vs 257 d) | Mild transient fever, nausea and vomiting (N = 1), generalized lymphadenopathy (N = 1) |
| Kikuchi et al (2001)[35] | 8[a] (phase I) | AA (N = 3) and GBM (N = 5) | Autologous DC-tumor fusion cells | PBMCs differentiated with GM-CSF, IL-4, and TNF-$\alpha$; one to nine injections i.d. every 3 wk | FACS assay: increased percentage of NK cells (N = 4 of 5 tested) ELISA: increased PBMC IFN-$\gamma$ release with autologous and allogeneic tumor (N = 6 of 6 tested) | Minor response (N = 2) (A) resolution of intractable headache (B) improved hemiparesis | Erythema at injection site (N = 1) |
| Kobayashi et al (2003)[36] | 5 | GBM (N = 5) | GFP transfected autologous tumor RNA with cationic lipid | PBMCs differentiated with GM-CSF and IL-4 | In vitro cytotoxicity against tumor by CD8+ (major) and NK-like T cells (minor) (significant in N = 3; minimal in N = 2) ELISA: increased IL-10 and decreased IFN-$\gamma$ production by CD8+ T cells in patients with minimal CD8 cytotoxicity | Not reported | None |

| | | | | Immune response | Clinical response | Toxicity |
|---|---|---|---|---|---|---|
| Yamanaka et al (2003)[37] | 10 (phase I and II) | AA (N = 3) or GBM (N = 7) | Autologous tumor lysate (with KLH) | PBMCs differentiated with GM-CSF and IL-4; one to ten injections i.d. (N = 5) or i.d and i.t. (N = 5), once every 3 wk | FACS assay: increased percentage of NK cells (N = 5 of 5 tested) and CD8, CD16-, and CD19-positive T cells (N = 4 of 5 tested) DTH: positive reaction to tumor lysate (N = 3 of 6 tested); ELISPOT: increased T-cell mediated antitumor activity (N = 2 of 5 tested) IHC: increased infiltration of CD4+ and CD8+ T cells in patients undergoing reoperation for tumor progression (N = 2 of 2) | Minor response (N = 2) (A) decreased contrast-enhancing portion of lesion (B) improvement in convulsions and decrease in contrast-enhancing portion of lesion | Mild headache (N = 1); erythema at injection site (N = 2) |
| Wheeler et al (2003)[39] | 17 (phase I and II) | New or recurrent GBM | Autologous tumor lysate | PBMCs differentiated with GM-CSF and IL-4; three injections s.c. biweekly (a fourth 6 wk after third in phase II patients) | Not reported; trial conducted to study the relationship between CD8+ recent thymic emigrants and survival | | |
| Caruso et al (2004)[40] | 9[a] (phase I) | PA (N = 1), AA (N = 1), GBM (N = 2), medulloblastomas (N = 1), ependymomas (N = 3), and pleomorphic xanthoastrocytomas (N = 1) | Autologous tumor RNA | PBMCs differentiated with GM-CSF and IL-4; zero to five injections i.v. and i.d. biweekly | ELISA: modest increase in specific antitumor antibodies (N = 2 of 5 tested) IFN-γ–producing assays: no significant antitumor response (N = 4 of 4 tested) T-cell proliferation assay: no significant antitumor response (N = 3 of 3 tested) | Tumor free, stable disease at 21, 6, and 2 mo follow-up (N = 3 of 7 treated) | None |

*(continued on next page)*

**Table 1** (*continued*)

| Series | Number of Patients (Type of Trial) | Tumor Characteristics | Antigen Source | Dendritic Cell Characteristics | Immunologic Response | Clinical Response | Toxicity |
|---|---|---|---|---|---|---|---|
| de Vleeschouwer et al (2004)[17] | 1[a] (case report) | Postradiation AA (N = 1) | Autologous tumor lysate | PBMCs differentiated with GM-CSF and IL-4; DCs matured with TNF-$\alpha$, IL-1$\beta$, and PGE$_2$; six injections i.d. first two every 2 wk, then every mo thereafter | DTH: positive reaction to tumor lysate (N = 1) MRI: transient contrast enhancement after fifth vaccine MET-PET: transient increased metabolic uptake around resection cavity | Tumor-free survival (60 mo following first vaccination) | None |
| Yu et al (2004)[41] | 14 (phase I and II) | Recurrent AA (N = 3) or GBM (N = 9) and new AA (N = 1) or GBM (N = 1) | Autologous tumor lysate | PBMCs differentiated with GM-CSF and IL-4; three injections s.c., biweekly | qPCR: IFN-$\gamma$ mRNA accumulation in PBMC (N = 6 of 10 tested) JAM assay: systemic T cell mediated antitumor cytotoxicity (N = 1 of 1 tested) Tetramer staining: increase in CD8+ antigen-specific T-cell clones (N = 4 of 9 tested) IHC: CD45RO+ memory T cells and CD8+ CTLs in resected progressive tumor (N = 3 of 6) | Increased median survival compared with controls (133 vs 30 wk, respectively) | Transient headache (N = 3), erythema at the injection site (N = 1), generalized seizures (N = 2) |
| Rutkowski et al (2004)[16] | 12[a] (phase I) | AA (N = 4) and GBM (N = 8) | Autologous tumor lysate | PBMCs differentiated with GM-CSF and IL-4; DCs matured with TNF-$\alpha$, IL-1$\beta$, and PGE$_2$; two to seven injections i.d., first two separated by 2 wk, then monthly thereafter | DTH: positive response to tumor lysate (N = 6 of 8 tested) | Following STR: stable disease (N = 1 of 6), partial response (N = 1 of 6) Following GTR: continuous complete remission 5 y after DC vaccine (N = 2 of 6) | Reversible grade IV neurologic deficits and lethargy (N = 1), grade II hematotoxicity (N = 2), transiently increased morning stiffness (N = 1), night sweats (N = 1), meningismus (N = 1) |

| Kikuchi et al (2004)[42] | 15 (phase I and II) AA (N = 9) and GBM (N = 6) | Autologous DC-tumor fusion cells | PBMCs differentiated with GM-CSF, IL-4, and TNF-α, three to nine injections i.d., once every 2 wk; systemic IL-12 given 2 and 5 d after each FC injection | FACS analysis: percentage of cell types did not change significantly (N = 7 of 7 tested) $^{51}$Cr release assay: increased cytotoxic activity (N = 2 of 8) Intracellular ELISA (CD8+ T cells): increased IFN-γ (N = 1 of 7) IHC: Robust infiltration CD8+ CTLs in patients undergoing reoperation for tumor progression (N = 2) | MRI/CT: Partial response (N = 4 of 15); mixed response (N = 1 of 15); stable disease (N = 2 of 15) | Transient grade I fever (N = 4), generalized convulsions (N = 1), erythema at injection site (N = 13), transient liver dysfunction (N = 6), leukocytopenia (N = 7) |
| Yamanaka et al (2005)[15] | 24 (phase I and II) Recurrent AA (N = 6) and GBM (N = 18) | Autologous tumor lysate (±KLH) | PBMCs differentiated with GM-CSF and IL-4; ±OK-432 for DC maturation (phase II); 1–22 injections i.d. or i.t. (by Ommaya) every 3 wk; immature DCs (phase I) and both immature and mature DCs (phase II) | DTH: Positive response to tumor lysate (N = 8 of 17 tested) ELISPOT assay: tumor-specific CTLs increased (N = 7 of 16) | MRI/CT: partial response (N = 1); minor response (N = 3); no change (N = 10); significantly increased median survival (480 vs 400 d) | Mild headache (N = 1); mild erythema at cervical injection site (N = 7) |

(continued on next page)

**Table 1**
*(continued)*

| Series | Number of Patients (Type of Trial) | Tumor Characteristics | Antigen Source | Dendritic Cell Characteristics | Immunologic Response | Clinical Response | Toxicity |
|---|---|---|---|---|---|---|---|
| Liau et al (2005)[33] | 12 (phase I) | New (N = 7) or recurrent (N = 5) GBM | Acid-eluted autologous tumor peptides | PBMCs differentiated with GM-CSF and IL-4; 3 injections i.d., once every 2–4 wk; dose escalation | Alamar blue CTL assay: systemic tumor specific CTL (N = 6 of 6 tested) IHC: CD8+/CD45RO+ memory T-cell infiltration in tumors of patients undergoing reoperation for progression who subsequently had >30 mo survival (N = 4 of 4); no increased TILs in tumors of patients undergoing reoperation who subsequently had <30 mo survival RT-PCR: lower expression of TGF$\beta_2$ in tumor of patients with detectable TILs | Partial response (N = 1); increased TTP (18.3 mo vs 8.2 mo in controls) and median survival (correlated with CTL response and minimal tumor burden) | Fever or flu-like symptoms (N = 4), nausea and vomiting (N = 3), erythema at injection site (N = 2), LAD (N = 2), fatigue (N = 5), seizures (N = 1) |
| Walker et al (2008)[43] | 13 (phase I) | AA (N = 4) and GBM (N = 9) | Irradiated tumor cells | PBMCs differentiated with GM-CSF and IL-4; 2–13 injections i.d., first six biweekly, thereafter every 6 wk | IHC: increased CD8+ and CD45RO+ T-cell infiltration in tumors of patients undergoing reoperation (N = 3 of 3) | Response to adjuvant chemotherapy: complete (N = 1 of 8 treated), partial (N = 4 of 8 treated), minimal/none (N = 3 of 8 treated) | None |

| Study | N | Tumor type | Antigen source | DC preparation and vaccination schedule | Immune response | Clinical outcome | Toxicity |
|---|---|---|---|---|---|---|---|
| de Vleeschouwer et al (2008)[14] | 56[a] | Recurrent GBM | Autologous tumor cell lysate | PBMCs differentiated with GM-CSF and IL-4; DCs matured with TNF-$\alpha$, IL-1$\beta$, and PGE$_2$; three to nine i.d. injections (A) wk 1 and 3 then every 4 wk thereafter (B) first five every 2 wk, then every 4 wk (C) four weekly; boosts with autologous tumor lysate | DTH: positive reaction to tumor lysate (N = 9 of 21 tested) before vaccination, with no correlation with survival | Significantly improved PFS in adults of cohort C; significantly improved overall survival in patients <35 y old and PFS in patients with GTR | Grade IV neurotoxicity (stupor) (N = 1), grade II hematotoxicity (N = 2), transient increase in focal neurologic signs (N = 6), headache (N = 9), vomiting (N = 2), flu-like symptoms (N = 3), increased frequency of seizures (N = 4), fatigue (N = 7), myalgias (N = 3), erythema around injection site (N = 56) |
| Wheeler et al (2008)[44] (phase II) | 34 | New (N = 11) or recurrent (N = 23) GBM | Autologous tumor lysate | PBMCs differentiated with GM-CSF and IL-4; 4 injections (three biweekly, then fourth 6 wk after third) s.c. | qPCR: progressively increased IFN-$\gamma$ after vaccinations, peaking after 3 vaccinations (significantly in 17 of 31 tested) | TTS and TTP significantly longer (but not in recurrent patients alone); TTS correlated logarithmically with postvaccine IFN-$\gamma$ response magnitudes exclusively in responders; significant increase in TTP during postvaccine chemotherapy interval compared with TTP following vaccine alone in both responders and nonresponders (N = 19) | Cutaneous GBM with single lymph node involvement at site of DTH testing |

*Abbreviations:* AA, anaplastic astrocytoma; CT, computerized tomography; CTLs, cytotoxic lymphocyte; DTH, delayed-type hypersensitivity; GBM, glioblastoma multiforme; GFP, green fluorescent protein; GM-CSF, granulocyte-macrophage colony–stimulating factor; GTR, gross total resection; IFN, interferon; IHC, immunohistochemistry; IL, interleukin; KLH, keyhole limpet hemocyanin; MRI, magnetic resonance imaging; PA, pilocytic astrocytoma; PBMCs, peripheral blood mononuclear cells; PFS, progression-free survival; PGE, prostaglandin E; TNF, tumor necrosis factor; TTP, time to progression; TTS, time to survival.

[a] Study includes pediatric patients.

phase I-II studies, including such measures as DTH,[14–16] the presence of TILs,[33,34,41–43] and antitumor immunity in vitro from systemic CTLs.[15,32–34,36,37,41] Results have been mixed, particularly with DTH, which was only shown to be predictive of improved survival in one study to date.[15] TILs in relapsed tumors and systemic antigen-specific CD8+ antitumor T cells following vaccination are ubiquitously found in patients who seem to respond to immunotherapy; however, they are not prognostically predictive because many nonresponders also present with such cells. It is thought that the microenvironment of the tumor itself, correlated with immunosuppressive cytokine release (eg, TGF-β), may inhibit the exacting of actual tumor killing despite sufficient cellular immunity.[33,36] Questions regarding which biologic indices are predictive of clinical outcome continue to be elucidated as larger cohorts are investigated in multicenter phase II clinical trials for glioblastomas (eg, DCVax). Presently, TTP and overall survival remain the best measures of efficacy in DC immunotherapy.

## Methods of DC Vaccine Development and Administration

Notwithstanding a decade of use, there still remains a great degree of variability in the development and administration of DC vaccines. Only a few studies have systematically examined these differences, resulting in a lack of data regarding the most effective means through which to carry out DC-based immunotherapy for CNS neoplasms. Some of these specifics have been resolved on account of information obtained from animal models or through empiric evidence gleaned from common practice. For example, although there are several different methods through which DC may be acquired, in all of the clinical trials involving DC immunotherapy for glioma to date, they were exclusively manufactured through the differentiation of PBMCs ex vivo. There now exists many methods through which DCs can be produced efficiently and in large enough quantities for clinical trials.[53–56]

Similarly, no studies exist comparing the efficacy of different sources of antigens in propagating antitumor immunity in human patients. The vast repertoire of antigen-loading strategies includes whole tumor cells,[27,35,42] apoptotic tumor cells,[43] acid-eluted tumor peptides,[19,32–34] synthetic peptides,[20,21] tumor lysate,[14–17,21–26,38,39,41,44] and tumor cDNA-RNA.[28,36,40,57] The effectiveness of these methods in stimulating DC-mediated antitumor immunity has primarily been studied in animal models for proof-of-principle rather than

comparative analyses. Although some animal studies have evaluated the efficacy of different sources of antigens in stimulating a DC-mediated antitumor response,[21,28] the choice of antigenic stimuli in clinical trials seems largely based on previous work with preclinical models and theoretical considerations. Clearly, prior experience with a particular DC vaccination protocol allows for ready transition from bench to bedside. Theoretically, however, methods using a wide range of autologous tumor antigens have been favored over peptide selection. This allows the vaccine to target all tumor-associated antigens without requisite characterization, helping avoid clonal selection of antigen-loss variants and subsequent tumor-escape.[58] Choice of antigen must also be considered for pragmatic reasons, because poor availability of resected tumor tissue may favor the use of cDNA-RNA to pulse DCs because these antigens are readily amplified through molecular techniques.[9] Because most of the antigen sources available to immunotherapy have been shown to prime DC appropriately, however, their use may remain largely an empiric choice until future studies comparatively examining their functionality and practicality are conducted.

It is well accepted that antigen loading is most effective when pulsing phenotypically immature DC. The maturation state in which to administer DCs to patients following this step, however, remains unclear. Numerous studies have shown that DC maturation is necessary for effective DC migration[59] and T-cell stimulation,[46,60] making them more effective in generating an antitumor response.[15] Given the need for an inflammatory stimulus or cytokine to induce DC maturation, DCs have been matured ex vivo to theoretically ensure proper functioning once they reach the lymph nodes of the host.[14–17] This is supported by work by Yamanaka and colleagues[15] who found that patients receiving mature DCs experienced a greater overall survival than patients receiving immature ones. Barratt-Boyes and colleagues,[18] however, were able to demonstrate that immature antigen-pulsed DC undergo natural maturation when injected intradermally and are quite capable of stimulating appropriate antitumor T-cell pathways in vivo. Moreover, they argue that the administration of immature DCs may even be superior to that of mature DCs, because the latter have relatively decreased emigration rates from the injection site. Because clinical trials have demonstrated clinical benefit with DC regimens using both immature and mature DC, future studies comparing the two preparations are needed to further evaluate the effect maturation status has on clinical efficacy and patient survival.[61]

The frequency of DC injections in clinical trials was initially modeled after administration schedules found to be effective in immunotherapy for non-CNS tumors.[19] Since then, most studies have roughly followed a biweekly injection regimen, with number of vaccinations varying from 1 to 22 times (see **Table 1**). Given the many differences in other aspects of the vaccination protocol, it is difficult to compare the efficacy of DC administration frequency between published studies. It has been argued that vaccination should be given expediently following maximal surgical cytoreduction, chemotherapy, or radiotherapy to fully benefit from the rebound in immune function following GTR before tumor recurrence.[52] Although early initiation of DC immunotherapy is encouraged, data from animal[26] and patient[14] studies suggest early follow-up vaccinations are not as critical and may hinder the immune response by causing activation-induced death of recently activated T cells. Instead, these studies have demonstrated that booster injections with tumor lysate alone may be more beneficial in stimulating an antitumor response. Interestingly, many studies have used the testing of DTH using tumor lysate,[14–17,37,44] which may have inadvertently served as a form of booster and improved antitumor immunity. Given the lack of controlled studies addressing these issues, the timing and frequency of DC vaccine administration remains largely based on empiric experience, and requires future studies to determine an optimal schedule.

The optimal dose of DC has similarly been questioned. Even from early preclinical studies, it was evident that low inoculations of DCs could stimulate an antitumor response.[16] Dose escalation protocols in clinical trials have substantiated the finding that DC-mediated immunity is an "on-off" rather than a dose-response phenomenon, because increasing numbers of these antigen-presenting cells do not affect the magnitude of the CTL response.[14,33] This is reassuring, because large quantities of autologous tumor lysate-pulsed DC were sometimes difficult to obtain during dose escalation protocols.[33,40]

Finally, the route of DC administration best for immunotherapy is still under investigation. DCs can be administered through a variety of ways, including subcutaneous, intradermal, intralymphatic, intranodal, and intratumoral injections. Several studies in mice and nonhuman primates have examined the differences in lymph node accumulation and T-cell stimulation with each route. Radioisotope tracing studies have shown that intravenous DC administration results in the accumulation of DC within the spleen and liver. This method results in the greatest humoral antitumor response, however, as indicated by increased tumor antigen-specific antibodies.[62–65] Conversely, intradermal,[62,65] intralymphatic,[62] intracranial,[66] intranodal,[59] and subcutaneous[63] injections of DCs have been shown to drain to lymph nodes and induce greater T cell–mediated immunity against tumor antigens compared with intravenous injections in preclinical models. Much attention has been given to the intranodal or perinodal administration of DCs, because lymph nodes are acknowledged as the processing centers responsible in mediating antigen presentation and T-cell activation.[67] Some investigators have questioned how the placement of these injections may alter the potency of the immune response. Recently, Calzascia and colleagues[68] were able to show that the distance from the cervical nodes was not as critical as the location of the tumor itself. Although there was some improved tissue tropism for the CNS when DCs were administered into cervical lymph nodes, they found that the ultimate determinant of homing signals was the residence of the actual tumor, as was evidenced by CNS-tropic T cells following inguinal node DC injection in an intracranial tumor model. To date, only one clinical trial has investigated the differences in patient outcome between two injection routes. Yamanaka and colleagues[15] found that patients who received both intratumoral and intradermal DCs had prolonged survival compared with those who received intradermal DCs alone. Further studies comparing injection sites and modalities in inducing antitumor immunity are still needed.

## Patient Selection for DC Vaccines

The increasing volume of studies reporting on the clinical response to DC-based immunotherapy has allowed for the analysis of patient demographics to better determine who may benefit the most from this novel treatment modality. As with traditional therapies for malignant brain tumors, younger patients (<40 years old) receiving DC vaccines seemed to do better in terms of overall survival compared with older patients with similar tumor histologies.[44,69] Although this may in part be attributable to the general trend for younger glioma patients to have better prognoses, one particular study was able to demonstrate that this was primarily because of associated declines in thymus function with increasing age.[39] They maintained that CD8+ T-cell production from the thymus was a prognostic indicator of response to DC immunotherapy independent and super-seding that of patient age.

Another critical patient characteristic that seems to have an effect on clinical outcome is surgical management. Those patients who underwent GTR of their brain tumor experienced significantly better progression-free survival compared with otherwise similar patients with appreciable residual tumor.[14] Moreover, bulky residual tumor or active tumor recurrence at the time of vaccination seems to debilitate the antitumor CTL response.[33]

Finally, patients with newly diagnosed malignant glioma seem to achieve greater response rates than those with recurrent tumors.[44] Although these findings remain to be validated by future studies, it seems that younger patients with newly diagnosed malignant glioma that are amenable to GTR stand to benefit the most from DC-based vaccines.

### Synergy of DC Vaccines with Other Therapies

Although much progress has been made in DC-based immunotherapy for CNS tumors, objective clinical responses for vaccinated brain tumor patients remains inconsistent. Consequently, some groups have examined the use of adjuvant treatments to augment the effects of DC vaccination. These methods include adjuvant chemotherapy, cytokine administration, and toll-like receptor agonists.

The use of cytokines to supplement DC-based immunotherapy in human patients is an extension of work done in preclinical animal studies.[24,27,29] Although systemic cytokine administration has only been used in one DC vaccine clinical trial to date,[42] studies conducted in vitro and with human patients have shown that cytokines, such as IL-10,[70] IL-18,[71] and IL-23,[72] may enhance the immune response of effector cells in DC immunotherapy. Because the data regarding this adjuvant modality are scarce, further studies are needed before routine clinical use of systemic cytokines can be considered.

The use of standard treatments, such as chemotherapy to aid immunotherapy, has also been considered. Chemotherapy has traditionally been regarded as an antagonist to the treatment effects of immunotherapy, because of its effects of bone marrow suppression causing lymphopenia. There has also been a belief that the dead apoptotic tumor cells produce immune tolerance, exacerbating the lymphopenic state that results. Mounting evidence argues that these apoptotic tumor cells may provide a rich antigen source for DC and that prompt DC vaccination following chemotherapy may actually provide greater benefit than delaying treatment.[48] Recently, studies have shown that when chemotherapy is used adjuvantly with DC-based immunotherapy, patients experience prolonged overall survival and increased time to disease progression.[43,44,47] Because evidence suggests that chemotherapy in the setting of DC immunotherapy may actually be beneficial rather than obstructive, it may be prudent to further investigate multimodality treatment strategies for the simultaneous treatment of brain tumor patients.

### SUMMARY

Over the past decade, DC-based immunotherapy for CNS tumors has progressed from preclinical rodent models and safety assessments to phase I-II clinical trials in over 200 patients, which have produced measurable immunologic responses and some prolonged survival rates. Many questions regarding the methods and molecular mechanisms behind this new treatment option remain unanswered. Results from currently ongoing and future studies will help to elucidate which DC preparations, treatment protocols, and adjuvant therapeutic regimens optimize the efficacy of DC vaccination. Additionally, it is important to characterize the pathways underlying the immunosuppressive microenvironment of brain tumors that currently hinder antitumor responses. Combined with further advances in the manipulation of various lymphocyte subsets, such as regulatory T cells and NK-like T cells, in addition to the usual armament of CD4+ and CD8+ T cells, understanding these immunologic intricacies will help maximize the cellular efficiency of immunotherapeutic techniques. As clinical studies continue to report results on DC-mediated immunotherapy, it will be critical to continue refining treatment methods and developing new ways to augment this promising form of glioma treatment.

### REFERENCES

1. Mitchell DA, Fecci PE, Sampson JH. Immunotherapy of malignant brain tumors. Immunol Rev 2008;222: 70–100.
2. Aloisi F, Ria F, Adorini L. Regulation of T-cell responses by CNS antigen-presenting cells: different roles for microglia and astrocytes. Immunol Today 2000;21:141–7.
3. Parajuli P, Sloan AE. Dendritic cell-based immunotherapy of malignant gliomas. Cancer Invest 2004; 22:405–16.
4. Rodriguez A, Regnault A, Kleijmeer M, et al. Selective transport of internalized antigens to the cytosol

for MHC class I presentation in dendritic cells. Nat Cell Biol 1999;1:362–8.

5. Albert ML, Sauter B, Bhardwaj N. Dendritic cells acquire antigen from apoptotic cells and induce class I-restricted CTLs. Nature 1998;392:86–9.

6. Watts C. Capture and processing of exogenous antigens for presentation on MHC molecules. Annu Rev Immunol 1997;15:821–50.

7. Albert ML, Jegathesan M, Darnell RB. Dendritic cell maturation is required for the cross-tolerization of CD8+ T cells. Nat Immunol 2001;2:1010–7.

8. Toes RE, Ossendorp F, Offringa R, et al. CD4 T cells and their role in antitumor immune responses. J Exp Med 1999;189:753–6.

9. Soling A, Rainov NG. Dendritic cell therapy of primary brain tumors. Mol Med 2001;7:659–67.

10. Yamanaka R. Cell- and peptide-based immunotherapeutic approaches for glioma. Trends Mol Med 2008;14:228–35.

11. Steinman RM, Dhodapkar M. Active immunization against cancer with dendritic cells: the near future. Int J Cancer 2001;94:459–73.

12. Figdor CG, de Vries IJ, Lesterhuis WJ, et al. Dendritic cell immunotherapy: mapping the way. Nat Med 2004;10:475–80.

13. Tschoep K, Manning TC, Harlin H, et al. Disparate functions of immature and mature human myeloid dendritic cells: implications for dendritic cell-based vaccines. J Leukoc Biol 2003;74:69–80.

14. De Vleeschouwer S, Fieuws S, Rutkowski S, et al. Postoperative adjuvant dendritic cell-based immunotherapy in patients with relapsed glioblastoma multiforme. Clin Cancer Res 2008;14:3098–104.

15. Yamanaka R, Homma J, Yajima N, et al. Clinical evaluation of dendritic cell vaccination for patients with recurrent glioma: results of a clinical phase I/II trial. Clin Cancer Res 2005;11:4160–7.

16. Rutkowski S, De Vleeschouwer S, Kaempgen E, et al. Surgery and adjuvant dendritic cell-based tumour vaccination for patients with relapsed malignant glioma, a feasibility study. Br J Cancer 2004;91:1656–62.

17. De Vleeschouwer S, Van Calenbergh F, Demaerel P, et al. Transient local response and persistent tumor control in a child with recurrent malignant glioma: treatment with combination therapy including dendritic cell therapy. Case report. J Neurosurg 2004;100:492–7.

18. Barratt-Boyes SM, Zimmer MI, Harshyne LA, et al. Maturation and trafficking of monocyte-derived dendritic cells in monkeys: implications for dendritic cell-based vaccines. J Immunol 2000;164:2487–95.

19. Liau LM, Black KL, Prins RM, et al. Treatment of intracranial gliomas with bone marrow-derived dendritic cells pulsed with tumor antigens. J Neurosurg 1999;90:1115–24.

20. Prins RM, Odesa SK, Liau LM. Immunotherapeutic targeting of shared melanoma-associated antigens in a murine glioma model. Cancer Res 2003;63:8487–91.

21. Grauer OM, Sutmuller RP, van Maren W, et al. Elimination of regulatory T cells is essential for an effective vaccination with tumor lysate-pulsed dendritic cells in a murine glioma model. Int J Cancer 2008;122:1794–802.

22. Heimberger AB, Crotty LE, Archer GE, et al. Bone marrow-derived dendritic cells pulsed with tumor homogenate induce immunity against syngeneic intracerebral glioma. J Neuroimmunol 2000;103:16–25.

23. Ni HT, Spellman SR, Jean WC, et al. Immunization with dendritic cells pulsed with tumor extract increases survival of mice bearing intracranial gliomas. J Neurooncol 2001;51:1–9.

24. Kim HS, Choo YS, Koo T, et al. Enhancement of antitumor immunity of dendritic cells pulsed with heat-treated tumor lysate in murine pancreatic cancer. Immunol Lett 2006;103:142–8.

25. Pellegatta S, Poliani PL, Corno D, et al. Dendritic cells pulsed with glioma lysates induce immunity against syngeneic intracranial gliomas and increase survival of tumor-bearing mice. Neurol Res 2006;28:527–31.

26. Jouanneau E, Poujol D, Gulia S, et al. Dendritic cells are essential for priming but inefficient for boosting antitumour immune response in an orthotopic murine glioma model. Cancer Immunol Immunother 2006;55:254–67.

27. Akasaki Y, Kikuchi T, Homma S, et al. Antitumor effect of immunizations with fusions of dendritic and glioma cells in a mouse brain tumor model. J Immunother (1991) 2001;24:106–13.

28. Yamanaka R, Zullo SA, Tanaka R, et al. Enhancement of antitumor immune response in glioma models in mice by genetically modified dendritic cells pulsed with Semliki forest virus-mediated complementary DNA. J Neurosurg 2001;94:474–81.

29. Yamanaka R, Yajima N, Tsuchiya N, et al. Administration of interleukin-12 and -18 enhancing the antitumor immunity of genetically modified dendritic cells that had been pulsed with Semliki forest virus-mediated tumor complementary DNA. J Neurosurg 2002;97:1184–90.

30. Aoki H, Mizuno M, Natsume A, et al. Dendritic cells pulsed with tumor extract-cationic liposome complex increase the induction of cytotoxic T lymphocytes in mouse brain tumor. Cancer Immunol Immunother 2001;50:463–8.

31. Bigner DD, Pitts OM, Wikstrand CJ. Induction of lethal experimental allergic encephalomyelitis in nonhuman primates and guinea pigs with human glioblastoma multiforme tissue. J Neurosurg 1981;55:32–42.

32. Liau LM, Black KL, Martin NA, et al. Treatment of a patient by vaccination with autologous dendritic

cells pulsed with allogeneic major histocompatibility complex class I-matched tumor peptides. Case report. Neurosurg Focus 2000;9:e8.

33. Liau LM, Prins RM, Kiertscher SM, et al. Dendritic cell vaccination in glioblastoma patients induces systemic and intracranial T-cell responses modulated by the local central nervous system tumor microenvironment. Clin Cancer Res 2005;11:5515–25.

34. Yu JS, Wheeler CJ, Zeltzer PM, et al. Vaccination of malignant glioma patients with peptide-pulsed dendritic cells elicits systemic cytotoxicity and intracranial T-cell infiltration. Cancer Res 2001;61: 842–7.

35. Kikuchi T, Akasaki Y, Irie M, et al. Results of a phase I clinical trial of vaccination of glioma patients with fusions of dendritic and glioma cells. Cancer Immunol Immunother 2001;50:337–44.

36. Kobayashi T, Yamanaka R, Homma J, et al. Tumor mRNA-loaded dendritic cells elicit tumor-specific CD8(+) cytotoxic T cells in patients with malignant glioma. Cancer Immunol Immunother 2003;52:632–7.

37. Yamanaka R, Abe T, Yajima N, et al. Vaccination of recurrent glioma patients with tumour lysate-pulsed dendritic cells elicits immune responses: results of a clinical phase I/II trial. Br J Cancer 2003;89:1172–9.

38. Yamanaka R, Tsuchiya N, Yajima N, et al. Induction of an antitumor immunological response by an intratumoral injection of dendritic cells pulsed with genetically engineered Semliki Forest virus to produce interleukin-18 combined with the systemic administration of interleukin-12. J Neurosurg 2003;99: 746–53.

39. Wheeler CJ, Black KL, Liu G, et al. Thymic CD8+ T cell production strongly influences tumor antigen recognition and age-dependent glioma mortality. J Immunol 2003;171:4927–33.

40. Caruso DA, Orme LM, Neale AM, et al. Results of a phase 1 study utilizing monocyte-derived dendritic cells pulsed with tumor RNA in children and young adults with brain cancer. Neuro Oncol 2004;6: 236–46.

41. Yu JS, Liu G, Ying H, et al. Vaccination with tumor lysate-pulsed dendritic cells elicits antigen-specific, cytotoxic T-cells in patients with malignant glioma. Cancer Res 2004;64:4973–9.

42. Kikuchi T, Akasaki Y, Abe T, et al. Vaccination of glioma patients with fusions of dendritic and glioma cells and recombinant human interleukin 12. J Immunother 2004;27:452–9.

43. Walker DG, Laherty R, Tomlinson FH, et al. Results of a phase I dendritic cell vaccine trial for malignant astrocytoma: potential interaction with adjuvant chemotherapy. J Clin Neurosci 2008;15:114–21.

44. Wheeler CJ, Black KL, Liu G, et al. Vaccination elicits correlated immune and clinical responses in glioblastoma multiforme patients. Cancer Res 2008;68:5955–64.

45. Schuler G, Schuler-Thurner B, Steinman RM. The use of dendritic cells in cancer immunotherapy. Curr Opin Immunol 2003;15:138–47.

46. Labeur MS, Roters B, Pers B, et al. Generation of tumor immunity by bone marrow-derived dendritic cells correlates with dendritic cell maturation stage. J Immunol 1999;162:168–75.

47. Wheeler CJ, Das A, Liu G, et al. Clinical responsiveness of glioblastoma multiforme to chemotherapy after vaccination. Clin Cancer Res 2004;10:5316–26.

48. Lake RA, Robinson BW. Immunotherapy and chemotherapy: a practical partnership. Nat Rev Cancer 2005;5:397–405.

49. Kammula US, Marincola FM, Rosenberg SA. Real-time quantitative polymerase chain reaction assessment of immune reactivity in melanoma patients after tumor peptide vaccination. J Natl Cancer Inst 2000; 92:1336–44.

50. Rosenberg SA, Yang JC, Restifo NP. Cancer immunotherapy: moving beyond current vaccines. Nat Med 2004;10:909–15.

51. Eisenhauer EA, Therasse P, Bogaerts J, et al. New response evaluation criteria in solid tumours: revised RECIST guideline (version 1.1). Eur J Cancer 2009; 45:228–47.

52. de Vleeschouwer S, Rapp M, Sorg RV, et al. Dendritic cell vaccination in patients with malignant gliomas: current status and future directions. Neurosurgery 2006;59:988–99 [discussion: 999–1000].

53. Sorg RV, Ozcan Z, Brefort T, et al. Clinical-scale generation of dendritic cells in a closed system. J Immunother 2003;26:374–83.

54. Thurner B, Roder C, Dieckmann D, et al. Generation of large numbers of fully mature and stable dendritic cells from leukapheresis products for clinical application. J Immunol Methods 1999;223:1–15.

55. Tuyaerts S, Noppe SM, Corthals J, et al. Generation of large numbers of dendritic cells in a closed system using cell factories. J Immunol Methods 2002;264:135–51.

56. Dauer M, Obermaier B, Herten J, et al. Mature dendritic cells derived from human monocytes within 48 hours: a novel strategy for dendritic cell differentiation from blood precursors. J Immunol 2003;170:4069–76.

57. Yamanaka R, Zullo SA, Ramsey J, et al. Marked enhancement of antitumor immune responses in mouse brain tumor models by genetically modified dendritic cells producing Semliki Forest virus-mediated interleukin-12. J Neurosurg 2002;97:611–8.

58. De Vleeschouwer S, Van Gool SW, Van Calenbergh F. Immunotherapy for malignant gliomas: emphasis on strategies of active specific immunotherapy using autologous dendritic cells. Childs Nerv Syst 2005;21:7–18.

59. De Vries IJ, Krooshoop DJ, Scharenborg NM, et al. Effective migration of antigen-pulsed dendritic cells

to lymph nodes in melanoma patients is determined by their maturation state. Cancer Res 2003;63:12–7.

60. Dhodapkar MV, Krasovsky J, Steinman RM, et al. Mature dendritic cells boost functionally superior CD8(+) T-cell in humans without foreign helper epitopes. J Clin Invest 2000;105:R9–14.

61. Engell-Noerregaard L, Hansen TH, Andersen MH, et al. Review of clinical studies on dendritic cell-based vaccination of patients with malignant melanoma: assessment of correlation between clinical response and vaccine parameters. Cancer Immunol Immunother 2009;58:1–14.

62. Fong L, Brockstedt D, Benike C, et al. Dendritic cells injected via different routes induce immunity in cancer patients. J Immunol 2001;166:4254–9.

63. Eggert AA, Schreurs MW, Boerman OC, et al. Biodistribution and vaccine efficiency of murine dendritic cells are dependent on the route of administration. Cancer Res 1999;59:3340–5.

64. Mackensen A, Krause T, Blum U, et al. Homing of intravenously and intralymphatically injected human dendritic cells generated in vitro from CD34+ hematopoietic progenitor cells. Cancer Immunol Immunother 1999;48:118–22.

65. Morse MA, Coleman RE, Akabani G, et al. Migration of human dendritic cells after injection in patients with metastatic malignancies. Cancer Res 1999;59:56–8.

66. Karman J, Ling C, Sandor M, et al. Initiation of immune responses in brain is promoted by local dendritic cells. J Immunol 2004;173:2353–61.

67. Barratt-Boyes SM, Figdor CG. Current issues in delivering DCs for immunotherapy. Cytotherapy 2004;6:105–10.

68. Calzascia T, Masson F, Di Berardino-Besson W, et al. Homing phenotypes of tumor-specific CD8 T cells are predetermined at the tumor site by crosspresenting APCs. Immunity 2005;22:175–84.

69. Ohgaki H, Kleihues P. Population-based studies on incidence, survival rates, and genetic alterations in astrocytic and oligodendroglial gliomas. J Neuropathol Exp Neurol 2005;64:479–89.

70. De Vleeschouwer S, Spencer Lopes I, Ceuppens JL, et al. Persistent IL-10 production is required for glioma growth suppressive activity by Th1-directed effector cells after stimulation with tumor lysate-loaded dendritic cells. J Neurooncol 2007;84:131–40.

71. Yamanaka R, Honma J, Tsuchiya N, et al. Tumor lysate and IL-18 loaded dendritic cells elicits Th1 response, tumor-specific CD8+ cytotoxic T cells in patients with malignant glioma. J Neurooncol 2005;72:107–13.

72. Hu J, Yuan X, Belladonna ML, et al. Induction of potent antitumor immunity by intratumoral injection of interleukin 23-transduced dendritic cells. Cancer Res 2006;66:8887–96.

# Glioma Stem Cell Research for the Development of Immunotherapy

Jianfei Ji, PhD[a], Keith L. Black, MD[a], John S. Yu, MD[b],*

## KEYWORDS

• Cancer stem cell • Glioma • CD133[+] • Immunotherapy

Human brain tumors are a diverse group of diseases characterized by the abnormal growth of brain cells contained within the skull, afflicting adults and children. According to the National Cancer Institute data, there are about 20,000 new cases of brain tumor and 13,000 deaths each year in the United States. In children, brain tumors are the leading cause of solid tumor cancer death; all forms of glioma make up about one-fifth of all childhood cancers (www.cancer.gov). In adults, the most common malignant brain tumor, glioblastoma multiforme (GBM), is also the most malignant primary tumor of the brain associated with one of the worst 5-year survival rates among all human cancers.[1,2] The median survival time is 14.6 months after first diagnosis.[3,4] Despite the advances in conventional treatments, composed of surgical resection, local radiotherapy, and systemic chemotherapy, the incidence and mortality rates for gliomas have changed little in the past decade. With greater understanding of the cellular and molecular mechanisms of cancer initiation and propagation, the cancer stem cell (CSC) hypothesis presents new insights for developing novel treatments that target this group of cells. In this article, the authors discuss the CSC hypothesis and its application to develop treatments for glioma.

## CSC BRAIN TUMOR STEM CELL AND CD133 CSCS

The first conclusive evidence for CSCs came from the studies of acute myeloid leukemia (AML).[5,6]

Bonnet and Dick[6] isolated a subpopulation of AML cells that were capable of initiating AML in immunodeficient NOD/SCID (nonobese diabetic/severe combined immunodeficient) mice. These leukemia cells (leukemia stem cells [LSCs]) express cell-surface markers that are similar to normal hematopoietic stem cells (HSCs). The AML that is established from these LSCs recapitulates the morphologic and immunophenotypic heterogeneity of the original tumor. These seminal studies opened the door for CSC study. Besides the properties shared with normal stem cells (self-renewal and the ability to differentiate into other cells), candidate cells must present the following properties to be considered as CSCs: (1) the unique ability to engraft, (2) the ability to recapitulate the tumor of origin morphologically and immunophenotypically in xenografts, and (3) the ability to be serially transplanted.[7] These criteria are the standard to identify other CSCs not only in hematopoietic tumors but also in solid tumors.

The first solid tumor CSCs were identified from breast cancer by isolating CD44[+]/CD24[−/low] cells from primary tumor cells.[8] The isolated CSCs can recapitulate the original breast cancer with the same morphologic and immunophenotypic features. CSCs could be isolated from these grafts and serially transplanted. For gliomas, several groups isolated brain tumor stem cells (BTSCs) from primary tumors based on the criteria mentioned earlier and the ability to form neurospheres as normal neural stem cells (NSCs)

[a] Department of Neurosurgery, Cedars-Sinai Medical Center, Maxine Dunitz Neurosurgical Institute, 8631 West Third Street, Suite 800 E, Los Angeles, CA 90048, USA
[b] Department of Neurosurgery, Gamma Knife Center, Maxine Dunitz Neurosurgical Institute, Los Angeles, CA, USA
* Corresponding author.
E-mail address: yuj@cshs.org (J.S. Yu).

Neurosurg Clin N Am 21 (2010) 159–166
doi:10.1016/j.nec.2009.08.006
1042-3680/09/$ – see front matter © 2010 Elsevier Inc. All rights reserved.

do.[9–16] In the authors' study, as few as 100 of these BTSCs could recapitulate the heterogeneity of GBM in immunocompromised rodents.[15] In addition to primary gliomas, the authors also isolated cancer stemlike cells from the commercial rat gliosarcoma cell line, 9L.[17] This cell line has been cultured in the laboratory over a long period under neurosphere conditions used for NSC expansion. Similar results were reported by Kondo and colleagues[18] for the rat GBM cell line, C6. These data indicate that glioma cell lines may retain the capacity for a stemlike phenotype even after years of in vitro culture. CSCs have also been identified in various other malignant primary tumors and cancer cell lines by using different cell-surface markers (**Table 1**).

Among the CSC-associated markers, CD133 (prominin-1) is one of the most important and well studied. It is a 120 kDa, 5-transmembrane-domain glycoprotein, with 2 cytoplasmic loops, 2 glycosylated extracellular domains, and a cytoplasmic C-terminal domain.[19–22] Despite mounting evidence that CD133 is an important marker for somatic stem cells and CSCs, its physiologic function is not known. Some studies suggested that CD133 is involved in neural-retinal development and phototransduction.[23,24] Due to its interaction with plasma membrane cholesterol and enrichment in cholesterol-based membrane microdomains, it may play some role in membrane topology.[25] Barcelos and colleagues[26] also demonstrated that CD133+ progenitor cells could promote the healing of diabetic ischemic ulcer through stimulating angiogenesis and activating the Wnt pathway. This observation may suggest a role for CD133+ CSCs in tumor angiogenesis and in related signaling pathways.

## GLIOMA CSCS AND CLINICAL TREATMENT

CSCs are often resistant to conventional chemotherapy and radiation therapy. Glioma CSCs are resistant to radiotherapy and chemotherapy. CD133+ glioma CSCs could preferentially activate the DNA damage checkpoint response under irradiation. The activation is Chk1 and Chk2 checkpoint kinase dependent.[27] Blazek and colleagues[28] also confirmed that CD133+ glioma cells are more radiation resistant than CD133− cells. This study also reported that CD133 expression is upregulated 1.6 fold under 2% $O_2$ (hypoxic conditions). Similar results had been reported by other groups also.[29,30] Because hypoxic conditions exist in most solid tumors, including gliomas,

**Table 1**
**Summary of identified cancer stem cells from different primary tumors and tumor cell lines**

| Tumor | Type | Isolation Markers | References |
|---|---|---|---|
| AML | Primary tumors | CD34+CD38− | 5,6,78 |
| Breast | Primary tumors | CD44+CD24−/LOW | 8 |
| Brain | Primary tumors | CD133+ | 9,10,13,27,32,79,80 |
| | Cell lines | CD133+/sphere formation | 17,28,81 |
| | Cell lines | Side population (SP) | 18 |
| Colon | Primary tumors | CD133+ | 61,82,83 |
| | Primary tumors | CD133+CD44+ | 84 |
| | Cell lines | CD133+ | 85 |
| Laryngeal | Cell lines | CD133+ | 86 |
| Leukemia | Primary tumors | CD34+CD10- | 87 |
| Liver | Primary tumors/cell line/blood | CD90+CD44+ | 88 |
| | Cell lines | CD133+ | 89–92 |
| Lung | Primary tumors | ALDH1 | 93 |
| | Primary tumors | CD133+ | 94 |
| Melanoma | Primary tumors | ABCB5+ | 57 |
| | Primary tumors | CD133+ABCG2+ | 95 |
| Ovarian | Primary tumors | CD133+ | 96 |
| Pancreas | Primary tumors | CD133+ | 97,98 |
| | Cell lines | CD133+ | 99 |
| Prostate | Primary tumors | CD133+ | 100 |

this upregulation of CD133 expression provides enhancement for specific targeting of glioma CSCs rather than NSCs.

An in vitro study showed that CD133$^+$ glioblastoma CSCs are more resistant to multiple chemotherapeutic agents than their CD133$^-$ counterparts.[31] The authors demonstrated that CD133$^+$ glioma CSCs express higher levels of the drug transporter gene, *BCRP*, combined with upregulation of the DNA repair protein, methylguanine DNA methyltransferase (MGMT) mRNA, and mRNAs of other genes that inhibit apoptosis, including *FLIP, Bcl-2, Bcl-X*, and some *IAP* family genes. These cells were significantly resistant to chemotherapeutic agents when compared with autologous CD133$^-$ cells.[32]

Glioma CSCs possess migration as an additional property to escape from conventional therapies. The authors and others reported that overexpression of chemokine receptors, such as CXCR4, is a common mechanism related to CSC migration.[32–34] As reviewed by Lefranc and colleagues,[35] glioma cell migration is a complex combination of multiple molecular processes, including the alteration of tumor cell adhesion to a modified extracellular matrix, the secretion of proteases by the cells, and modifications to the actin cytoskeleton. Intracellular signaling pathways involved in the acquisition of resistance to apoptosis by migrating glioma cells include PI3K, Akt, mTOR, NF-κB, and autophagy (programmed cell death type II).

## TARGETING SIGNALING PATHWAYS IN CSCS

Signaling pathways, including Wnt, hedgehog, Notch, HOX family members, Bmi-1, phosphatase and tensin (PTEN) homolog, telomerase, and efflux transporters, are involved in balancing self-renewal and differentiation of NSCs and CSCs.[36–39] Newer studies also show that Notch, hedgehog, and bone morphogenic protein (BMP) pathways are involved in controlling CD133$^+$ CSC functions in glioma.[40–42] Bao and colleagues[43] showed that glioma CSCs generate vascular tumors through overexpression of vascular endothelial growth factor (VEGF). Because VEGF is a validated therapeutic target for glioma therapy,[44–46] this finding may indicate more favorable targeting of CSCs in glioma therapy.

Due to the common pathways and cell-surface markers shared by NSCs and CSCs, it is important to develop CSC-specific therapies that avoid potential toxicities to NSCs. Selective targeting of AML CSCs by Guzman and colleagues[47] demonstrated the possibility of such selectivity. They showed that LSCs, but not normal HSCs, were susceptible to the apoptotic effects of the proteasome inhibitor MG-132 combined with the anthracycline idarubicin through NF-κB activity. NF-κB inhibitors could induce LSC apoptosis but spare normal HSCs.[48] In a subsequent study, the same group also showed that 4-benzyl-2-methyl-1,2,4-thiadiazolidine-3,5-dione (TDZD-8) treatment could induce oxidative stress and selectively kill LSCs in vitro but not HSCs.[49] Other studies demonstrated that AML is PTEN pathway dependent. Rapamycin, a PI3K/PTEN signaling pathway inhibitor, could dramatically decrease leukemia burden.[50] In addition, this treatment appeared to be specific for the LSCs because normal HSCs were unaffected.

When selective targeting of CSCs becomes possible, another strategy to target CSCs is by forcing them to differentiate and become more sensitive to conventional chemo-radiotherapies. Differentiation therapy is based on this concept, and several agents had been tested in recent years.[51,52] All-trans retinoic acid (ATRA) is the most studied differentiation therapy molecule. Sell[53] reported that about 90% of newly diagnosed patients with acute promyelocytic leukemia achieved complete remission and more than 70% were cured by ATRA therapy. Differentiation with ATRA was also reported in early-stage mouse embryonic stem cells,[54] rat C6 glioma cells,[55] and human embryonic NSCs.[56] These studies opened up the possibility of using ATRA to induce differentiation of glioma CSCs as a therapeutic technique. Besides ATRA, other agents have also been tested for this approach of differentiation therapy. Piccirillo and colleagues[42] have shown that treating CSCs with differentiation factors can effectively deplete CSCs in human glioma. In this study, researchers reported that BMPs, especially BMP4, activate BMP receptors and trigger the Smad signaling cascade in cells isolated from human glioblastomas. This activated signaling pathway leads to a reduction in proliferation and increased expression of differentiated neural markers in both CD133$^+$ CSCs and normal glioma cells. When xenotransplanted BMP4–pretreated glioma CSCs were transplanted into mice, invasive glioma was not detected. These data provided evidence that differentiation therapy is a promising noncytotoxic strategy to deplete CSCs.

## TARGETING CSCS USING PASSIVE IMMUNOTHERAPY

Antibody therapy (passive immunotherapy) directed against CSCs has resulted in several experimental therapeutic successes. Schatton and colleagues[57] identified melanoma CSCs with the expression of the chemoresistance mediator ABCB5+ (ATP binding cassette B5+). Treatment with anti-ABCB5 antibody for xenografted melanomas resulted in significant reduction of tumor size. Moreover, this direct targeting of the CSC antigen induced tumor cell death through antibody-dependent cell-mediated cytotoxicity. Another encouraging result of antibody therapy was reported by Jin and colleagues.[58] In their study, CD44 had been identified as an AML CSC surface marker. Although the same marker is expressed on normal bone marrow HSCs at a lower level, treatment with anti-CD44 antibody before transplant can selectively block engraftment of AML LSCs but not normal HSCs. Treatment of previously engrafted AML LSCs with the same antibody led to a significant reduction in disease burden by 83% to 100%. In vivo treated AML CSCs resulted in lower engraftment, suggesting that anti-CD44 antibody treatment directly altered the fate of CSCs either by inducing differentiation or by inhibiting their repopulation ability. This study provided evidence that passive immunotherapy with antibodies targeting CSC antigens could be effective even when the same antigen is shared with NSCs. Krause and colleagues[59] also reported that the expression of CD44 is required on leukemic cells that initiate chronic myeloid leukemia (CML). Anti-CD44 antibody treatment attenuated the induction of CML-like leukemia in recipients, suggesting that CD44 blockade may be beneficial in autologous transplantation in CML.

Passive immunotherapy targeting solid tumor CSCs has also been reported. Smith and colleagues[60] demonstrated that antibody-drug conjugates (ADCs) could be used for both hepatocellular and gastric cancers. When an anti-CD133 antibody was conjugated to a potent cytotoxic drug, monomethyl auristatin F, this conjugate effectively inhibited the growth of Hep3B hepatocellular and KATO III gastric cancer cells in vitro by inducing apoptosis in CD133+ CSCs. In vivo administration of this ADC also resulted in significant delay of tumor growth in SCID mice.

In addition to directly targeting CSC surface antigens, antibody therapy has also been used as sensitizing agents combined with chemotherapy. Todaro and colleagues[61] showed that treatment of CD133+ colon CSCs with anti-IL-4 antibody before treatment with oxaliplatin, 5-FU (fluorouracil), or TRAIL (tumor necrosis factor–related apoptosis-inducing ligand) resulted in increased cell death. In vivo injection of IL-4 neutralizing antibodies followed by oxiplatin effectively reduced tumor burden.

## TARGETING CSCS USING ACTIVE IMMUNOTHERAPY

Active immunotherapy is designed to generate vaccines that could stimulate the host's intrinsic immune response to the tumor. Early-stage active immunotherapy vaccines for glioma treatment used irradiated whole tumor cells for inoculation, cells that are either engineered to secrete cytokines[62] or combined with cytokine secreting cells[63] or cytokine itself.[64] Although promising data have been obtained from those tumor cell–based vaccination strategies, the success of this approach was limited by the poor inherent antigen-presenting capacity of glioma cells. The use of professional antigen-presenting cells, such as dendritic cells (DCs), to initiate tumor-specific T-cell responses may be a more promising strategy for cancer vaccination. Emerging evidence showed that DC-mediated antigen presentation might be more effective than using irradiated tumor cells because DCs abundantly express many of the costimulatory molecules that are essential for appropriate activation of naive T cells. Also, they have the ability to efficiently process and present antigenic peptides in combination with cell-surface MHC (major histocompatibility complex).[65–70] For glioma immunotherapy with DC vaccines, different tumor-associated antigens (TAAs), including specific tumor-associated peptides, tumor RNA and cDNA, tumor cell lysate, or apoptotic tumor cells, have been tested in various studies.[71]

In the authors' phase I study using DC vaccines in patients with newly diagnosed high-grade glioma,[72] DC vaccine was generated with the patients' peripheral blood mononuclear cell–derived DCs that are pulsed ex vivo with autologous tumor cell–surface peptides isolated by means of acid elution. After surgical resection and external beam radiotherapy, 9 patients were given DC vaccination intradermally every other week over a 6-week period. Four patients, who showed disease progression, underwent surgery again after receiving the third DC vaccination. The harvested tumor tissue samples from 2 of the 4 patients showed robust infiltration with CD8+ and CD45RO+ T cells, which was not apparent in the same patients' tumor specimens before the vaccination. The median survival period for the study group was 455 days, which was longer than the 257 days for the matched control population. As the results were promising and without any observed destructive autoimmune responses, this study was expanded into a phase II trial.

In another phase I study using DCs pulsed with tumor lysate as antigen,[73] 14 patients with malignant glioma were given 3 vaccinations over a 6-week period and were followed with immunomonitor assay using an HLA-restricted tetramer staining protocol. Results in 4 patients showed that at least 1 or more TAA-specific cytotoxic lymphocytes (CTL) were activated against specific glioma antigens, including melanoma antigen-encoding gene-1, gp-100, and human epidermal growth factor receptor-2. The median survival period of the study group was significantly longer than the control group of recurrent glioblastoma patients, 133 weeks versus 30 weeks.

In a study by Liau and colleagues,[74] 12 glioma patients were treated with DC vaccination by using autologous DCs pulsed with acid-eluted autologous tumor peptides. Results showed that 6 patients generated peripheral tumor-specific CTL postvaccination, without major adverse events and autoimmune reactions. The patients who developed systemic antitumor cytotoxicity had longer survival times than patients with a negative response. All the patients who had stable disease generated a positive CTL response, whereas those with active progressive disease did not show statistically significant CTL response.

With encouraging data generated from these DC vaccine clinical trials, current studies are attempting to further improve the efficacy of this strategy not only by inducing glioma specific CTL but also by depleting inhibitory $T_{reg}$ (regulatory T) cells.[75,76] Two European group studies showed that depletion of $T_{reg}$ cells before DC vaccination could boost antiglioma immune response, leading to tumor rejection and long-term immunity. The 2 studies thus suggested that combination of $T_{reg}$ depletion and DC vaccination is a more effective option to generate antiglioma immunity.

## SUMMARY

With emerging evidence that glioma CSCs play an important role in tumor initiation, one can escape from conventional surgical and chemotherapies and target glioma CSCs with different therapeutic strategies, providing new hope for treatment of glioma. Studies that used immunotherapy to target glioma have achieved promising results. But because of the complex and divergent mechanisms with which glioma evades immune surveillance and the genetic instability of CSCs,[77] a combination of therapies with 2 or more immunotherapy strategies may be more effective in eliminating gliomas. With a better understanding of stem cell biology (especially CSC biology), glioma CSC-specific immunotherapy (based on

the new discovery) combined with other therapeutic strategies may eventually provide new approaches to treat gliomas.

## REFERENCES

1. Walid MS, Smisson HF 3rd, Robinson JS Jr. Long-term survival after glioblastoma multiforme. South Med J 2008;101:971–2.
2. Krex D, Klink B, Hartmann C, et al. Long-term survival with glioblastoma multiforme. Brain 2007; 130:2596–606.
3. Ohgaki H, Dessen P, Jourde B, et al. Genetic pathways to glioblastoma: a population-based study. Cancer Res 2004;64:6892–9.
4. Smith JS, Jenkins RB. Genetic alterations in adult diffuse glioma: occurrence, significance, and prognostic implications. Front Biosci 2000;5:D213–31.
5. Lapidot T, Sirard C, Vormoor J, et al. A cell initiating human acute myeloid leukaemia after transplantation into SCID mice. Nature 1994;367:645–8.
6. Bonnet D, Dick JE. Human acute myeloid leukemia is organized as a hierarchy that originates from a primitive hematopoietic cell. Nat Med 1997;3:730–7.
7. Park CY, Tseng D, Weissman IL. Cancer stem cell-directed therapies: recent data from the laboratory and clinic. Mol Ther 2009;17:219–30.
8. Al-Hajj M, Wicha MS, Benito-Hernandez A, et al. Prospective identification of tumorigenic breast cancer cells. Proc Natl Acad Sci U S A 2003;100: 3983–8.
9. Singh SK, Clarke ID, Terasaki M, et al. Identification of a cancer stem cell in human brain tumors. Cancer Res 2003;63:5821–8.
10. Singh SK, Hawkins C, Clarke ID, et al. Identification of human brain tumour initiating cells. Nature 2004; 432:396–401.
11. Galli R, Binda E, Orfanelli U, et al. Isolation and characterization of tumorigenic, stem-like neural precursors from human glioblastoma. Cancer Res 2004;64:7011–21.
12. Ignatova TN, Kukekov VG, Laywell ED, et al. Human cortical glial tumors contain neural stem-like cells expressing astroglial and neuronal markers in vitro. Glia 2002;39:193–206.
13. Hemmati HD, Nakano I, Lazareff JA, et al. Cancerous stem cells can arise from pediatric brain tumors. Proc Natl Acad Sci U S A 2003;100: 15178–83.
14. Lee J, Kotliarova S, Kotliarov Y, et al. Tumor stem cells derived from glioblastomas cultured in bFGF and EGF more closely mirror the phenotype and genotype of primary tumors than do serum-cultured cell lines. Cancer Cell 2006;9:391–403.
15. Yuan X, Curtin J, Xiong Y, et al. Isolation of cancer stem cells from adult glioblastoma multiforme. Oncogene 2004;23:9392–400.

16. Uchida N, Buck DW, He D, et al. Direct isolation of human central nervous system stem cells. Proc Natl Acad Sci U S A 2000;97:14720–5.

17. Ghods AJ, Irvin D, Liu G, et al. Spheres isolated from 9L gliosarcoma rat cell line possess chemoresistant and aggressive cancer stem-like cells. Stem Cells 2007;25:1645–53.

18. Kondo T, Setoguchi T, Taga T. Persistence of a small subpopulation of cancer stem-like cells in the C6 glioma cell line. Proc Natl Acad Sci U S A 2004; 101:781–6.

19. Corbeil D, Roper K, Hellwig A, et al. The human AC133 hematopoietic stem cell antigen is also expressed in epithelial cells and targeted to plasma membrane protrusions. J Biol Chem 2000;275: 5512–20.

20. Miraglia S, Godfrey W, Yin AH, et al. A novel five-transmembrane hematopoietic stem cell antigen: isolation, characterization, and molecular cloning. Blood 1997;90:5013–21.

21. Yin AH, Miraglia S, Zanjani ED, et al. AC133, a novel marker for human hematopoietic stem and progenitor cells. Blood 1997;90:5002–12.

22. Bidlingmaier S, Zhu X, Liu B. The utility and limitations of glycosylated human CD133 epitopes in defining cancer stem cells. J Mol Med 2008;86: 1025–32.

23. Maw MA, Corbeil D, Koch J, et al. A frameshift mutation in prominin (mouse)-like 1 causes human retinal degeneration. Hum Mol Genet 2000;9:27–34.

24. Zacchigna S, Oh H, Wilsch-Brauninger M, et al. Loss of the cholesterol-binding protein prominin-1/CD133 causes disk dysmorphogenesis and photoreceptor degeneration. J Neurosci 2009;29: 2297–308.

25. Shmelkov SV, St Clair R, Lyden D, et al. AC133/CD133/Prominin-1. Int J Biochem Cell Biol 2005; 37:715–9.

26. Barcelos LS, Duplaa C, Krankel N, et al. Human CD133+ progenitor cells promote the healing of diabetic ischemic ulcers by paracrine stimulation of angiogenesis and activation of Wnt signaling. Circ Res 2009;104:1095–102.

27. Bao S, Wu Q, McLendon RE, et al. Glioma stem cells promote radioresistance by preferential activation of the DNA damage response. Nature 2006;444:756–60.

28. Blazek ER, Foutch JL, Maki G. Daoy medulloblastoma cells that express CD133 are radioresistant relative to CD133– cells, and the CD133+ sector is enlarged by hypoxia. Int J Radiat Oncol Biol Phys 2007;67:1–5.

29. Potgens AJ, Schmitz U, Kaufmann P, et al. Monoclonal antibody CD133-2 (AC141) against hematopoietic stem cell antigen CD133 shows crossreactivity with cytokeratin 18. J Histochem Cytochem 2002;50: 1131–4.

30. Griguer CE, Oliva CR, Gobin E, et al. CD133 is a marker of bioenergetic stress in human glioma. PLoS One 2008;3:e3655.

31. Eramo A, Ricci-Vitiani L, Zeuner A, et al. Chemotherapy resistance of glioblastoma stem cells. Cell Death Differ 2006;13:1238–41.

32. Liu G, Yuan X, Zeng Z, et al. Analysis of gene expression and chemoresistance of CD133+ cancer stem cells in glioblastoma. Mol Cancer 2006;5:67.

33. Salmaggi A, Boiardi A, Gelati M, et al. Glioblastoma-derived tumorospheres identify a population of tumor stem-like cells with angiogenic potential and enhanced multidrug resistance phenotype. Glia 2006;54:850–60.

34. Dirks PB. Glioma migration: clues from the biology of neural progenitor cells and embryonic CNS cell migration. J Neurooncol 2001;53:203–12.

35. Lefranc F, Brotchi J, Kiss R. Possible future issues in the treatment of glioblastomas: special emphasis on cell migration and the resistance of migrating glioblastoma cells to apoptosis. J Clin Oncol 2005;23:2411–22.

36. Reya T, Morrison SJ, Clarke MF, et al. Stem cells, cancer, and cancer stem cells. Nature 2001;414: 105–11.

37. Lobo NA, Shimono Y, Qian D, et al. The biology of cancer stem cells. Annu Rev Cell Dev Biol 2007;23: 675–99.

38. Huntly BJ, Gilliland DG. Leukaemia stem cells and the evolution of cancer-stem-cell research. Nat Rev Cancer 2005;5:311–21.

39. Krause DS, Van Etten RA. Right on target: eradicating leukemic stem cells. Trends Mol Med 2007; 13:470–81.

40. Fan X, Matsui W, Khaki L, et al. Notch pathway inhibition depletes stem-like cells and blocks engraftment in embryonal brain tumors. Cancer Res 2006;66:7445–52.

41. Clement V, Sanchez P, de Tribolet N, et al. HEDGEHOG-GLI1 signaling regulates human glioma growth, cancer stem cell self-renewal, and tumorigenicity. Curr Biol 2007;17:165–72.

42. Piccirillo SG, Reynolds BA, Zanetti N, et al. Bone morphogenetic proteins inhibit the tumorigenic potential of human brain tumour-initiating cells. Nature 2006;444:761–5.

43. Bao S, Wu Q, Sathornsumetee S, et al. Stem cell-like glioma cells promote tumor angiogenesis through vascular endothelial growth factor. Cancer Res 2006;66:7843–8.

44. Vredenburgh JJ, Desjardins A, Herndon JE 2nd, et al. Bevacizumab plus irinotecan in recurrent glioblastoma multiforme. J Clin Oncol 2007;25: 4722–9.

45. Vredenburgh JJ, Desjardins A, Herndon JE 2nd, et al. Phase II trial of bevacizumab and irinotecan

in recurrent malignant glioma. Clin Cancer Res 2007;13:1253–9.

46. Batchelor TT, Sorensen AG, di Tomaso E, et al. AZD2171, a pan-VEGF receptor tyrosine kinase inhibitor, normalizes tumor vasculature and alleviates edema in glioblastoma patients. Cancer Cell 2007;11:83–95.

47. Guzman ML, Swiderski CF, Howard CS, et al. Preferential induction of apoptosis for primary human leukemic stem cells. Proc Natl Acad Sci U S A 2002;99:16220–5.

48. Guzman ML, Rossi RM, Neelakantan S, et al. An orally bioavailable parthenolide analog selectively eradicates acute myelogenous leukemia stem and progenitor cells. Blood 2007;110:4427–35.

49. Guzman ML, Li X, Corbett CA, et al. Rapid and selective death of leukemia stem and progenitor cells induced by the compound 4-benzyl, 2-methyl, 1,2,4-thiadiazolidine, 3,5 dione (TDZD-8). Blood 2007;110:4436–44.

50. Yilmaz OH, Valdez R, Theisen BK, et al. Pten dependence distinguishes haematopoietic stem cells from leukaemia-initiating cells. Nature 2006; 441:475–82.

51. Sell S. Cancer stem cells and differentiation therapy. Tumour Biol 2006;27:59–70.

52. Sell S. Leukemia: stem cells, maturation arrest, and differentiation therapy. Stem Cell Rev 2005;1: 197–205.

53. Sell S. Stem cell origin of cancer and differentiation therapy. Crit Rev Oncol Hematol 2004;51: 1–28.

54. Guo X, Ying W, Wan J, et al. Proteomic characterization of early-stage differentiation of mouse embryonic stem cells into neural cells induced by all-trans retinoic acid in vitro. Electrophoresis 2001;22:3067–75.

55. Bianchi MG, Gazzola GC, Tognazzi L, et al. C6 glioma cells differentiated by retinoic acid overexpress the glutamate transporter excitatory amino acid carrier 1 (EAAC1). Neuroscience 2008;151: 1042–52.

56. Wang F, Li ST, Huang Q, et al. [Expression of Notch1 gene in the differentiation of the human embryonic neural stem cells to neurons]. Xi Bao Yu Fen Zi Mian Yi Xue Za Zhi 2004;20:769–72 [in Chinese].

57. Schatton T, Murphy GF, Frank NY, et al. Identification of cells initiating human melanomas. Nature 2008;451:345–9.

58. Jin L, Hope KJ, Zhai Q, et al. Targeting of CD44 eradicates human acute myeloid leukemic stem cells. Nat Med 2006;12:1167–74.

59. Krause DS, Lazarides K, von Andrian UH, et al. Requirement for CD44 in homing and engraftment of BCR-ABL-expressing leukemic stem cells. Nat Med 2006;12:1175–80.

60. Smith LM, Nesterova A, Ryan MC, et al. CD/133/prominin-1 is a potential therapeutic target for antibody-drug conjugates in hepatocellular and gastric cancers. Br J Cancer 2008;9:100–9.

61. Todaro M, Alea MP, Stefano AB, et al. Colon cancer stem cells dictate tumor growth and resist cell death by production of interleukin-4. Cell Stem Cell 2007;1:389–402.

62. Herrlinger U, Kramm CM, Johnston KM, et al. Vaccination for experimental gliomas using GM-CSF-transduced glioma cells. Cancer Gene Ther 1997;4:345–52.

63. Sobol RE, Fakhrai H, Shawler D, et al. Interleukin-2 gene therapy in a patient with glioblastoma. Gene Ther 1995;2:164–7.

64. Plautz GE, Miller DW, Barnett GH, et al. T cell adoptive immunotherapy of newly diagnosed gliomas. Clin Cancer Res 2000;6:2209–18.

65. Ashley DM, Faiola B, Nair S, et al. Bone marrow-generated dendritic cells pulsed with tumor extracts or tumor RNA induce antitumor immunity against central nervous system tumors. J Exp Med 1997;186:1177–82.

66. Heimberger AB, Crotty LE, Archer GE, et al. Bone marrow-derived dendritic cells pulsed with tumor homogenate induce immunity against syngeneic intracerebral glioma. J Neuroimmunol 2000;103: 16–25.

67. Liau LM, Black KL, Prins RM, et al. Treatment of intracranial gliomas with bone marrow-derived dendritic cells pulsed with tumor antigens. J Neurosurg 1999;90:1115–24.

68. Ni HT, Spellman SR, Jean WC, et al. Immunization with dendritic cells pulsed with tumor extract increases survival of mice bearing intracranial gliomas. J Neurooncol 2001;51:1–9.

69. Okada H, Tahara H, Shurin MR, et al. Bone marrow-derived dendritic cells pulsed with a tumor-specific peptide elicit effective anti-tumor immunity against intracranial neoplasms. Int J Cancer 1998;78: 196–201.

70. Yamanaka R, Zullo SA, Tanaka R, et al. Enhancement of antitumor immune response in glioma models in mice by genetically modified dendritic cells pulsed with Semliki forest virus-mediated complementary DNA. J Neurosurg 2001;94: 474–81.

71. Soling A, Rainov NG. Dendritic cell therapy of primary brain tumors. Mol Med 2001;7:659–67.

72. Yu JS, Wheeler CJ, Zeltzer PM, et al. Vaccination of malignant glioma patients with peptide-pulsed dendritic cells elicits systemic cytotoxicity and intracranial T-cell infiltration. Cancer Res 2001;61:842–7.

73. Yu JS, Liu G, Ying H, et al. Vaccination with tumor lysate-pulsed dendritic cells elicits antigen-specific, cytotoxic T-cells in patients with malignant glioma. Cancer Res 2004;64:4973–9.

74. Liau LM, Prins RM, Kiertscher SM, et al. Dendritic cell vaccination in glioblastoma patients induces systemic and intracranial T-cell responses modulated by the local central nervous system tumor microenvironment. Clin Cancer Res 2005;11:5515–25.

75. Maes W, Rosas GG, Verbinnen B, et al. DC vaccination with anti-CD25 treatment leads to long-term immunity against experimental glioma. Neuro Oncol 2009;11:529–42.

76. Grauer OM, Sutmuller RP, van Maren W, et al. Elimination of regulatory T cells is essential for an effective vaccination with tumor lysate-pulsed dendritic cells in a murine glioma model. Int J Cancer 2008;122:1794–802.

77. Lagasse E. Cancer stem cells with genetic instability: the best vehicle with the best engine for cancer. Gene Ther 2008;15:136–42.

78. Ishikawa F, Yoshida S, Saito Y, et al. Chemotherapy-resistant human AML stem cells home to and engraft within the bone-marrow endosteal region. Nat Biotechnol 2007;25:1315–21.

79. Taylor MD, Poppleton H, Fuller C, et al. Radial glia cells are candidate stem cells of ependymoma. Cancer Cell 2005;8:323–35.

80. Zeppernick F, Ahmadi R, Campos B, et al. Stem cell marker CD133 affects clinical outcome in glioma patients. Clin Cancer Res 2008;14:123–9.

81. Bexell D, Gunnarsson S, Siesjo P, et al. CD133+ and nestin+ tumor-initiating cells dominate in N29 and N32 experimental gliomas. Int J Cancer 2009;125:15–22.

82. Ricci-Vitiani L, Lombardi DG, Pilozzi E, et al. Identification and expansion of human colon-cancer-initiating cells. Nature 2007;445:111–5.

83. O'Brien CA, Pollett A, Gallinger S, et al. A human colon cancer cell capable of initiating tumour growth in immunodeficient mice. Nature 2007;445:106–10.

84. Dallas NA, Xia L, Fan F, et al. Chemoresistant colorectal cancer cells, the cancer stem cell phenotype, and increased sensitivity to insulin-like growth factor-I receptor inhibition. Cancer Res 2009;69:1951–7.

85. Ieta K, Tanaka F, Haraguchi N, et al. Biological and genetic characteristics of tumor-initiating cells in colon cancer. Ann Surg Oncol 2008;15:638–48.

86. Wei XD, Zhou L, Cheng L, et al. In vivo investigation of CD133 as a putative marker of cancer stem cells in Hep-2 cell line. Head Neck 2009;31:94–101.

87. Cox CV, Evely RS, Oakhill A, et al. Characterization of acute lymphoblastic leukemia progenitor cells. Blood 2004;104:2919–25.

88. Yang ZF, Ho DW, Ng MN, et al. Significance of CD90+ cancer stem cells in human liver cancer. Cancer Cell 2008;13:153–66.

89. Suetsugu A, Nagaki M, Aoki H, et al. Characterization of CD133+ hepatocellular carcinoma cells as cancer stem/progenitor cells. Biochem Biophys Res Commun 2006;351:820–4.

90. Ma S, Lee TK, Zheng BJ, et al. CD133+ HCC cancer stem cells confer chemoresistance by preferential expression of the Akt/PKB survival pathway. Oncogene 2008;27:1749–58.

91. Ma S, Chan KW, Hu L, et al. Identification and characterization of tumorigenic liver cancer stem/progenitor cells. Gastroenterology 2007;132:2542–56.

92. Yin S, Li J, Hu C, et al. CD133 positive hepatocellular carcinoma cells possess high capacity for tumorigenicity. Int J Cancer 2007;120:1444–50.

93. Jiang F, Qiu Q, Khanna A, et al. Aldehyde dehydrogenase 1 is a tumor stem cell-associated marker in lung cancer. Mol Cancer Res 2009;7:330–8.

94. Eramo A, Lotti F, Sette G, et al. Identification and expansion of the tumorigenic lung cancer stem cell population. Cell Death Differ 2008;15:504–14.

95. Monzani E, Facchetti F, Galmozzi E, et al. Melanoma contains CD133 and ABCG2 positive cells with enhanced tumourigenic potential. Eur J Cancer 2007;43:935–46.

96. Ferrandina G, Bonanno G, Pierelli L, et al. Expression of CD133-1 and CD133-2 in ovarian cancer. Int J Gynecol Cancer 2008;18:506–14.

97. Hermann PC, Huber SL, Herrler T, et al. Distinct populations of cancer stem cells determine tumor growth and metastatic activity in human pancreatic cancer. Cell Stem Cell 2007;1:313–23.

98. Li C, Heidt DG, Dalerba P, et al. Identification of pancreatic cancer stem cells. Cancer Res 2007;67:1030–7.

99. Olempska M, Eisenach PA, Ammerpohl O, et al. Detection of tumor stem cell markers in pancreatic carcinoma cell lines. Hepatobiliary Pancreat Dis Int 2007;6:92–7.

100. Collins AT, Berry PA, Hyde C, et al. Prospective identification of tumorigenic prostate cancer stem cells. Cancer Res 2005;65:10946–51.

# Virally Mediated Immunotherapy for Brain Tumors

Pankaj K. Agarwalla, MSt[a], Zachary R. Barnard, MS[b],
William T. Curry Jr, MD[b,c],*

**KEYWORDS**

- Glioblastoma • Immunotherapy • Oncolytic virus
- Brain cancer • Immunosuppression • Gene therapy

Brain tumors are a leading cause of mortality and morbidity in the United States. Malignant brain tumors occur in approximately 80,000 adults.[1] Furthermore, the average 5-year survival rate for malignant brain tumors across all ages and races is approximately 30% and has remained relatively static over the past few decades, showing the need for continued research and progress in brain tumor therapy.[1] Improved techniques in molecular biology have allowed expansion in understanding of tumor genetics and have permitted viral engineering and the anticancer therapeutic use of viruses as directly cytotoxic agents and as gene vectors. Preclinical models have shown promising antitumor effects, and generation of clinical grade vectors is feasible. In parallel to these developments, better understanding of antitumor immunity has been accompanied by progress in cancer immunotherapy, the goal of which is to stimulate host rejection of a growing tumor. This article reviews the intersection between the use of viral therapy and immunotherapy in the treatment of malignant gliomas. Each approach shows great promise on its own and in combined or integrated forms.

This article initially reviews the fundamental concepts of viral therapy for brain tumors and traces how these have developed. Next, how viruses, wild-type and oncolytic, interact with the immune system is examined, followed by how immunomodulation, both positively and negatively, can augment antitumor effects of viruses. The final sections briefly review how the immune-modifying capacity of an oncolytic virus can be used to enhance a standard immunotherapy vaccine approach.

## VIRAL THERAPY FOR BRAIN TUMORS

Viral therapy for brain tumors can be considered in two main categories: (1) the use of replication-defective viruses, which do not multiply or propagate progeny at the site of inoculation, and (2) the use of replication-selective viruses, which divide in tumor cells and lyse them (oncolysis), and whose progeny infect and kill neighboring cells, continuing the cycle.[2] Although these approaches have yielded promising data in preclinical studies, more recent work, particularly in combination with immunotherapy, has focused on the use of oncolytic (replicating) viruses. The therapeutic effect of replication-defective viral vectors is not produced through direct killing, but rather through the expression of transgenes.

The types of genes inserted and expressed can be divided into five categories based on mechanism of purpose[2,3]:

a Brain Tumor Immunotherapy Laboratory, Department of Neurosurgery, Massachusetts General Hospital/Harvard Medical School, Boston, MA, USA
b Department of Neurosurgery, Stephen E. and Catherine Pappas Center for Neuro-oncology, Massachusetts General Hospital, 55 Fruit Street/Y9E, Boston, MA 02114, USA
c Department of Neurosurgery, Harvard Medical School, Boston, MA, USA
* Corresponding author. Department of Neurosurgery, Stephen E. and Catherine Pappas Center for Neuro-oncology, Massachusetts General Hospital, 55 Fruit Street/Y9E, Boston, MA 02114, USA.
E-mail address: wcurry@partners.org (W. T. Curry).

Neurosurg Clin N Am 21 (2010) 167–179
doi:10.1016/j.nec.2009.08.013
1042-3680/09/$ – see front matter © 2010 Published by Elsevier Inc.

1. Correction of genetic defects in cancer, such as replacement of wild-type *p53* in glioma, which often contains *p53* mutations.
2. Expression of antiangiogenic gene products, such as decoy vascular endothelial growth factor receptors.
3. Immune-modifying genes, particularly cytokines, designed to stimulate the immune system.
4. Drug resistance–modifying genes that help prevent the development of resistance to commonly used chemotherapeutics.
5. Prodrug-activating enzymes that enhance chemotherapeutic targeting of tumors.

Challenges in treating malignant brain tumors with replication-defective viruses have included delivering the agent to a sufficient number of cells within a tumor and in achieving adequate viral titers. For example, retrovirus was initially a commonly used vector in cancer gene therapy models because it infects actively mitotic cells (eg, tumor cells and tumor-associated vascular endothelium).

To increase the intratumoral retroviral load, vector-producing cells (VPCs), typically fibroblasts, have been infected with retrovirus and implanted intratumorally, with the goal of generating higher and effective titers in the tumor microenvironment. However, initial studies showed very little spread of the virus through the tumor, with activity limited to a small zone at the injection site.[4] More recent advances, particularly with alternative vectors such as adenovirus and lentivirus, have streamlined this approach, but significant limitations in transduction efficiency remain.[5] Contributing factors include a lack of expression on many tumors of the adenovirus receptor (eg, Coxsackie adenovirus receptor [CAR]) and the natural host immune response against the vectors, as is discussed later.[6]

In contrast, oncolytic viruses infect and kill tumor cells, selectively allowing spread of viral progeny into adjacent tumor cells.[2] In 1991, Martuza and colleagues[7] showed that a genetically engineered herpes simplex virus type 1(HSV-1) effectively and safely treated xenografted glioma tumors in mice. Since then, several oncolytic viruses have been studied and used in preclinical models and patients who have gliomas. These viruses are modified to replicate selectively in tumor cells, conferring specificity and safety.

Although their principal effect may be through direct oncolysis, oncolytic viruses may be designed to simultaneously deliver gene products that enhance antitumor activity. The most commonly used oncolytic virus backbones have been adenovirus and HSV-1. Clinical trials in malignant glioma have also been performed with reovirus.[8]

Human adenoviruses belong to a family of non-enveloped DNA viruses, of which serotypes Ad5 and Ad2 have been most commonly studied and used in oncolytic therapy.[9] Adenoviruses bind to cells through a fiber protein and penton base, which mediate cell-binding by way of specific receptors on cells, depending on the serotype.[10] A common receptor for many oncolytic adenoviruses is CAR, which is expressed on human glioma, thereby allowing efficient transduction of these tumor cells.[6] Onyx-015 is an early-developed oncolytic adenoviral vector. Onyx-015 carries a mutation in the *E1B* gene, the 55kD product of which inactivates normal p53 function in cells, thus resulting in a replication-selective oncolytic virus. Initial studies of this mutated virus suggested that it can replicate selectively in tumor cells deficient in p53 function, which is a common feature in many tumors, including gliomas. Further investigation has shown that Onyx-015 tumor selectivity may actually be conferred through tumor substitution of another *E1B* function; that is, late viral mRNA export.[5,11–14]

Delta-24 adenovirus is a well-developed vector currently in clinical trials for glioma (http://clinicaltrials.gov/ct2/show/NCT00805376, accessed June 3, 2009). Delta-24 adenovirus has a 24-bp deletion in the viral gene *E1A*.[11,15] The *E1A* gene product normally stabilizes the Rb protein so that E2F (a transcription factor) is released from E2F–Rb complexes and is free to activate the E2 promoter of the adenovirus, and several other cell-cycle genes.

In cells with normal Rb function, the viral gene *E1A* allows wild-type adenoviral infection and replication. Normal cells are, however, resistant to infection by Delta-24 adenovirus. The *E1A* mutation prevents binding of Rb and the subsequent transcription of viral genes by way of E2F in normal cells. In tumor cells that are defective in Rb and its upstream tumor suppressor, p16, Delta-24 is able to replicate, which is the basis for its tumor cell selectivity. Enhancements related to this basic premise have been made to increase selectivity for glioma cells.[16,17]

HSV-1 is a particularly well-developed asset as an oncolytic virus against brain tumors. HSV-1 is an enveloped, double-stranded DNA virus with several advantages for use in gene and oncolytic therapy: (1) it is a large genome suitable for insertion of foreign genes; (2) its tropism for neural cells; (3) it has a safety mechanism in its sensitivity to agents such as ganciclovir; (4) high titers can be generated; and (5) it does not integrate into the host genome, so it is unlikely to be oncogenic.[2]

The first engineered HSV-1 oncolytic virus had a mutation in the viral thymidine kinase (TK) gene, and showed killing of glioma cells in vitro and in in vivo models of glioma.[7,18] Tumor specificity of this mutant is achieved through the virus' dependence for replication on up-regulated human TK, present in rapidly dividing tumor cells. Viral TK is the substrate for the antiviral efficacy of nucleoside analogs, such as ganciclovir, which interrupts DNA synthesis when incorporated as ganciclovir triphosphate.

HSV-TK is much more efficient than human nucleoside kinases at monophosphorylating ganciclovir, which is subsequently converted by other cellular kinases into the toxic triphosphate form.[2] Ganciclovir, therefore, has specificity against the HSV, which serves as a potential "shut-off" mechanism. Transduction of tumor cells with the HSV-TK gene (either through HSV itself or other vectors such as adenovirus) in conjunction with systemic ganciclovir administration is a potent mechanism for tumor killing, with important immune consequences.[2]

The inability to use nucleoside analogs as a safety mechanism for this first-generation viral TK–mutated vector raised significant safety concerns, and, in fact, neurotoxicity was seen at high doses.[18] In an alternative HSV-1 vector, a mutation in the $\gamma_1 34.5$ gene was introduced. The $\gamma_1 34.5$ gene and its product, ICP34.5, allow normal HSV to subvert the host's shut-off response against infection.

Once infected with HSV, a normal cell will activate protein kinase R (PKR), which in turn phosphorylates and inactivates eukaryotic initiation factor-2α (eIF-2α), thereby shutting down protein synthesis in the normal host cell. ICP34.5 restores protein synthesis through activating protein phosphatase-1α which dephosphorylates and restores eIF-2α function.[18] Mutations in this gene, $\gamma_1 34.5$, result in an HSV that cannot replicate in normal cells, which abrogate protein-synthesis machinery. In malignant cells, however, the activation of PKR is less pronounced, likely because of other mutations, and therefore the ICP34.5-mutant HSV can selectively replicate.

A second mutation was added that confers tumor selectivity—the interruption of the gene for the large subunit of ribonucleotide reductase (ICP6). Double-mutant viruses are theoretically safer because the chances of in vivo recombination and restoration of wild-type HSV phenotype are decreased.[18,19] This second-generation virus, termed *G207*, harbors an insertion of the *Escherichia Coli lacZ* gene into the *ICP6* gene, which also allows immunohistochemical detection of the virus in tumor cells.[19] Using the G207 backbone, a third-generation oncolytic HSV-1, G47Δ, was developed through deleting the viral *α47* gene. *α47* encodes a protein that inhibits transporter associated with antigen presentation (TAP). Wild-type HSV-1 evades immune detection partially through inhibiting TAP in infected cells, thereby interfering with peptide assembly with major histocompatibility complex class I (MHC-I) molecules in the endoplasmic reticulum and preventing antigen presentation.[20]

Recently, bacterial artificial chromosome (BAC)–mediated systems have improved the efficiency of inserting transgenes into the HSV-1 backbones, including with G47Δ, which may have particular relevance for immunotherapy.[21,22]

## IMMUNE COMPARTMENTS, BRAIN TUMORS, AND VIRUSES

Recently, understanding of cancer immunology has advanced dramatically. A model illustrating the dynamic and complex relationship between tumor cells and the immune system is that of cancer immunoediting. In this framework, newly transformed cancer cells are initially subject to immunosurveillance, which may result in their elimination. In response, developing tumor cells may acquire mutations that allow them to avoid being fully eliminated, but they remain quiescent, existing in a tenuous equilibrium state, because the immune response prevents uncontrolled proliferation and spread.

Eventually, this balance is tipped in favor of the malignant cells, because they secrete cytokines or cause proliferation of cellular subsets that result in immunosuppression and ultimately immune escape.[23–25] For instance, mechanisms of escape may include secretion of soluble natural killer (NK) cell ligands, recruitment and activation of regulatory T cells, and release of immunosuppressive cytokines.

Human immunity can be broadly divided into innate and adaptive arms. Innate immunity is antigen-nonspecific, provides a crucial barrier against many foreign antigens, and stimulates the development of adaptive immunity.[26] Adaptive immunity is specific to certain antigens and includes direct cell killing through specifically activated cytotoxic lymphocytes, and activation of lymphocytes that generate specific antibody responses. Antigen-presenting cells (APCs) link the innate and adaptive immune systems; the most efficient APC in the dendritic cell (DC). Precursors in the bone marrow give rise to immature DCs, which circulate throughout the body, or are resident in tissues, and act as immunologic sensors for foreign antigen. These immature DCs express specific Pattern-Recognition Receptors (PRRs) that are capable of recognizing pathogenic epitopes.

The most well-studied group of PRRs are the toll-like receptors (TLRs), which identify and bind to evolutionarily conserved patterns from microbes, including viruses.[27] For example, TLR9 is expressed on the nuclear membrane of APCs and binds unmethylated CpG motifs in DNA, which are often derived from viral infection.[27] TLRs are also found on NK cells, which are important effectors of the innate immune system that can help inhibit viral replication. Once a TLR-bearing immature DC is activated by an immune danger signal, such as mediators released after viral or bacterial infection, it migrates to lymphoid tissue as it matures and activates effectors of the adaptive immune system, including T cells and B cells.[28]

Efficient antigen presentation requires high expression of MHC class I and II molecules. Stimulation of T lymphocytes by APCs also requires surface expression of costimulatory molecules, such as CD80 and CD86, and ligation of cognate receptors (eg, CD28) on the lymphocyte side of the immune synapse. Activated DCs up-regulate expression of MHC and costimulatory molecules and also secrete immunostimulatory cytokines, such as interleukin (IL)-12. Antigen presentation without concomitant costimulation can actually result in immune anergy.[26,28]

The expression of immunostimulatory cytokines in the immune environment is critical for activating the relevant cellular entities, and many immuno-therapeutic and oncolytic viral approaches drive cytokine overexpression, creating a more stimulatory milieu to shift the immune system toward an antitumor immune response. Although many cytokines and chemokines are involved, some of the most prominent with respect to the response to oncolytic viruses include granulocyte macrophage colony-stimulating factor (GM-CSF), IL-1, IL-2, IL-4, IL-12, IL-17, IL-18, interferon (IFN)-$\gamma$, and FMS-like tyrosine kinase 3 ligand (FLT3L).[26]

IFN-$\gamma$, FLT3L, and GM-CSF are important mediators for improving tumor cell antigen presentation and DC function. IL-2 and IL-4 activate T cells, whereas IL-12 and IL-18 shift the T-cell response to a type 1 helper T cell ($T_H1$) rather than a type 2 helper T cell ($T_H2$) response.[26] Although the array of cytokines involved in the immune response can be complex, this is one of the primary mechanisms through which oncolytic viral therapy and immunotherapy are intertwined. Genetically modifying oncolytic viruses to carry genes for immune-modulating cytokines may enhance stimulation of antitumor immunity. Viral infection itself results in the cellular elaboration of cytokines, some of

which are involved in DC maturation and activation.

Although immunostimulatory activity may be productive for strengthening antitumor immunity, the normal immune response to viruses can significantly inhibit viral spread and subsequent tumor cell lysis. Wild-type HSV, for example, activates strong innate and then adaptive antiviral immune responses. Players in the innate immune system, including complement, NK cells, and type 1 IFNs, are activated early in the infection.[29] The complement cascade activates the immune system against oncolytic viruses; complement depletion, in fact, allows better oncolytic viral replication in animal hosts.[30]

Type 1 IFNs play an important role in activating innate immune responses. Although all cell types can express type I IFNs, plasmacytoid DCs, also activated through toll-like receptors, are the heaviest producers of type 1 IFNs. Oncolytic viruses, including HSV-1 and vesicular stomatitis virus (VSV), clearly induce strong type 1 IFN responses.[31,32] NK cells, stimulated by the postinfectious inflammatory cytokine environment, bind to up-regulated receptors on infected cells and kill them.[33]

Shortly after this innate response to oncolytic viral infection, the adaptive immune system is activated and the developing $T_H1$ immune response causes activation of CD4+ T lymphocytes and release of IFN-$\gamma$ and IL-12. $T_H1$ responses are more likely effective against tumors themselves, although usually the response to viral infection is skewed toward $T_H2$, with expression of IL-4 and IL-10.[29]

In summary, viral infection causes a strong innate immune response, largely characterized by a type I IFN response, followed by adaptive ($T_H1$ and $T_H2$) antiviral responses, which are associated with cell-mediated humoral immunity, and then the virus may be eradicated or driven into latency (**Fig. 1**).

## IMMUNITY AND THERAPEUTIC ANTICANCER VIRUSES

Direct viral oncolysis and the virally mediated delivery of immune-modifying transgenes impact the host immune system in separate, related, and complementary ways. Although antiviral immunity is provoked after infection, oncolysis also initiates a cascade through which danger signals are released within the tumor microenvironment at the same time as lethal damage occurs to tumor cells, with exposure of previously hidden tumor-associated antigens in the midst of this inflammatory milieu. Therefore, antitumor immunity accompanies antiviral immunity.

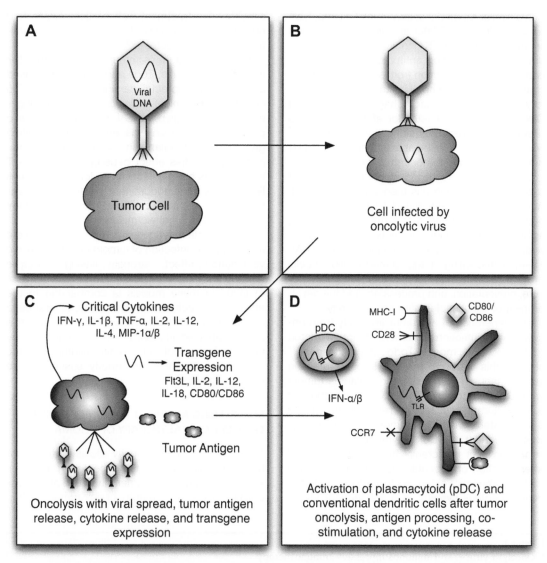

**Fig. 1.** Mechanism of therapeutic anticancer virus and immunity shows viral oncolysis and subsequent stimulation of dendritic cells. (*A*) Anticancer virus introduced to tumor cell. (*B*) Infection of tumor cell with viral DNA. (*C*) Viral infection of tumor cell permits viral replication and spread. Simultaneously, tumor antigens, immunostimulatory type I interferons, and other cytokines critical to mount an antiviral and antitumor immune response are released. If transgenes are inserted into viral DNA, these products will be expressed, including immunostimulatory molecules. (*D*) Viral infection creates inflammatory milieu of "danger signals" with cytokines, costimulatory molecules (CD80/CD86 with CD28), and viral activation of nuclear toll-like receptors, facilitating major histocompatibility complex I tumor antigen presentation and dendritic cell activation with CCR7 chemokine receptor up-regulation, for example.

Although this vaccine effect of oncolytic viral infection of tumors was a somewhat serendipitous finding, it may be invaluable in extending the therapeutic effect beyond tumor cells that are directly infected and may allow for durability of response.

The following discussion delineates the understanding of how an oncolytic virus can stimulate sustained antitumor immunity and antivector immunity that constrains oncolytic viral efficacy.

Early studies on the model of virally delivered HSV-TK in brain tumors described an interesting phenomenon of enhanced tumor killing beyond the area of infection.[34] Culver and colleagues[34] first showed this enhanced tumor killing in a rat model of glioma and termed it a *bystander effect*, wherein tumor cells that were not transduced with HSV-TK were still killed, perhaps because of contact with neighboring transduced cells.

In a similar rat model of intracranial glioma, Barba and colleagues[35] later showed that long-term survivors after HSV-TK/ganciclovir gene therapy developed long-lasting antitumor immunity, confirmed through protection from subsequent tumor challenge and intratumoral infiltration of inflammatory cells, including macrophages/microglia and CD8+ T cells. This bystander effect, which was previously believed to require cell-to-cell contact,[2] was thereby shown to be at least partly caused by development of antitumor immunity.

Okada and colleagues[36] conducted a series of experiments in which this theory was confirmed. Adenoviral and TK-mediated killing of subcutaneous tumors led to antitumor immune responses, again shown through protection against secondary intracranial tumor challenge. The HSV-TK–mediated killing of subcutaneous glioma cells provided a mechanism for improved antigen exposure, presentation, and processing, and the development of sustainable antitumor immunity.

The generation of antitumor immunity from oncolytic viral infection of tumors is not restricted to the HSV-TK model. Todo and colleagues[37] showed this vaccination effect through infecting subcutaneous N18 murine neuroblastoma tumors with G207 oncolytic HSV-1. G207 infection of a flank tumor resulted in reduced growth in a contralateral uninfected tumor, in a manner that was dependent on CD8+ T lymphocytes. In addition, growth of intracranial tumors was reduced after infection of subcutaneous tumors, showing that this immunity extended to tumors within the central nervous system. In a subsequent study,

simultaneous treatment with corticosteroids had no impact on oncolysis but abrogated the antitumor immune effects.[37,38]

To confirm that these immune effects with G207 were tumor-specific, Toda and colleagues[39] used a syngeneic colorectal carcinoma model (CT26 cells in BALB/c mice), which has poor immunogenicity but a known MHC-I restricted antigenic peptide. G207 again was effective in inhibiting growth in injected flank and contralateral tumors. Not only was this effect dependent on CD8+ T lymphocytes but also specificity for the CT26 cell line and its immunodominant peptide was clarified. Similar results were seen in the same study using the M3 syngeneic melanoma model.

In multiple syngeneic, immunocompetent models, G207 infection of tumors drives a specific vaccination effect, strongly linking oncolytic therapy with immunotherapy. This vaccine effect of G207 in these models is comparable to the efficacy of active cellular immunotherapeutic approaches. More recent work shows that this antigen-specific immunity can be generated by G207 infection of intracranial glioma tumors, even when the cells are poorly susceptible to direct oncolysis.[40]

## SUPPRESSING ANTIVIRAL IMMUNITY DURING ONCOLYTIC VIRAL THERAPY OF GLIOMA

Suppressing innate immunity allows better oncolytic viral replication and tumor cell killing (**Table 1**). Although blood–brain barrier disruption allows oncolytic HSV-1 to reach brain tumors when

| Table 1 | | | |
|---|---|---|---|
| Oncolytic viruses and immunosuppressive immunotherapy | | | |
| Oncolytic Virus Type | Oncolytic Virus Variant | Immunosuppressive Agent | Action/Mechanism |
| HSV | hrR3 | Cyclophosphamide | Reduction in microglia/macrophages and intratumoral IFN-γ[44,45] Depletion of complement and pre-immune IgM[42,43] |
| HSV | hrR3 and MGH-1 | Cobra venom factor and cyclophosphamide | Depletion of complement[30] |
| VSV | VSV-ΔM51 | HDIs and carrier cells | HDIs inhibit IFN-mediated antiviral response in normal cells and carrier cells shield the virus from the immune system for improved local delivery[49,50,52] |

*Abbreviations:* HDI, histone deacetylase inhibitors; HSV, herpes simplex virus; IFN, interferon; VSV, vesicular stomatitis virus.

administered intravascularly, its effect is attenuated by innate immunity, shown in the rat to be related to preimmune IgM.[41] Cyclophosphamide, a strongly immunosuppressive alkylating agent, substantially increases viral efficacy and limits the inactivation of virus by IgM.[42] The initial hypothesis was that preimmune IgM causes aggregation of viral particles, allowing activation of the classical pathway of complement. Cyclophosphamide, however, affects B cells primarily in their production of preimmune IgM and IgG, while leaving the complement system intact.[42]

Ikeda and colleagues[43] examined the effects of complement depletion on the efficacies of oncolytic adenovirus and HSV. After exposing these viruses to rat plasma pretreated with complement-depleting cobra venom factor, they showed improved virus activity, which was further augmented by addition of cyclophosphamide.[43]

Although innate immunoglobulins such as IgM and their resulting activation of the complement cascade might provide an initial immune response to oncolytic viruses, other effectors of the innate immune system, including natural killer cells and cells of monocyte lineage (macrophages/microglia), play a significant role, particularly in the brain.

To investigate the mechanism of cyclophosphamide and its enhancement of oncolytic viral therapy, Fulci and colleagues[44] studied a rat model of glioma with intratumoral injection of oncolytic HSV-1 and showed a rapid increase in the number of intratumoral NK cells, intratumoral IFN-γ, and intratumoral microglia and macrophages. Pretreatment with cyclophosphamide significantly reduced infiltration of these innate immune effectors, allowing for increased oncolytic virus replication and spread. In later work, both peripheral macrophages and brain-resident microglia were depleted from rodents to confirm that these innate immune effectors significantly decreased the titer of oncolytic virus in the brain (**Fig. 2**).[45]

VSV is another oncolytic virus whose efficacy is impacted by innate immunity. Although primarily studied in tumor models other than glioma, oncolytic VSV shows the importance of innate immunity in shaping the activity of therapeutic viruses. VSV is a single-stranded, negative-sense RNA virus that is neurotropic and very sensitive to the host type-1 IFN response.[46] In fact, type-1 interferons are primarily responsible for preventing central nervous system VSV infection from progressing to encephalitis.[47] Cancer cell selectivity is conferred, therefore, by the fact that several malignancies are deficient in their interferon response to viral infection.[46] An attenuated version of wild-type

VSV is safer and more selective, because normal cells fully arrest viral replication, whereas malignant cells are unable to do so.[48] One attenuated VSV has an insertion in the gene for the viral matrix (M) protein and is denoted *VSV-ΔM51*.[49] One of the M protein's functions is to block intracellular interferon mRNA; a mutated M protein allows restoration of the normal type-1 IFN response of infected cells.

Using this attenuated virus, Lun and colleagues[49] showed significant tumor inhibition against 14 human glioma cell lines in vivo. Systemic delivery of VSV-ΔM51 prolonged survival against orthotopic U87 invasive glioma in nude mice.[49] Significant neurotoxicity from inflammation was seen when the virus was delivered intracranially, suggesting that further engineering may be necessary to control the innate immune response for safer and more selective VSV replication. In response, the investigators treated colon and breast cancer cell lines in nude mice with VSV-ΔM51 and histone deacetylase inhibitors (HDIs). HDIs are known to depress the IFN-based antiviral immune response, suppressing innate immunity.[50]

Power and colleagues[51,52] explored another method to escape antivector immunity with VSV. Nonimmunogenic carrier cells were designed to convey VSV to the tumor site and release the virus there, extending the period of immune evasion in a syngeneic mouse model.

## ENHANCING ANTIGLIOMA IMMUNITY THROUGH ONCOLYTIC VIRAL TREATMENT

The potential downside of using immunosuppression to improve viral load and replication is the possible depression of antitumor immune effects. Rather than immunosuppressive modification of the tumor microenvironment, an alternative approach to glioma therapy is to bolster the antitumor immune effects seen with oncolytic viral infection (**Table 2**). Several variations of this have been used, with the most common approach being insertion of immunostimulatory transgenes or cotreatment with helper viruses engineered to express immune-active agents.

A rat glioma model showed that intratumoral adenoviral (nonlytic) delivery of the immune-stimulatory gene Flt3L was ineffective by itself but caused significantly prolonged survival when combined with an oncolytic viral system (ie, with expression of HSV-TK and systemic administration of ganciclovir).[53] This effect was lost with depletion of CD4+ T lymphocytes or macrophages, but depletion of CD8+ cells or NK cells had no effect.

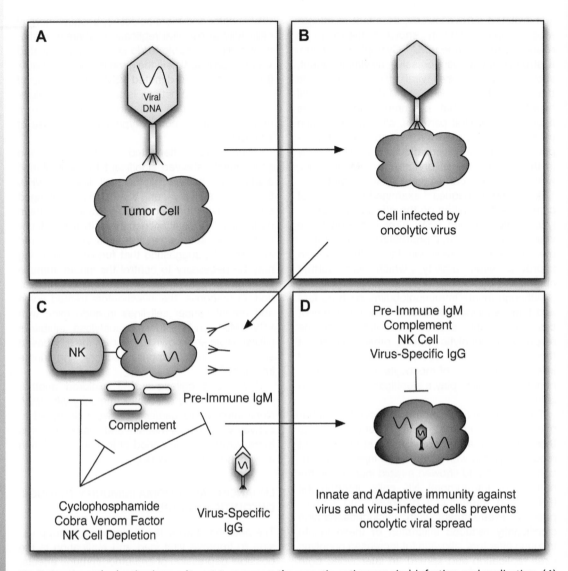

**Fig. 2.** Innate and adaptive immunity act to suppress therapeutic anticancer viral infection and replication. (*A*) Anticancer virus introduced to tumor cell. (*B*) Infection of tumor cell with viral DNA. (*C*) Strategies to limit antiviral immune response include cyclophosphamide, cobra venom factor, and natural killer cell depletion. (*D*) Without specific immunosuppressive strategies to allow viral replication and oncolysis, natural killer cells, complement, preimmune IgM, and virus-specific IgG act in concert to limit anticancer viral infection and replication.

A likely mechanism for these effects is Flt3L stimulation of antigen-presenting cells, which may be attracted to the environment by chemokines and other danger signals associated with viral infection and HSV-TK–mediated cell death. DCs are the most important link between the introduction of tumor-associated antigens and the activation of the adaptive immune system.[28] DCs express several receptors for pathogen-associated molecular patterns, including toll-like receptors, which can activate a DC to up-regulate

costimulatory molecules, such as CD80 and CD86 (B7-1 and B7-2, respectively), that assist in activating an immune response.

At the heart of combination oncolytic viral therapy and immunotherapy is the goal of augmenting this natural DC activation and function, which can be achieved not only using viral particles, which activate toll-like receptors, but also using tumor cell necrotic and apoptotic death, associated with release of antigens for processing by APCs. Oncolytic viruses that express cytokines

**Table 2**
**Oncolytic virus and immunostimulatory immunotherapy**

| Oncolytic Virus Type | Oncolytic Virus Variant | Immunostimulatory Agent | Action/Mechanism |
|---|---|---|---|
| Adeno | Ad5 | FLT3L and HSV-TK | FLT3L stimulates antigen presentation by DCs and HSV-TK with systemic ganciclovir eradicates tumor with additional bystander effect[53,54] |
| Adeno | Ad5 | IFN-alpha and DCs | IFN-alpha and DCs were injected intratumorally, which helps present antigen derives from oncolytic virus killing[71] |
| HSV | MGH-1-BAC | Soluble B7-1 (CD80), IL-12, IL-18 | B7-1 improves costimulation, whereas IL-12 and IL-18 stimulate T-cell–based adaptive immunity[22] |
| HSV | G47Δ-BAC | Soluble B7-1 (CD80) and IL-18 | Improved costimulation and T-cell adaptive immunity[21] |
| HSV | G47Δ | Intratumoral DC injection | Improved presentation of antigen by DCs after tumor cell lysis by oncolytic virus[56] |
| Vaccinia | rVV | IL-2 and IL-12 | IL-2 stimulates expansion of cytotoxic T cells and IL-12 enhances NK cells and T-cell–based adaptive immunity[72,73] |
| VSV | VSV-ΔM51 | DCs infected by VSV-ΔM51 | DCs are infected with VSV-ΔM51 and the virus itself is used as an immunostimulatory adjuvant for costimulation with antigen presentation[49,74] |
| NDV | NDV | Autologous glioma vaccine infected with NDV | NDV infection of glioma vaccine functions as immune adjuvant to elicit interferon response[58] |

*Abbreviations:* DC, dendritic cell; FLT3L, FMS-like tyrosine kinase 3 ligand; HSV, herpes simplex virus; IFN, interferon; IL, interleukin; NDV, Newcastle disease virus; NK, natural killer; TK, thymidine kinase; VSV, vesicular stomatitis virus.

such as Flt3L, which helps maturation of DCs, further augment the stimulation of antitumor immunity against tumors. Ultimately, this therapy can generate a powerful and effective antitumor response against intracranial glioma.[53]

To simulate invasive and diffusely infiltrating human malignant glioma, the same group used this Flt3L/TK treatment system in a multifocal glioma model.[54] Brain tumors that were not directly inoculated with virus were controlled, confirming that distant, infiltrating glioma cells can be tracked by the effectors of oncolytic gene therapy.

Consistent with this approach, other transgenes whose products enhance antigen presentation have been used to arm oncolytic viruses. In an immunocompetent mouse model of neuroblastoma, oncolytic HSV-1 was modified through a BAC system to express IL-18 and soluble B7-1 (CD80). IL-18 is an important cytokine that induces the release of IFN-$\gamma$, which helps stimulate T-cell immunity. Soluble B7-1 is an important costimulatory molecule that binds to CD28 on T lymphocytes to activate the immune response.[21] Combined expression of IL-18 and release of this soluble B7-1 showed significant efficacy against prostate cancer and neuroblastoma tumors.[21] The capacity for engineering viral vectors with multiple complementary immunostimulatory genes was shown through the triple arming of oncolytic HSV-1 with genes for IL-12, IL-18, and soluble B7-1.[22]

The intra- or peritumoral presence of DCs is associated with improved survival in some human cancers. Oncolytic virus infection itself may increase the number of DCs in the tumor environment.[55] Likewise, viral expression of chemokines or Flt3L further increases the number of intratumoral DCs. We have shown that combining intratumoral injection of oncolytic HSV-1 with direct injection of immature DCs establishes powerful curative immunity in mice with subcutaneous tumors.[56] This model has a specific requirement for immature DCs, because injecting mature cells does not augment the effects of virus alone. This research suggests that oncolytic HSV-1 infection of tumors provides the antigenic material for processing by immature DCs and the activating signals required for DC maturation and subsequent migration and antigen presentation in lymph nodes.

Newcastle disease virus (NDV) has been shown to be safe and feasible for use in patients who have recurrent malignant glioma.[57] NDV is an oncolytic paramyxovirus that replicates selectively in tumor cells. Cellular response to infection by NDV is characterized by up-regulated expression of immune danger signals, such as double-stranded RNA, IFNs, and chemokines. This property has been exploited in an autologous tumor cell vaccination clinical trial. Glioma cells were harvested at surgery and infected with NDV, before being injected intradermally into patients.[58]

Results of this phase I trial were promising, because biologic activity was seen in essentially every patient, partly shown through positive delayed-type hypersensitivity reactions. Later preclinical work in a rat model used active specific immunization with NDV–glioma vaccine plus transforming growth factor (TGF)-$\beta$ antisense oligonucleotides in the form of nanoparticles to show increased survival in treated rats and an increase in effector immune cells.[59]

In something of a twist, the immunostimulatory properties of an oncolytic virus were used for ex vivo modification of a tumor vaccine, promoting better in situ immune recognition and activation.

As oncolytic viral therapy and immunotherapy become confluent, one can envision scenarios for specific targeting of various aspects of the immune system. For instance, the neuroblastoma microenvironment is particularly suppressive to DC maturation.[60] The combination of intratumoral oncolytic HSV-1 and intratumoral injection of ex vivo–generated immature DCs may be particularly well suited for these tumors. In the case of glioma, the proportion of regulatory T cells (expressing the transcription factor Foxp3) and high expression of TGF-$\beta$ contribute to tumor-derived immunosuppression, and, therefore, combining oncolytic viral infection with T-regulatory cell depletion or targeting would be rational.[61] These areas are being actively studied, and this type of work is already being translated into clinical applications. In a small trial of patients who had recurrent glioblastoma, gene therapy with HSV-TK and IL-2 was shown to be safe and feasible, and achieved objective tumor responses.[62]

## IMMUNOTHERAPEUTIC TARGETING OF VIRAL ANTIGENS AS THERAPY

This article has focused on the use of viruses as vectors for gene therapy or as oncolytic agents. Human cytomegalovirus (HCMV) is a herpes virus that seems to be highly expressed in gliomas, perhaps because of a natural tropism for glial cells.[63] In addition, HCMV gene products have been implicated in the disruption of cellular pathways that could lead to cellular transformation.[64–66] HCMV viral DNA was also noted to be shed in the blood of patients who have malignant glioma.[67]

In one study involving vaccinations of DCs pulsed with autologous tumor lysate, a patient who had glioblastoma developed a strong CD8+ T-cell response to the pp65 epitope of HCMV, which was found to be expressed in the patient's tumor.[68] Ongoing clinical studies involve vaccinating malignant glioma patients with DCs pulsed with tumor antigens (http://clinicaltrials.gov/ct2/show/NCT00639639).

## SUMMARY

Although much remains to be learned about the mechanisms, virus-mediated death of tumor cells seems to be associated with development of real antitumor immunity. From an immunotherapy point of view, viral vectors were initially considered carriers of immunostimulatory cytokines, with the goal of activating better tumor cell expression of MHC, activating T lymphocytes in the tumor milieu, or attracting circulating immune cells into the tumor. Through immunoediting, cancer cells have effectively hidden themselves from immune detection.

Effective immunotherapy requires two achievements: (1) tumor-associated antigens must be exposed or unmasked and (2) negative immune regulation must be overcome. Oncolytic viral infection has promise as cancer therapy based on viral killing alone; furthermore, virus-associated cell death may provide the charge to the system required for initiating an antitumor immune response that has specificity and durability. In a clinical scenario, this immune activity itself is unlikely to cure advanced malignancies; however, if intelligently integrated among other therapies that may be synergistic (eg, low-dose chemotherapy, VEGF blockade, other immunotherapies), clinical benefit may be realized. Experts continue to explore combining oncolytic virus infection of tumors with other therapies in preclinical glioma models, with the specific intent of maximizing antitumor immunity.

Although pretreatment with immunosuppressive agents such as cyclophosphamide would seem to impair postviral inoculation antitumor immunity, this may not true, and increasing intratumoral viral spread is a rational goal. Low-dose cyclophosphamide may act as an immune adjuvant, perhaps because of selective suppression of regulatory T lymphocytes.[69] If timed properly, vaccination efforts may benefit from some degree of myeloablation, because effector cells reconstitute at a different pace than do regulatory cells.[70] Clearly, details of dose, schedule, and agent must be worked out, but a strategy that will optimize viral replication without compromising postinfectious antiglioma immunity is envisioned. Clinical trials designed to address these issues are critical to maintaining momentum toward these goals.

## REFERENCES

1. CBTRUS. Statistical report: primary brain tumors in the United States 2000–2004. Chicago: Central Brain Tumor Registry of the United States; 2008.
2. Chiocca EA, Aghi M, Fulci G. Viral therapy for glioblastoma. Cancer J 2003;9:167–79.
3. Selznick LA, Shamji MF, Fecci P, et al. Molecular strategies for the treatment of malignant glioma–genes, viruses, and vaccines. Neurosurg Rev 2008;31:141–55.
4. Rainov NG, Ren H. Gene therapy for human malignant brain tumors. Cancer J 2003;9:180–8.
5. Bischoff JR, Kirn DH, Williams A, et al. An adenovirus mutant that replicates selectively in p53-deficient human tumor cells. Science 1996;274:373–6.
6. Asaoka K, Tada M, Sawamura Y, et al. Dependence of efficient adenoviral gene delivery in malignant glioma cells on the expression levels of the Coxsackievirus and adenovirus receptor. J Neurosurg 2000;92:1002–8.
7. Martuza RL, Malick A, Markert JM, et al. Experimental therapy of human glioma by means of a genetically engineered virus mutant. Science 1991;252:854–6.
8. Forsyth P, Roldan G, George D, et al. A phase I trial of intratumoral administration of reovirus in patients with histologically confirmed recurrent malignant gliomas. Mol Ther 2008;16:627–32.
9. Vecil GG, Lang FF. Clinical trials of adenoviruses in brain tumors: a review of Ad-p53 and oncolytic adenoviruses. J Neurooncol 2003;65:237–46.
10. Cattaneo R, Miest T, Shashkova EV, et al. Reprogrammed viruses as cancer therapeutics: targeted, armed and shielded. Nat Rev Microbiol 2008;6:529–40.
11. Chiocca EA. Oncolytic viruses. Nat Rev Cancer 2002;2:938–50.
12. Geoerger B, Grill J, Opolon P, et al. Oncolytic activity of the E1B-55 kDa-deleted adenovirus ONYX-015 is independent of cellular p53 status in human malignant glioma xenografts. Cancer Res 2002;62:764–72.
13. O'Shea CC, Johnson L, Bagus B, et al. Late viral RNA export, rather than p53 inactivation, determines ONYX-015 tumor selectivity. Cancer Cell 2004;6:611–23.
14. O'Shea CC, Soria C, Bagus B, et al. Heat shock phenocopies E1B-55K late functions and selectively sensitizes refractory tumor cells to ONYX-015 oncolytic viral therapy. Cancer Cell 2005;8:61–74.
15. Fueyo J, Gomez-Manzano C, Alemany R, et al. A mutant oncolytic adenovirus targeting the Rb pathway produces anti-glioma effect in vivo. Oncogene 2000;19:2–12.
16. Heise C, Hermiston T, Johnson L, et al. An adenovirus E1A mutant that demonstrates potent and selective systemic anti-tumoral efficacy. Nat Med 2000;6:1134–9.
17. Johnson L, Shen A, Boyle L, et al. Selectively replicating adenoviruses targeting deregulated E2F activity are potent, systemic antitumor agents. Cancer Cell 2002;1:325–37.
18. Markert JM, Parker JN, Buchsbaum DJ, et al. Oncolytic HSV-1 for the treatment of brain tumours. Herpes 2006;13:66–71.
19. Mineta T, Rabkin SD, Yazaki T, et al. Attenuated multi-mutated herpes simplex virus-1 for the treatment of malignant gliomas. Nat Med 1995;1:938–43.
20. Todo T, Martuza RL, Rabkin SD, et al. Oncolytic herpes simplex virus vector with enhanced MHC class I presentation and tumor cell killing. Proc Natl Acad Sci U S A 2001;98:6396–401.

21. Fukuhara H, Ino Y, Kuroda T, et al. Triple gene-deleted oncolytic herpes simplex virus vector double-armed with interleukin 18 and soluble B7-1 constructed by bacterial artificial chromosome-mediated system. Cancer Res 2005;65:10663–8.

22. Ino Y, Saeki Y, Fukuhara H, et al. Triple combination of oncolytic herpes simplex virus-1 vectors armed with interleukin-12, interleukin-18, or soluble B7-1 results in enhanced antitumor efficacy. Clin Cancer Res 2006;12:643–52.

23. Dunn GP, Bruce AT, Ikeda H, et al. Cancer immunoediting: from immunosurveillance to tumor escape. Nat Immunol 2002;3:991–8.

24. Dunn GP, Old LJ, Schreiber RD. The immunobiology of cancer immunosurveillance and immunoediting. Immunity 2004;21:137–48.

25. Dunn GP, Old LJ, Schreiber RD. The three Es of cancer immunoediting. Annu Rev Immunol 2004; 22:329–60.

26. Dranoff G. Cytokines in cancer pathogenesis and cancer therapy. Nat Rev Cancer 2004;4:11–22.

27. Rakoff-Nahoum S, Medzhitov R. Toll-like receptors and cancer. Nat Rev Cancer 2009;9:57–63.

28. Pulendran B. Modulating vaccine responses with dendritic cells and Toll-like receptors. Immunol Rev 2004;199:227–50.

29. Broberg EK, Hukkanen V. Immune response to herpes simplex virus and gamma134.5 deleted HSV vectors. Curr Gene Ther 2005;5:523–30.

30. Wakimoto H, Ikeda K, Abe T, et al. The complement response against an oncolytic virus is species-specific in its activation pathways. Mol Ther 2002; 5:275–82.

31. Balachandran S, Barber GN. Defective translational control facilitates vesicular stomatitis virus oncolysis. Cancer Cell 2004;5:51–65.

32. Balachandran S, Thomas E, Barber GN. A FADD-dependent innate immune mechanism in mammalian cells. Nature 2004;432:401–5.

33. Lanier LL. Evolutionary struggles between NK cells and viruses. Nat Rev Immunol 2008;8:259–68.

34. Culver KW, Ram Z, Wallbridge S, et al. In vivo gene transfer with retroviral vector-producer cells for treatment of experimental brain tumors. Science 1992; 256:1550–2.

35. Barba D, Hardin J, Sadelain M, et al. Development of anti-tumor immunity following thymidine kinase-mediated killing of experimental brain tumors. Proc Natl Acad Sci U S A 1994;91:4348–52.

36. Okada T, Shah M, Higginbotham JN, et al. AV.TK-mediated killing of subcutaneous tumors in situ results in effective immunization against established secondary intracranial tumor deposits. Gene Ther 2001;8:1315–22.

37. Todo T, Rabkin SD, Sundaresan P, et al. Systemic antitumor immunity in experimental brain tumor therapy using a multimutated, replication-competent herpes simplex virus. Hum Gene Ther 1999;10: 2741–55.

38. Todo T, Rabkin SD, Chahlavi A, et al. Corticosteroid administration does not affect viral oncolytic activity, but inhibits antitumor immunity in replication-competent herpes simplex virus tumor therapy. Hum Gene Ther 1999;10:2869–78.

39. Toda M, Rabkin SD, Kojima H, et al. Herpes simplex virus as an in situ cancer vaccine for the induction of specific anti-tumor immunity. Hum Gene Ther 1999; 10:385–93.

40. Iizuka Y, Kojima H, Kobata T, et al. Identification of a glioma antigen, GARC-1, using cytotoxic T lymphocytes induced by HSV cancer vaccine. Int J Cancer 2006;118:942–9.

41. Rainov NG, Zimmer C, Chase M, et al. Selective uptake of viral and monocrystalline particles delivered intra-arterially to experimental brain neoplasms. Hum Gene Ther 1995;6:1543–52.

42. Ikeda K, Ichikawa T, Wakimoto H, et al. Oncolytic virus therapy of multiple tumors in the brain requires suppression of innate and elicited antiviral responses. Nat Med 1999;5:881–7.

43. Ikeda K, Wakimoto H, Ichikawa T, et al. Complement depletion facilitates the infection of multiple brain tumors by an intravascular, replication-conditional herpes simplex virus mutant. J Virol 2000;74: 4765–75.

44. Fulci G, Breymann L, Gianni D, et al. Cyclophosphamide enhances glioma virotherapy by inhibiting innate immune responses. Proc Natl Acad Sci U S A 2006;103:12873–8.

45. Fulci G, Dmitrieva N, Gianni D, et al. Depletion of peripheral macrophages and brain microglia increases brain tumor titers of oncolytic viruses. Cancer Res 2007;67:9398–406.

46. Stojdl DF, Lichty B, Knowles S, et al. Exploiting tumor-specific defects in the interferon pathway with a previously unknown oncolytic virus. Nat Med 2000;6:821–5.

47. Detje CN, Meyer T, Schmidt H, et al. Local type I IFN receptor signaling protects against virus spread within the central nervous system. J Immunol 2009; 182:2297–304.

48. Stojdl DF, Lichty BD, tenOever BR, et al. VSV strains with defects in their ability to shutdown innate immunity are potent systemic anti-cancer agents. Cancer Cell 2003;4:263–75.

49. Lun X, Senger DL, Alain T, et al. Effects of intravenously administered recombinant vesicular stomatitis virus (VSV(deltaM51)) on multifocal and invasive gliomas. J Natl Cancer Inst 2006;98:1546–57.

50. Nguyen TL, Abdelbary H, Arguello M, et al. Chemical targeting of the innate antiviral response by histone deacetylase inhibitors renders refractory cancers sensitive to viral oncolysis. Proc Natl Acad Sci U S A 2008;105:14981–6.

51. Power AT, Bell JC. Taming the Trojan horse: optimizing dynamic carrier cell/oncolytic virus systems for cancer biotherapy. Gene Ther 2008;15:772–9.

52. Power AT, Wang J, Falls TJ, et al. Carrier cell-based delivery of an oncolytic virus circumvents antiviral immunity. Mol Ther 2007;15:123–30.

53. Ali S, King GD, Curtin JF, et al. Combined immunostimulation and conditional cytotoxic gene therapy provide long-term survival in a large glioma model. Cancer Res 2005;65:7194–204.

54. King GD, Muhammad AK, Curtin JF, et al. Flt3L and TK gene therapy eradicate multifocal glioma in a syngeneic glioblastoma model. Neuro Oncol 2008;10:19–31.

55. Benencia F, Courreges MC, Conejo-Garcia JR, et al. HSV oncolytic therapy upregulates interferon-inducible chemokines and recruits immune effector cells in ovarian cancer. Mol Ther 2005;12:789–802.

56. Farrell CJ, Zaupa C, Barnard Z, et al. Combination immunotherapy for tumors via sequential intratumoral injections of oncolytic herpes simplex virus 1 and immature dendritic cells. Clin Cancer Res 2008;14: 7711–6.

57. Freeman AI, Zakay-Rones Z, Gomori JM, et al. Phase I/II trial of intravenous NDV-HUJ oncolytic virus in recurrent glioblastoma multiforme. Mol Ther 2006;13:221–8.

58. Schneider T, Gerhards R, Kirches E, et al. Preliminary results of active specific immunization with modified tumor cell vaccine in glioblastoma multiforme. J Neurooncol 2001;53:39–46.

59. Schneider T, Becker A, Ringe K, et al. Brain tumor therapy by combined vaccination and antisense oligonucleotide delivery with nanoparticles. J Neuroimmunol 2008;195:21–7.

60. Shurin GV, Shurin MR, Bykovskaia S, et al. Neuroblastoma-derived gangliosides inhibit dendritic cell generation and function. Cancer Res 2001;61:363–9.

61. Mitchell DA, Fecci PE, Sampson JH. Immunotherapy of malignant brain tumors. Immunol Rev 2008;222: 70–100.

62. Colombo F, Barzon L, Franchin E, et al. Combined HSV-TK/IL-2 gene therapy in patients with recurrent glioblastoma multiforme: biological and clinical results. Cancer Gene Ther 2005;12:835–48.

63. Cobbs CS, Harkins L, Samanta M, et al. Human cytomegalovirus infection and expression in human malignant glioma. Cancer Res 2002;62:3347–50.

64. Loenen WA, Bruggeman CA, Wiertz EJ. Immune evasion by human cytomegalovirus: lessons in immunology and cell biology. Semin Immunol 2001;13:41–9.

65. Lokensgard JR, Cheeran MC, Gekker G, et al. Human cytomegalovirus replication and modulation of apoptosis in astrocytes. J Hum Virol 1999; 2:91–101.

66. Salvant BS, Fortunato EA, Spector DH. Cell cycle dysregulation by human cytomegalovirus: influence of the cell cycle phase at the time of infection and effects on cyclin transcription. J Virol 1998;72:3729–41.

67. Mitchell DA, Xie W, Schmittling R, et al. Sensitive detection of human cytomegalovirus in tumors and peripheral blood of patients diagnosed with glioblastoma. Neuro Oncol 2008;10:10–8.

68. Prins RM, Cloughesy TF, Liau LM. Cytomegalovirus immunity after vaccination with autologous glioblastoma lysate. N Engl J Med 2008;359: 539–41.

69. Liu J-Y, Wu Y, Zhang X-S, et al. Single administration of low dose cyclophosphamide augments the antitumor effect of dendritic cell vaccine. Cancer Immunol Immunother 2007;56:1597–604.

70. Heimberger AB, Sun W, Hussain SF, et al. Immunological responses in a patient with glioblastoma multiforme treated with sequential courses of temozolomide and immunotherapy: case study. Neuro Oncol 2008;10:98–103.

71. Tsugawa T, Kuwashima N, Sato H, et al. Sequential delivery of interferon-alpha gene and DCs to intracranial gliomas promotes an effective antitumor response. Gene Ther 2004;11:1551–8.

72. Chen B, Timiryasova TM, Andres ML, et al. Evaluation of combined vaccinia virus-mediated antitumor gene therapy with p53, IL-2, and IL-12 in a glioma model. Cancer Gene Ther 2000;7:1437–47.

73. Chen B, Timiryasova TM, Gridley DS, et al. Evaluation of cytokine toxicity induced by vaccinia virus-mediated IL-2 and IL-12 antitumour immunotherapy. Cytokine 2001;15:305–14.

74. Boudreau JE, Bridle BW, Stephenson KB, et al. Recombinant vesicular stomatitis virus transduction of dendritic cells enhances their ability to prime innate and adaptive antitumor immunity. Mol Ther 2009;17: 1465–72.

# Distinguishing Glioma Recurrence from Treatment Effect After Radiochemotherapy and Immunotherapy

Isaac Yang, MD[a],*, Nancy G. Huh, MD[a], Zachary A. Smith, MD[b],
Seunggu J. Han, BS[a], Andrew T. Parsa, MD, PhD[a]

**KEYWORDS**

- Immunotherapy • Tumor recurrence • Pseudoprogression
- Radiation-induced necrosis • Bevacizumab
- Temozolomide • Glioma

Despite advances in treatment for glioblastoma (GBM), the survival of patients with malignant gliomas has not significantly improved over the past 2 decades.[1–4] Radiotherapy and chemotherapy (radiochemotherapy) is currently the standard of care for patients with GBM, followed by serial imaging to monitor posttreatment GBM progression.[5–7] Increased posttreatment imaging has led to incidental diagnosis and awareness of progressive imaging lesions with or without clinical sequelae that do not clinically behave longterm as glioma recurrence.[3,5,8,9] Imaging findings of treatment effect and GBM tumor recurrence are not easily distinguishable with conventional contrast-enhanced standard MRI and hence present challenges to investigators and clinicians.[3,5,10–18] This article reviews the recent advances in radiology imaging modalities that have the potential to distinguish GBM recurrence from treatment effect after radiochemotherapy and immunotherapy.

## TREATMENT-EFFECT NECROSIS

Since randomized trials in the 1970s showed the clinical benefits of radiotherapy in malignant gliomas, a total of 60 Gy fractionated radiation to the target glioma and tumor margins has become standard care for these glioblastomas.[2,6,19] Radiation-induced necrosis is the necrotic damage associated with radiation-based treatment modalities of malignant glioblastomas and is frequently identified in patients who undergo surgical treatment of progressive lesions within 6 months after radiochemotherapy.[3,8] The clinical course for radionecrosis is highly variable and can present with focal deficits, increased intracranial pressure, or can be asymptomatic.[3] Typically, radiation-induced necrosis occurs 3 to 12 months after radiochemotherapy, but occasionally does occur years after radiation treatment.[12,20]

On MRI, treatment-effect necrosis commonly appears as a contrast-enhancing mass lesion on T1-weighted imaging with gadolinium, and on

All authors declare no potential conflicts of interest. IY was partially supported by a UCSF Clinical and Translational Scientist Training Research Award and a NIH National Research Service Award grant. SJH was funded by a Howard Hughes Medical Institute Research Training Fellowship. ATP was partially funded by a Reza and Georgianna Khatib Endowed Chair in Skull Base Tumor Surgery.

[a] Department of Neurological Surgery, University of California at San Francisco, 505 Parnassus Avenue, San Francisco, CA 94143, USA

[b] Department of Neurological Surgery, University of California at Los Angeles, 757 Westwood Plaza, Los Angeles, CA 90095, USA

* Corresponding author.

*E-mail address:* yangi@neurosurg.ucsf (I. Yang).

Neurosurg Clin N Am 21 (2010) 181–186
doi:10.1016/j.nec.2009.08.003
1042-3680/09/$ – see front matter © 2010 Published by Elsevier Inc.

T2-weighted imaging with increased signal intensity in the necrotic central component of the mass lesion.[3,12] This appearance on conventional MRI is indistinguishable from tumor progression or pseudoprogression using standard imaging techniques.[3,11–18] Treatment-effect necrosis does appear to have an increased incidence in the periventricular white matter, which may be due to the vulnerability of frail blood supply to these areas.[3]

The reported incidence of treatment-effect necrosis is approximately 3% to 24% after radiochemotherapy for glioblastomas with a direct association to increased radiation dose and larger irradiated brain tissue volume.[3,11,21] Treatment-effect necrosis occurs most commonly at the site of maximal radiation exposure, typically in the surrounding area near the tumor or resection cavity.[3] After 50 Gy radiation to two-thirds of the total brain volume or 60 Gy to one-third of the brain using fractionation, the approximate five-year risk for radiation induced necrosis is 5%.[3,21] However, the real risk of treatment-effect necrosis may be underestimated because many of these patients die earlier than 5 years due to GBM tumor progression.[3] Several clinical factors such as higher radiation doses, hyperfractionation, interstitial brachytherapy, reirradiation, and radiochemotherapy have been reported to increase the risk for treatment-effect necrosis.[2,3,8,12,21–26]

Treatment-effect necrosis is a severe local tissue reaction to adjuvant radiochemotherapy, which manifests as a concomitant disruption of the blood brain barrier, necrosis, edema, and mass effect on MRI.[3,17] Histopathologic characteristics in addition to the necrosis include gliosis, endothelial thickening, hyalinization, and fibroid deposition.[3] Furthermore, these areas of necrosis are commonly scattered with tumor cells with uncertain viability on histologic review.[3,27]

## PSEUDOPROGRESSION

Pseudoprogression is the early subacute treatment reaction with edema, contrast enhancement, mass effect, and sometimes with associated clinical symptoms, which suggests GBM progression—but these lesions and their associated clinical symptoms resolve and recover spontaneously without intervention.[3,5,8,9,28,29] In early reports, pseudoprogression was identified and defined when, after radiochemotherapy, patients with malignant GBM were found to have new areas of contrast-enhancing lesions on MR imaging, mimicking glioma progression—but these lesions would subsequently improve without any further treatment.[3,5,8,9] Because these lesions appeared as tumor progression, these early subacute effects

of treatment were coined pseudoprogression.[3,5,8,9,28,29] Pseudoprogression lesions differ from treatment-effect necrosis in that pseudoprogression typically is identified on early MRI done within the first 2 months after adjuvant treatment.[5,8,9] Conversely, treatment-effect necrosis is a more late effect, typically occurring 3 months to a year after treatment.[3,9,21]

The reported incidence of pseudoprogression in patients with malignant GBM treated with radiation alone is roughly 10%, with a significant increase in incidence when radiochemotherapy treatment is used.[5,8,9] On follow-up imaging, these pseudoprogression lesions usually stabilize or shrink in size and contrast enhancement.[3]

It has been suggested that pseudoprogression represents a spectrum of treatment-induced injury to neuronal tissue. With milder forms of injury, this mechanism may produce pseudoprogression on subacute MRI that will resolve without treatment, but more severe levels of treatment-effect injury may lead to true necrosis.[3] Both pseudoprogression and treatment-effect necrosis have been noted to increase in frequency with the combination of chemotherapy with radiation.[8]

## IDENTIFYING TREATMENT EFFECT ON IMAGING AFTER IMMUNOTHERAPY

With the development of novel clinical trials using immunotherapy as a potential treatment modality, evaluation of posttreatment enhancement on MRI is problematic. Contrast-enhancing pseudoprogression and treatment-effect necrosis is increased with multimodality radiochemotherapy, and these problems with poor diagnostic specificity of contrast enhancement will likely increase with addition of other novel modalities such as immunotherapy, anti-vascular therapy, and gene therapy.[10,30–35] Addition of immunotherapy and other novel treatment modalities to the standard radiochemotherapy may synergistically enhance multiple apoptotic pathways through several metabolic pathways, which may explain the increased incidence of contrast-enhancing pseudoprogression and treatment-effect necrosis with multimodality therapy. Recent cases of dramatic early onset contrast-enhancing pseudoprogression in the first 2 months after immunotherapy and radiochemotherapy have been reported to present with dramatic size and contrast enhancement, followed with almost complete regression in 6 months—consistent with pseudoprogression.[10]

Because pseudoprogression may represent a local inflammatory or immune response, immunotherapy posttreatment lesions might be more likely to present as pseudoprogression or treatment-effect necrosis. Immunotherapy specifically with immune stimulation may be ultimately found to increase the incidence of contrast-enhancing pseudoprogression lesions, which ultimately regress without altering treatment. Careful posttreatment imaging is then critical because these pseudoprogression and treatment-effect, contrast-enhancing lesions are more common with multimodality therapies and possibly further elicited by immunotherapy. Radiographic advances in imaging modalities are critical, if not even more important, for patients receiving immunotherapy to accurately distinguish glioma recurrence from treatment effect with greater sensitivity.

## RADIOGRAPHIC ADVANCES IN DISTINGUISHING TUMOR RECURRENCE FROM TREATMENT EFFECT

Standard conventional MRI cannot reliably distinguish between the similar imaging characteristics of glioma tumor recurrence and treatment-effect necrosis or pseudoprogression.[3,11-18] The determination of active tumor infiltration and recurrence is of utmost clinical importance, and making this radiographic distinction has important consequences.[3,11-13,36] As novel therapies such as immunotherapy are investigated and developed, the incidence of treatment-effect necrosis and pseudoprogression may increase as more modalities are added to the standard multimodality of radiochemotherapy. Several recent advancements in radiographic modalities have shown promise in the noninvasive differentiation between glioma tumor recurrence and treatment effects, but these techniques have yet to be proven in large prospective trials.

Diffusion-weighted MRI (DWI) using the differences in apparent diffusion coefficients (ADC) is a nonstandard MR sequence that has shown promise in distinguishing treatment-effect necrosis from tumor recurrence after radiochemotherapy, but the specificity for DWI has yet to be fully characterized.[14,16,17,36-40] This DWI is a physiology based technique that measures the diffusion of Brownian water movement in vivo.[15,41-43] Increased cellularity decreases ADC values, which has been suggested as a method to distinguish glioma recurrence from treatment effects. A recent prospective study of 44 patient using DWI indicates that DWI-positive imaging in the immediate postoperative period is associated with imaging findings consistent with pseudoprogression or radiation necrosis in MRI scans 2 to 4 months later.[15] A recent retrospective review of 18 patients with contrast enhancement indicated that lower ADC and ADC ratios were significantly more associated with glioma recurrence than treatment

effect.[38] This imaging differentiation suggests some role for DWI to help distinguish tumor recurrence from treatment effect, but the full clinical application of DWI requires further investigations.

Noninvasive, functional imaging using proton-based magnetic resonance spectroscopy (MRS) has also been used to distinguish necrosis from tumor residual or recurrence by characterizing the metabolic properties of the lesion on MRS imaging.[16,44-48] Single voxel, early applications of MRS have had difficulty in heterogeneous lesions and differentiating between glioma and tumor mixed with necrosis.[11,16,44] Recent multivoxel, three-dimensional proton MRS techniques have been applied to the brain and demonstrate the feasibility of MRS to distinguish between treatment effects and glioma.[11,16,49-52] Using the most modern three-dimensional multivoxel application of MRS, a sensitivity of 94% and specificity of 100% was reported in an MRS evaluation of 28 glioma patients.[11] Floeth and colleagues[10] have demonstrated the feasibility and usefulness of MRS imaging to also distinguish between pseudoprogression and tumor recurrence after radiochemotherapy and immunotherapy. Although this functional proton-based MRS has shown promise, further investigations with larger samples are needed to confirm its reliability, feasibility with longer scan times, and usefulness in posterior fossa lesions, and sensitivity in distinguishing glioma recurrence from treatment effects.[11,44,53] These advances in radiographic imaging are used to distinguish tumor recurrence from treatment effect in other novel treatment modalities, such as immunotherapy, and exhibit great promise for this clinical utility in all brain tumor treatments.[10]

It has been suggested that a combination of two-dimensional MRS and DWI may increase the accuracy of distinguishing between tumor and treatment effect.[14,16,37,38] In a study of 55 patients, the addition of ADC ratios permitted a more broad analysis, not possible with MRS alone, with a 96% rate of correctly differentiating between tumor recurrence and treatment-effect injury.[14] Verma and colleagues[36] have demonstrated this feasibility of combining several MR modalities, including DWI, to improve the tissue characterization of brain neoplasms.

Recently, biologic functional scanning with positron emission tomography (PET) has shown potential in identifying tumor recurrence. 18-Fluorodeoxyglucose PET can be used to distinguish tumor from necrosis—although with limited sensitivity and specificity because of the baseline high glucose use of the normal brain.[54,55] Use of amino acid tracers and PET imaging improve on this inherent biology and have shown potential in discriminating between tumor and necrosis.[18,56] This imaging modality shows as much promise or specificity as the MRS-imaging modality described above.

## MANAGEMENT OF PATIENTS WITH RADIOGRAPHIC CHANGES AFTER GBM RESECTIONS

Because of the frequent incidence of pseudoprogression within the first 3 months after radiochemotherapy, the management of early progressive lesions remains problematic for clinicians because treatment decisions are difficult without identifying these posttreatment lesions. These difficult clinical decisions may be made more difficult by the addition of increasing modalities such as immunotherapy, which potentially increase the incidence of contrast-enhancing treatment effects. If there is early tumor progression, temozolomide is not effective; but, in the case of pseudoprogression or treatment-effect necrosis, temozolomide should be continued in asymptomatic patients with early progressive lesions.[3,57] Steroids can be used to mitigate the effects of the edema, but patients with early progressive lesions and clinical symptoms, should be managed surgically in the hopes of improving their clinical condition and determining a tissue and histologic diagnosis of the lesion.[3] This histopathology is further complicated because areas of radiation-induced necrosis are commonly scattered with tumor cells with uncertain viability.[3,27] Temozolomide should be continued if only necrosis is seen in these surgical treatments.[3,57] MRI scans with DWI and MRS should be seriously considered in patients receiving immunotherapy and multimodality adjuvant therapy to increase the sensitivity and specificity of imaging and to distinguish between glioma recurrence and pseudoprogression or treatment-effect necrosis.

## SUMMARY

Recent advances with multimodality radiation and chemotherapy have become standard of care for malignant gliomas with minimal improvements in survival. The increased efficacy of these multimodality therapies has likely manifested with the increasing incidence and diagnosis of pseudoprogression and treatment-effect necrosis. With the development of ever-increasing treatment modalities such as immunotherapy, the incidence of pseudoprogression and treatment-effect necrosis is likely to increase.

Accurately diagnosing these contrast-enhancing lesions as either tumor recurrence or treatment effect is of critical importance to prognosis and glioma treatment algorithms. Current standard MRI techniques are inadequate to reliably differentiate between tumor recurrence and pseudoprogression or treatment effects. Modern advancements with MRS, DWI, and functional PET scans have shown the promise to accurately identify tumor recurrence from treatment effect and may soon become part of the standard of care for posttreatment imaging. Conventional standards of evaluating contrast enhancement will be even less applicable to novel modalities such as immunotherapy, and these modern techniques of MRS, DWI, and PET scanning will become even more critical to discriminate tumor recurrence as newly developed therapeutic modalities emerge. Finally, these radiographic imaging advances can be applied clinically to decrease the misdiagnosis of contrast-enhancing lesions as tumor recurrence and improve posttreatment therapy with more accurate differentiation between tumor recurrence and treatment effects from multimodal adjuvant therapies.

## REFERENCES

1. Nieder C, Grosu AL, Mehta MP, et al. Treatment of malignant gliomas: radiotherapy, chemotherapy and integration of new targeted agents. Expert Rev Neurother 2004;4(4):691–703.
2. Nieder C, Andratschke N, Wiedenmann N, et al. Radiotherapy for high-grade gliomas. Does altered fractionation improve the outcome? Strahlenther Onkol 2004;180(7):401–7.
3. Brandsma D, Stalpers L, Taal W, et al. Clinical features, mechanisms, and management of pseudoprogression in malignant gliomas. Lancet Oncol 2008;9(5):453–61.
4. Yang I, Kremen TJ, Giovannone AJ, et al. Modulation of major histocompatibility complex Class I molecules and major histocompatibility complex-bound immunogenic peptides induced by interferon-alpha and interferon-gamma treatment of human glioblastoma multiforme. J Neurosurg 2004;100(2):310–9.
5. Brandes AA, Franceschi E, Tosoni A, et al. MGMT promoter methylation status can predict the incidence and outcome of pseudoprogression after concomitant radiochemotherapy in newly diagnosed glioblastoma patients. J Clin Oncol 2008;26(13):2192–7.
6. Stupp R, Mason WP, van den Bent MJ, et al. Radiotherapy plus concomitant and adjuvant temozolomide for glioblastoma. N Engl J Med 2005;352(10):987–96.

7. Mirimanoff RO, Gorlia T, Mason W, et al. Radio-therapy and temozolomide for newly diagnosed glio-blastoma: recursive partitioning analysis of the EORTC 26981/22981-NCIC CE3 phase III random-ized trial. J Clin Oncol 2006;24(16):2563–9.

8. Chamberlain MC, Glantz MJ, Chalmers L, et al. Early necrosis following concurrent Temodar and radio-therapy in patients with glioblastoma. J Neurooncol 2007;82(1):81–3.

9. de Wit MC, de Bruin HG, Eijkenboom W, et al. Imme-diate post-radiotherapy changes in malignant glioma can mimic tumor progression. Neurology 2004;63(3):535–7.

10. Floeth FW, Wittsack HJ, Engelbrecht V, et al. Comparative follow-up of enhancement phenomena with MRI and Proton MR Spectroscopic Imaging after intralesional immunotherapy in glioblastoma–Report of two exceptional cases. Zentralbl Neurochir 2002;63(1):23–8.

11. Zeng QS, Li CF, Zhang K, et al. Multivoxel 3D proton MR spectroscopy in the distinction of recurrent glioma from radiation injury. J Neurooncol 2007; 84(1):63–9.

12. Kumar AJ, Leeds NE, Fuller GN, et al. Malignant gliomas: MR imaging spectrum of radiation therapy- and chemotherapy-induced necrosis of the brain after treatment. Radiology 2000;217(2): 377–84.

13. Mullins ME, Barest GD, Schaefer PW, et al. Radiation necrosis versus glioma recurrence: conventional MR imaging clues to diagnosis. AJNR Am J Neuroradiol 2005;26(8):1967–72.

14. Zeng QS, Li CF, Liu H, et al. Distinction between recurrent glioma and radiation injury using magnetic resonance spectroscopy in combination with diffu-sion-weighted imaging. Int J Radiat Oncol Biol Phys 2007;68(1):151–8.

15. Smith JS, Cha S, Mayo MC, et al. Serial diffusion-weighted magnetic resonance imaging in cases of glioma: distinguishing tumor recurrence from post-resection injury. J Neurosurg 2005;103(3):428–38.

16. Rock JP, Scarpace L, Hearshen D, et al. Associa-tions among magnetic resonance spectroscopy, apparent diffusion coefficients, and image-guided histopathology with special attention to radiation necrosis. Neurosurgery 2004;54(5):1111–7 [discus-sion: 1117–9].

17. Kashimura H, Inoue T, Beppu T, et al. Diffusion tensor imaging for differentiation of recurrent brain tumor and radiation necrosis after radiotherapy—three case reports. Clin Neurol Neurosurg 2007; 109(1):106–10.

18. Rachinger W, Goetz C, Popperl G, et al. Positron emission tomography with O-(2-[18F]fluoroethyl)-l-tyrosine versus magnetic resonance imaging in the diagnosis of recurrent gliomas. Neurosurgery 2005;57(3):505–11 [discussion: 505–11].

19. Herfarth KK, Gutwein S, Debus J. Postoperative radiotherapy of astrocytomas. Semin Surg Oncol 2001;20(1):13–23.

20. Giglio P, Gilbert MR. Cerebral radiation necrosis. Neurologist 2003;9(4):180–8.

21. Ruben JD, Dally M, Bailey M, et al. Cerebral radia-tion necrosis: incidence, outcomes, and risk factors with emphasis on radiation parameters and chemo-therapy. Int J Radiat Oncol Biol Phys 2006;65(2): 499–508.

22. Bauman GS, Sneed PK, Wara WM, et al. Reirradia-tion of primary CNS tumors. Int J Radiat Oncol Biol Phys 1996;36(2):433–41.

23. Floyd NS, Woo SY, Teh BS, et al. Hypofractionated intensity-modulated radiotherapy for primary glio-blastoma multiforme. Int J Radiat Oncol Biol Phys 2004;58(3):721–6.

24. Mayer R, Sminia P. Reirradiation tolerance of the human brain. Int J Radiat Oncol Biol Phys 2008; 70(5):1350–60.

25. McDermott MW, Sneed PK, Gutin PH. Interstitial bra-chytherapy for malignant brain tumors. Semin Surg Oncol 1998;14(1):79–87.

26. Soffietti R, Sciolla R, Giordana MT, et al. Delayed adverse effects after irradiation of gliomas: clinico-pathological analysis. J Neurooncol 1985;3(2): 187–92.

27. Perry A, Schmidt RE. Cancer therapy-associated CNS neuropathology: an update and review of the literature. Acta Neuropathol 2006;111(3):197–212.

28. Griebel M, Friedman HS, Halperin EC, et al. Revers-ible neurotoxicity following hyperfractionated radia-tion therapy of brain stem glioma. Med Pediatr Oncol 1991;19(3):182–6.

29. Watne K, Hager B, Heier M, et al. Reversible oedema and necrosis after irradiation of the brain. Diagnostic procedures and clinical manifestations. Acta Oncol 1990;29(7):891–5.

30. Zimmerman RA. Imaging of adult central nervous system primary malignant gliomas. Staging and follow-up. Cancer 1991;67(Suppl 4):1278–83.

31. Albert FK, Forsting M, Sartor K, et al. Early postoper-ative magnetic resonance imaging after resection of malignant glioma: objective evaluation of residual tumor and its influence on regrowth and prognosis. Neurosurgery 1994;34(1):45–60 [discussion: 60–1].

32. Preul MC, Leblanc R, Caramanos Z, et al. Magnetic resonance spectroscopy guided brain tumor resec-tion: differentiation between recurrent glioma and radiation change in two diagnostically difficult cases. Can J Neurol Sci 1998;25(1):13–22.

33. Smith MM, Thompson JE, Castillo M, et al. MR of recurrent high-grade astrocytomas after intralesional immunotherapy. AJNR Am J Neuroradiol 1996;17(6): 1065–71.

34. Deliganis AV, Baxter AB, Berger MS, et al. Serial MR in gene therapy for recurrent glioblastoma: initial

experience and work in progress. AJNR Am J Neuroradiol 1997;18(8):1401–6.

35. Ram Z, Culver KW, Oshiro EM, et al. Therapy of malignant brain tumors by intratumoral implantation of retroviral vector-producing cells. Nat Med 1997; 3(12):1354–61.

36. Verma R, Zacharaki EI, Ou Y, et al. Multiparametric tissue characterization of brain neoplasms and their recurrence using pattern classification of MR images. Acad Radiol 2008;15(8):966–77.

37. Chan YL, Yeung DK, Leung SF, et al. Diffusion-weighted magnetic resonance imaging in radiation-induced cerebral necrosis. Apparent diffusion coefficient in lesion components. J Comput Assist Tomogr 2003;27(5):674–80.

38. Hein PA, Eskey CJ, Dunn JF, et al. Diffusion-weighted imaging in the follow-up of treated high-grade gliomas: tumor recurrence versus radiation injury. AJNR Am J Neuroradiol 2004;25(2):201–9.

39. Asao C, Korogi Y, Kitajima M, et al. Diffusion-weighted imaging of radiation-induced brain injury for differentiation from tumor recurrence. AJNR Am J Neuroradiol 2005;26(6):1455–60.

40. Castillo M, Smith JK, Kwock L, et al. Apparent diffusion coefficients in the evaluation of high-grade cerebral gliomas. AJNR Am J Neuroradiol 2001; 22(1):60–4.

41. Bammer R. Basic principles of diffusion-weighted imaging. Eur J Radiol 2003;45(3):169–84.

42. Luypaert R, Boujraf S, Sourbron S, et al. Diffusion and perfusion MRI: basic physics. Eur J Radiol 2001;38(1):19–27.

43. Mukherji SK, Chenevert TL, Castillo M. Diffusion-weighted magnetic resonance imaging. J Neuro-ophthalmol 2002;22(2):118–22.

44. Schlemmer HP, Bachert P, Herfarth KK, et al. Proton MR spectroscopic evaluation of suspicious brain lesions after stereotactic radiotherapy. AJNR Am J Neuroradiol 2001;22(7):1316–24.

45. Rabinov JD, Lee PL, Barker FG, et al. In vivo 3-T MR spectroscopy in the distinction of recurrent glioma versus radiation effects: initial experience. Radiology 2002;225(3):871–9.

46. Schlemmer HP, Bachert P, Henze M, et al. Differentiation of radiation necrosis from tumor progression using proton magnetic resonance spectroscopy. Neuroradiology 2002;44(3):216–22.

47. Weybright P, Sundgren PC, Maly P, et al. Differentiation between brain tumor recurrence and radiation injury using MR spectroscopy. AJR Am J Roentgenol 2005;185(6):1471–6.

48. Yang D, Korogi Y, Sugahara T, et al. Cerebral gliomas: prospective comparison of multivoxel 2D chemical-shift imaging proton MR spectroscopy, echoplanar perfusion and diffusion-weighted MRI. Neuroradiology 2002;44(8):656–66.

49. Nelson SJ. Multivoxel magnetic resonance spectroscopy of brain tumors. Mol Cancer Ther 2003;2(5): 497–507.

50. McKnight TR, von dem Bussche MH, Vigneron DB, et al. Histopathological validation of a three-dimensional magnetic resonance spectroscopy index as a predictor of tumor presence. J Neurosurg 2002; 97(4):794–802.

51. Gonen O, Gruber S, Li BS, et al. Multivoxel 3D proton spectroscopy in the brain at 1.5 versus 3.0 T: signal-to-noise ratio and resolution comparison. AJNR Am J Neuroradiol 2001;22(9):1727–31.

52. Inglese M, Liu S, Babb JS, et al. Three-dimensional proton spectroscopy of deep gray matter nuclei in relapsing-remitting MS. Neurology 2004;63(1): 170–2.

53. Lichy MP, Plathow C, Schulz-Ertner D, et al. Follow-up gliomas after radiotherapy: 1H MR spectroscopic imaging for increasing diagnostic accuracy. Neuroradiology 2005;47(11):826–34.

54. Ricci PE, Karis JP, Heiserman JE, et al. Differentiating recurrent tumor from radiation necrosis: time for re-evaluation of positron emission tomography? AJNR Am J Neuroradiol 1998;19(3):407–13.

55. Wong TZ, van der Westhuizen GJ, Coleman RE. Positron emission tomography imaging of brain tumors. Neuroimaging Clin N Am 2002;12(4): 615–26.

56. Tsuyuguchi N, Takami T, Sunada I, et al. Methionine positron emission tomography for differentiation of recurrent brain tumor and radiation necrosis after stereotactic radiosurgery–in malignant glioma. Ann Nucl Med 2004;18(4):291–6.

57. Brandes AA, Tosoni A, Cavallo G, et al. Temozolomide 3 weeks on and 1 week off as first-line therapy for recurrent glioblastoma: phase II study from Gruppo Italiano Cooperativo di Neuro-Oncologia (GICNO). Br J Cancer 2006;95(9):1155–60.

# Immunotherapy Combined with Chemotherapy in the Treatment of Tumors

James L. Frazier, MD, James E. Han, BS, Michael Lim, MD,
Alessandro Olivi, MD*

## KEYWORDS

- Immunotherapy • Chemotherapy • Immunosuppression
- Blood-brain barrier

Chemotherapy and immunotherapy, as dual treatment modalities for cancer, have been viewed as incompatible in the past, because chemotherapy has been known to cause immunosuppression in patients. Chemotherapy may induce immunosuppression by

> Immunosuppressive cytokines
> Anergy, whereby tumor cells lose targeted antigens
> Lymphopenia
> Impaired antibody production
> Inhibition of immune effector cell function
> Reduction of major histocompatability complex expression
> Or inhibition of costimulatory proteins[1,2]

In addition, intrinsic defects in cell-mediated immunity have been found in patients harboring malignant gliomas, although purified T-cell populations have been demonstrated to respond to mitogenic stimulation.[2] Some chemotherapeutic agents at low doses have been shown to potentiate an immune response against tumor cells, however, and this has been demonstrated in a murine leukemia model.[3–5]

This article provides a broad overview of the data, including laboratory and clinical studies, currently available on the combination of immunotherapy and chemotherapy for treating cancer. The various forms of immunotherapy combined with chemotherapy include monoclonal antibodies

(mAb), adoptive lymphocyte transfer, or active specific immunotherapy, such as tumor proteins, irradiated tumor cells, tumor cell lysates, dendritic cells pulsed with peptides or lysates, or tumor antigens expressed in plasmids or viral vectors. This discussion is not limited to malignant brain tumors, because many of the studies have been conducted on various cancer types, thereby providing a comprehensive perspective that may encourage further studies that combine chemotherapy and immunotherapy for treating brain tumors.

It must be noted, however, that unlike most forms of systemic cancer, the blood–brain barrier (BBB) poses a formidable challenge when attempting to devise effective treatments for tumors of the central nervous system (CNS). When treating malignant tumors of the CNS, chemotherapeutic agents must have the ability to permeate the BBB, or it can be circumvented with the use of local drug delivery mechanisms such as convection-enhanced delivery or biodegradable polymers.[6–18] Additionally, the CNS has been viewed as an immune-privileged site, and the methods utilized to elicit an immune response against many forms of systemic cancer may not have the same efficacy when treating CNS tumors. For example, it has been thought that antibodies do not permeate the BBB effectively unless an inflammatory process disrupts it. Experimental studies in animals have demonstrated that peripheral immunization can lead to the accumulation of

Department of Neurosurgery, The Johns Hopkins University School of Medicine, The Johns Hopkins Hospital, 600 North Wolfe Street, Phipps 100, Baltimore, MD 21224, USA
* Corresponding author.
*E-mail address:* aolivi@jhmi.edu (A. Olivi).

Neurosurg Clin N Am 21 (2010) 187–194
doi:10.1016/j.nec.2009.09.003
1042-3680/09/$ – see front matter © 2010 Published by Elsevier Inc.

antibodies in the cerebrospinal fluid and brain parenchyma at a ratio of 0.1% to 1% to the titer level found in the serum.[2] It remains debatable whether antibodies can accumulate to levels within the CNS to effectively function against pathological processes, such as tumor cells. A local delivery mechanism, such as convection-enhanced delivery, may deliver optimal amounts of antibodies to CNS tumors.

## POSSIBLE MECHANISMS OF ACTION OF COMBINED CHEMOTHERAPY AND IMMUNOTHERAPY

Various mechanisms have been postulated in an attempt to explain the synergistic effects of chemotherapy and immunotherapy. Chemotherapeutic drugs may enhance the antitumor effects of immunotherapy by acting directly on the tumor and host environment, minimizing the drugs' immunosuppressive effects.[19] Some studies have demonstrated that certain drugs may modify the immunogenicity of tumor cells.[1,20–26] Some chemotherapeutic agents may cause tumor cells to become highly immunogenic, such as increasing the expression of major histocompatability complex molecules (MHC) with tumor antigens. Chemotherapy may cause tumor cell death directly with the release of a multitude of epitopes for recognition by the immune system. The induction of tumor cell death by chemotherapy may lead to phagocytosis of the dead cells by antigen-presenting cells, which may present tumor antigens to lymphocytes and incite an immune response against tumor cells, such as lysis by cytotoxic T-lymphocytes (CTLs). Moreover, chemotherapy may eliminate or reduce the activity of regulatory T-cells, in addition to its tumoricidal activity.[1,27–32] Another strategy is the causation of transient lymphopenia with chemotherapy, which may eliminate the activity of regulatory T-cells among other potential mechanisms, including the stimulation of antitumor CTLs.[33]

Administering immunotherapy may sensitize tumor cells to chemotherapy. Monoclonal antibodies may inhibit DNA repair mechanisms after DNA damage caused by chemotherapy. Also, mAbs may cause chemo-resistant tumor cells to become chemosensitive.[34–36]

The exact molecular and cellular mechanisms underlying the synergistic effects of each form of immunotherapy combined with chemotherapy have not been elucidated fully. It is also possible that the effects of each treatment modality may be independent of each other, and synergism may be contingent upon the timing and scheduling of the administration of each treatment.

## LABORATORY STUDIES
### Chemotherapy and mAb

Several studies have been conducted in mice to investigate the efficacy of the combination of chemotherapy and mAb against tumors.[37–43] Many of these studies administered chemotherapy and immunotherapy concurrently with some success in prolonging survival compared with either treatment modality given alone. In addition, the combination treatment was able to inhibit the growth of established tumors. Ciardiello and colleagues[42] investigated the efficacy of topotecan and an mAb against the epidermal growth factor receptor (EGFR) in a murine model of human colon carcinoma and demonstrated an enhancement in survival in the mice. The observed efficacy may have resulted from the blockade of EGFR activation and the inhibition of topoisomerase. Another study of a murine model of human breast adenocarcinoma and squamous cell carcinoma resulted in a prolongation of survival after treatment with anti-EGFR antibodies and doxorubicin, which likely led to apoptosis of tumor cells.[40] A murine mesothelioma model resulted in improvement in survival when mice were treated with anti-CD40 antibodies and gemcitabine, and a similar finding was demonstrated in a mouse model of human prostate cancer when Taxol and an mAb against herceptin were utilized.[44]

Moreover, laboratories have investigated the efficacy of immunotherapy administered before or after chemotherapy. McMillin and colleagues[45] tested the effects of trimetrexate given to mice 4 days after anti-CD137 in a murine sarcoma model. They were able to demonstrate prolongation in survival.

### Chemotherapy and Active Specific Immunotherapy

Various forms of active specific immunotherapy have been combined with chemotherapy and studied in animal models.[46–56] Tumor cell lysates, tumor proteins, irradiated tumor cells, and tumor antigens expressed in viral vectors or plasmids have been utilized as modes of vaccine delivery. Many of the experimental studies involved the administration of the immunotherapy after chemotherapy, and some of them resulted in survival prolongation or inhibition of established tumors. Jeglum and colleagues[53] used a canine lymphoma model in which irradiated lymphoma cells were administered 2 weeks after vincristine and cyclophosphamide and showed an increase in survival. In a murine model of glioma, survivin RNA-transfected dendritic cells were injected subcutaneously 7 days after temozolomide was given to the mice.[26,57] The mice lived longer when compared with mice treated with either therapy alone.

Studies also have been conducted in which active specific immunotherapy was given prior to chemotherapy. A study involving murine models of colon and lung carcinoma demonstrated inhibition of established tumor growth and prolongation in survival when the mice were treated with recombinant endoglin 7 days before cisplatin.[58] Murine models of lung carcinoma and hepatoma produced similar results when gemcitabine was administered 7 days after recombinant vascular endothelial growth factor receptor was given subcutaneously.[59] Both anti-endoglin and anti-vascular endothelial growth factor receptor antibodies in the former and latter studies, respectively, likely inhibited tumor angiogenesis. In an attempt to increase the number of tumor infiltrating lymphocytes, Hayakawa and colleagues[60] administered irradiated mouse tumor cells transduced with the costimulatory protein B7-1 4 weeks before methotrexate in a rat osteosarcoma model. The treatment resulted in inhibition of tumor growth and an increase in survival.

### Chemotherapy and Adoptive Lymphocyte Immunotherapy

It has been hypothesized that the tumor microenvironment plays a vital role in the effects of the combination of chemotherapy and adoptive lymphocyte immunotherapy. In a murine model of fibrosarcoma, antigen-specific T-cells were transferred to the mice with established tumors 2 days after the administration of gemcitabine.[19] This treatment resulted in rejection of the tumors in seven out of eight mice. Pretreatment with a chemotherapeutic agent may have caused a strong release of antigens, which normally may be expressed in low levels. The increased levels of antigen likely sensitized the stromal cells for eradication by CTLs that were transferred adoptively.

### CLINICAL STUDIES
### Chemotherapy and mAb

Clinical trials of chemotherapy and mAb have resulted in some efficacy against cancer in patients.[61–72] A few studies have been conducted in which both treatments were administered simultaneously for pancreatic cancer, B-cell lymphoma, breast cancer, and acute myeloid leukemia (AML). In one study involving 101 AML patients, gemtuzumab was linked to calicheamicin, and complete responses, remission with incomplete platelet recovery, and no responses were observed in 13,

15, and 73 patients, respectively.[69] Bouzani and colleagues[63] administered anti-CD20 mAb, cyclophosphamide, doxorubicin, vincristine, prednisone, and methotrexate to three patients with B-cell lymphoma and observed complete responses in each of them. Two studies evaluated the effects of anti-EGFR mAb and gemcitabine in patients with pancreatic cancer. Graeven and colleagues[73] demonstrated a partial response, stable disease, and progressive disease in three, five, and four patients, respectively. The other larger study resulted in stable disease, progressive disease, and partial responses in 26, 6, and 5 patients, respectively.[74] There were no follow-up data available for four patients. In a trial of 22 patients with breast cancer, mAb specific for herceptin combined with methotrexate and cyclophosphamide were administered simultaneously.[75] Partial responses, stable disease, and progressive disease were seen in 4, 10, and 8 patients, respectively.

A larger proportion of the clinical trials involved the administration of chemotherapy after the mAb. Shin and colleagues[71] administered cisplatin 1 day after an anti-EGFR mAb in nine patients with head and neck cancer, and complete responses, partial responses, and progressive disease were observed in two, four, and three patients, respectively. In another study, 96 patients with head and neck cancer were treated with cisplatin and carboplatin 1 hour after anti-EGFR mAb.[76] Partial responses, stable disease, and progressive disease were observed in 10, 41, and 27 patients, respectively. A large study involving 202 patients with non-Hodgkin's lymphoma investigated the efficacy of anti-CD20 administered 1 day prior to cyclophosphamide, doxorubicin, vincristine, and prednisone.[64,65] Interestingly, 152 patients experienced a complete response, while 31 had progressive disease. Slamon and colleagues[77] treated a group of 235 metastatic breast cancer patients with doxorubicin, cyclophosphamide, epirubicin, and paclitaxel 7 days after an antiherceptin mAb. Progressive disease was seen in 117 patients, while partial responses and complete responses were observed in 100 and 18 patients, respectively.

### Chemotherapy and Active Specific Immunotherapy

Clinical trials utilizing both chemotherapy and vaccine therapy also have been performed in patients with different cancer types, including glioblastoma multiforme (GBM), colon cancer, pancreatic cancer, prostate cancer, and small cell lung cancer.[78–85] Wheeler and colleagues[84]

investigated the clinical responsiveness of GBM to chemotherapy after vaccination. Three groups of patients were treated with chemotherapy alone (13), vaccination alone (12), or chemotherapy after vaccination (13). All patients underwent a craniotomy and received radiation. The vaccination consisted of autologous dendritic cells loaded with either peptides from cultured tumor cells or autologous tumor lysate. There were three vaccines administered 2 weeks apart, and vaccination commenced approximately 15 weeks after surgery. In the vaccine/chemotherapy and chemotherapy alone groups, temozolomide and 1,3-bis (2-chloroehthyl)-1-nitrosourea (BCNU) were administered to patients. Three patients received Gliadel wafers, which are biodegradable polymers that slowly release BCNU. The mean survival time for the chemotherapy alone, vaccine alone, and vaccine/chemotherapy groups were 16 months, 18 months, and 26 months, respectively. An analysis demonstrated a 2-year survival in 1 of 12 patients in the chemotherapy alone group, 1 of 12 patients in the vaccine alone group, and 5 of 12 patients in the vaccine/chemotherapy group. Only the vaccine/chemotherapy group had 3-year survivors; 2 out of 11 remaining patients were 3-year survivors. These results demonstrated a significantly longer postchemotherapy survival in the vaccine/chemotherapy group when compared with the vaccine and chemotherapy groups in isolation. These results are promising for the future development of vaccine trials for GBM patients.

### Chemotherapy and Adoptive Lymphocyte Immunotherapy

Lymphodepletion by chemotherapy followed by the adoptive transfer of lymphocytes has been evaluated in small-scale studies in melanoma cancer patients.[86–90] In a study of 35 patients, Dudley and colleagues[89] adoptively transferred autologous cytotoxic lymphocytes with the administration of interleukin-2 1 day after cyclophosphamide and fludarabine administration. They observed a complete response in only 3 patients, partial responses in 15, and no response to the treatment in 17 patients. Larger-scale studies are needed to assess the efficacy of this treatment modality in cancer patients.

A study by Peres and colleagues[91] investigated the efficacy of high-dose chemotherapy followed by the adoptive transfer of lymphocytes in three pediatric patients with recurrent brain tumors. Two patients were diagnosed with a GBM, and the pathology revealed an ependymoma in the other patient. All three patients underwent

resection of the tumors, and the tumor was used the source of antigen. The patients were treated with high-dose chemotherapy using cyclophosphamide, cisplatin, carmustine, and Taxol followed by stem cell rescue. T-cells were generated from peripheral blood after immunization with autologous cancer cells. The T-cells were expanded ex vivo and adoptively transferred to the patients. Survival was 16 months, 23 months, and 48 months, respectively. Survival in two of the patients was markedly prolonged when compared with historical controls. More studies with a larger number of patients will have to be conducted to assess the efficacy of this treatment in children with malignant brain tumors.

### SUMMARY

In summary, the combination of chemotherapy and immunotherapy for treating cancer holds promise for patients suffering from this disease. Optimal treatment paradigms need to be devised to fine-tune the scheduling and timing of the administration of each treatment along with the discovery of the most effective chemotherapeutic and immunotherapeutic modalities for each type of cancer. The treatment of CNS malignancies is a more formidable task given the immune-privileged status of the CNS and the BBB. The BBB may be circumvented by local delivery mechanisms, such as convection-enhanced delivery and biodegradable polymers. Larger randomized, controlled phase 3 trials are needed to ascertain the efficacy of the combination of chemotherapy and immunotherapy.

### REFERENCES

1. Andersen MH, Sorensen RB, Schrama D, et al. Cancer treatment: the combination of vaccination with other therapies. Cancer Immunol Immunother 2008;57:1735–43.
2. Mitchell DA, Fecci PE, Sampson JH. Immunotherapy of malignant brain tumors. Immunol Rev 2008;222: 70–100.
3. Mihich E. Combined effects of chemotherapy and immunity against leukemia L1210 in DBA-2 mice. Cancer Res 1969;29:848–54.
4. Mihich E. Modification of tumor regression by immunologic means. Cancer Res 1969;29:2345–50.
5. Mihich E. Preclinical evaluation of the inter-relationships between cancer chemotherapy and immunity. Natl Cancer Inst Monogr 1971;34:90–102.
6. Bobo RH, Laske DW, Akbasak A, et al. Convection-enhanced delivery of macromolecules in the brain. Proc Natl Acad Sci U S A 1994;91:2076–80.

7. Brem H, Kader A, Epstein JI, et al. Biocompatibility of a biodegradable, controlled-release polymer in the rabbit brain. Sel Cancer Ther 1989;5:55–65.

8. Degen JW, Walbridge S, Vortmeyer AO, et al. Safety and efficacy of convection-enhanced delivery of gemcitabine or carboplatin in a malignant glioma model in rats. J Neurosurg 2003;99:893–8.

9. Groothuis DR. The blood–brain and blood–tumor barriers: a review of strategies for increasing drug delivery. Neuro Oncol 2000;2:45–59.

10. Hall WA, Rustamzadeh E, Asher AL. Convection-enhanced delivery in clinical trials. Neurosurg Focus 2003;14:e2.

11. Haroun RI, Brem H. Local drug delivery. Curr Opin Oncol 2000;12:187–93.

12. Kroll RA, Pagel MA, Muldoon LL, et al. Increasing volume of distribution to the brain with interstitial infusion: dose, rather than convection, might be the most important factor. Neurosurgery 1996;38:746–52 [discussion: 752–4].

13. Lopez KA, Waziri AE, Canoll PD, et al. Convection-enhanced delivery in the treatment of malignant glioma. Neurol Res 2006;28:542–8.

14. Mamelak AN. Locoregional therapies for glioma. Oncology (Williston Park) 2005;19:1803–10 [discussion: 1810, 1816–7, 1821–2].

15. Pollack IF, Keating R. New delivery approaches for pediatric brain tumors. J Neurooncol 2005;75:315–26.

16. Raghavan R, Brady ML, Rodriguez-Ponce MI, et al. Convection-enhanced delivery of therapeutics for brain disease, and its optimization. Neurosurg Focus 2006;20:E12.

17. Read TA, Thorsen F, Bjerkvig R. Localised delivery of therapeutic agents to CNS malignancies: old and new approaches. Curr Pharm Biotechnol 2002;3:257–73.

18. Vogelbaum MA. Convection enhanced delivery for the treatment of malignant gliomas: symposium review. J Neurooncol 2005;73:57–69.

19. Zhang B, Bowerman NA, Salama JK, et al. Induced sensitization of tumor stroma leads to eradication of established cancer by T-cells. J Exp Med 2007;204:49–55.

20. Bonmassar E, Testorelli C, Franco P, et al. Changes of the immunogenic properties of a radiation-induced mouse lymphoma following treatment with antitumor drugs. Cancer Res 1975;35:1957–62.

21. Casares N, Pequignot MO, Tesniere A, et al. Caspase-dependent immunogenicity of doxorubicin-induced tumor cell death. J Exp Med 2005;202:1691–701.

22. Fioretti MC, Bianchi R, Romani L, et al. Drug-induced immunogenic changes of murine leukemia cells: dissociation of onset of resistance and emergence of novel immunogenicity. J Natl Cancer Inst 1983;71:1247–51.

23. Fioretti MC, Romani L, Bonmassar E. Antigenic changes related to drug action. Prog Clin Biol Res 1983;132B:435–45.

24. Giampietri A, Fioretti MC, Goldin A, et al. Drug-mediated antigenic changes in murine leukemia cells: antagonistic effects of quinacrine, an antimutagenic compound. J Natl Cancer Inst 1980;64:297–301.

25. Nowak AK, Lake RA, Marzo AL, et al. Induction of tumor cell apoptosis in vivo increases tumor antigen cross-presentation, cross-priming rather than cross-tolerizing host tumor-specific CD8 T cells. J Immunol 2003;170:4905–13.

26. Park SD, Kim CH, Kim CK, et al. Cross-priming by temozolomide enhances antitumor immunity of dendritic cell vaccination in murine brain tumor model. Vaccine 2007;25:3485–91.

27. Berd D. Low doses of chemotherapy to inhibit suppressor T-cells. Prog Clin Biol Res 1989;288:449–58.

28. Berd D, Mastrangelo MJ. Effect of low-dose cyclophosphamide on the immune system of cancer patients: depletion of CD4+, 2H4+ suppressor-inducer T-cells. Cancer Res 1988;48:1671–5.

29. Liu JY, Wu Y, Zhang XS, et al. Single administration of low dose cyclophosphamide augments the antitumor effect of dendritic cell vaccine. Cancer Immunol Immunother 2007;56:1597–604.

30. Mokyr MB, Dray S. Some advantages of curing mice bearing a large subcutaneous MOPC-315 tumor with a low dose rather than a high dose of cyclophosphamide. Cancer Res 1983;43:3112–9.

31. Mokyr MB, Hengst JC, Dray S. Role of antitumor immunity in cyclophosphamide-induced rejection of subcutaneous nonpalpable MOPC-315 tumors. Cancer Res 1982;42:974–9.

32. Motoyoshi Y, Kaminoda K, Saitoh O, et al. Different mechanisms for antitumor effects of low- and high-dose cyclophosphamide. Oncol Rep 2006;16:141–6.

33. Muranski P, Boni A, Wrzesinski C, et al. Increased intensity lymphodepletion and adoptive immunotherapy—how far can we go? Nat Clin Pract Oncol 2006;3:668–81.

34. Demidem A, Lam T, Alas S, et al. Chimeric anti-CD20 (IDEC-C2B8) monoclonal antibody sensitizes a B-cell lymphoma cell line to cell killing by cytotoxic drugs. Cancer Biother Radiopharm 1997;12:177–86.

35. Hancock MC, Langton BC, Chan T, et al. A monoclonal antibody against the c-erbB-2 protein enhances the cytotoxicity of cis-diamminedichloroplatinum against human breast and ovarian tumor cell lines. Cancer Res 1991;51:4575–80.

36. Pietras RJ, Fendly BM, Chazin VR, et al. Antibody to HER-2/neu receptor blocks DNA repair after cisplatin in human breast and ovarian cancer cells. Oncogene 1994;9:1829–38.

37. Agus DB, Scher HI, Higgins B, et al. Response of prostate cancer to anti-Her-2/neu antibody in androgen-dependent and -independent human xenograft models. Cancer Res 1999;59:4761–4.

38. Balin-Gauthier D, Delord JP, Rochaix P, et al. In vivo and in vitro antitumor activity of oxaliplatin in combination with cetuximab in human colorectal tumor cell lines expressing different level of EGFR. Cancer Chemother Pharmacol 2006;57: 709–18.

39. Baselga J, Norton L, Albanell J, et al. Recombinant humanized anti-HER2 antibody (Herceptin) enhances the antitumor activity of paclitaxel and doxorubicin against HER2/neu overexpressing human breast cancer xenografts. Cancer Res 1998;58:2825–31.

40. Baselga J, Norton L, Masui H, et al. Antitumor effects of doxorubicin in combination with antiepidermal growth factor receptor monoclonal antibodies. J Natl Cancer Inst 1993;85:1327–33.

41. Chalandon Y, Mach JP, Pelegrin A, et al. Combined radioimmunotherapy and chemotherapy of human colon carcinoma grafted in nude mice: advantages and limitations. Anticancer Res 1992;12:1131–9.

42. Ciardiello F, Bianco R, Damiano V, et al. Antitumor activity of sequential treatment with topotecan and antiepidermal growth factor receptor monoclonal antibody C225. Clin Cancer Res 1999;5:909–16.

43. Ciardiello F, Damiano V, Bianco R, et al. Antitumor activity of combined blockade of epidermal growth factor receptor and protein kinase A. J Natl Cancer Inst 1996;88:1770–6.

44. Nowak AK, Robinson BW, Lake RA. Synergy between chemotherapy and immunotherapy in the treatment of established murine solid tumors. Cancer Res 2003;63:4490–6.

45. McMillin DW, Hewes B, Gangadharan B, et al. Complete regression of large solid tumors using engineered drug-resistant hematopoietic cells and anti-CD137 immunotherapy. Hum Gene Ther 2006; 17:798–806.

46. Akbulut H, Tang Y, Akbulut KG, et al. Antitumor immune response induced by i.t. injection of vector-activated dendritic cells and chemotherapy suppresses metastatic breast cancer. Mol Cancer Ther 2006;5:1975–85.

47. Cantrell JL, Killion JJ, Kollmorgen GM. Correlations between humoral immunity and successful chemotherapy–immunotherapy. Cancer Res 1976;36: 3051–7.

48. Correale P, Del Vecchio MT, Di Genova G, et al. 5-fluorouracil-based chemotherapy enhances the antitumor activity of a thymidylate synthase-directed polyepitopic peptide vaccine. J Natl Cancer Inst 2005;97:1437–45.

49. Correale P, Del Vecchio MT, La Placa M, et al. Chemotherapeutic drugs may be used to enhance the killing efficacy of human tumor antigen peptide-specific CTLs. J Immunother 2008;31: 132–47.

50. Dunussi-Joannopoulos K, Krenger W, Weinstein HJ, et al. CD8+ T-cells activated during the course of murine acute myelogenous leukemia elicit therapeutic responses to late B7 vaccines after cytoreductive treatment. Blood 1997;89:2915–24.

51. Eralp Y, Wang X, Wang JP, et al. Doxorubicin and paclitaxel enhance the antitumor efficacy of vaccines directed against HER 2/neu in a murine mammary carcinoma model. Breast Cancer Res 2004;6:R275–83.

52. Han HD, Song CK, Park YS, et al. A chitosan hydrogel-based cancer drug delivery system exhibits synergistic antitumor effects by combining with a vaccinia viral vaccine. Int J Pharm 2008;350: 27–34.

53. Jeglum KA, Young KM, Barnsley K, et al. Chemotherapy versus chemotherapy with intralymphatic tumor cell vaccine in canine lymphoma. Cancer 1988;61:2042–50.

54. Machiels JP, Reilly RT, Emens LA, et al. Cyclophosphamide, doxorubicin, and paclitaxel enhance the antitumor immune response of granulocyte/macrophage colony-stimulating factor-secreting whole-cell vaccines in HER-2/neu tolerized mice. Cancer Res 2001;61:3689–97.

55. Zheng SJ, Zheng SP, Huang FY, et al. Synergistic antitumor effect of recombinant chicken fibroblast growth factor receptor-1-mediated antiangiogenesis and low-dose gemcitabine in a mouse colon adenocarcinoma model. World J Gastroenterol 2007;13: 2484–9.

56. Zheng SP, Zheng SJ, Wu RL, et al. Enhanced efficacy in anti-tumour activity by combined therapy of recombinant FGFR-1 related angiogenesis and low-dose cytotoxic agent. Eur J Cancer 2007;43: 2134–9.

57. Kim CH, Woo SJ, Park JS, et al. Enhanced antitumour immunity by combined use of temozolomide and TAT-survivin pulsed dendritic cells in a murine glioma. Immunology 2007;122:615–22.

58. Tan GH, Tian L, Wei YQ, et al. Combination of low-dose cisplatin and recombinant xenogeneic endoglin as a vaccine induces synergistic antitumor activities. Int J Cancer 2004;112:701–6.

59. Hou JM, Liu JY, Yang L, et al. Combination of low-dose gemcitabine and recombinant quail vascular endothelial growth factor receptor-2 as a vaccine induces synergistic antitumor activities. Oncology 2005;69:81–7.

60. Hayakawa M, Kawaguchi S, Ishii S, et al. B7-1-transfected tumor vaccine counteracts chemotherapy-induced immunosuppression and prolongs the survival of rats bearing highly metastatic osteosarcoma cells. Int J Cancer 1997;71:1091–102.

61. Baselga J, Pfister D, Cooper MR, et al. Phase I studies of antiepidermal growth factor receptor chimeric antibody C225 alone and in combination with cisplatin. J Clin Oncol 2000;18:904–14.

62. Bianchi G, Albanell J, Eiermann W, et al. Pilot trial of trastuzumab starting with or after the doxorubicin component of a doxorubicin plus paclitaxel regimen for women with HER2-positive advanced breast cancer. Clin Cancer Res 2003; 9:5944–51.

63. Bouzani M, Karmiris T, Rontogianni D, et al. Disseminated intravascular B-cell lymphoma: clinicopathological features and outcome of three cases treated with anthracycline-based immunochemotherapy. Oncologist 2006;11:923–8.

64. Coiffier B. Rituximab in combination with CHOP improves survival in elderly patients with aggressive non-Hodgkin's lymphoma. Tumori 2002;88: S26–8.

65. Coiffier B, Lepage E, Briere J, et al. CHOP chemotherapy plus rituximab compared with CHOP alone in elderly patients with diffuse large B-cell lymphoma. N Engl J Med 2002;346:235–42.

66. Czuczman MS. CHOP plus rituximab chemoimmunotherapy of indolent B-cell lymphoma. Semin Oncol 1999;26:88–96.

67. Czuczman MS. Immunochemotherapy in indolent non-Hodgkin's lymphoma. Semin Oncol 2002;29: 11–7.

68. Czuczman MS, Grillo-Lopez AJ, White CA, et al. Treatment of patients with low-grade B-cell lymphoma with the combination of chimeric anti-CD20 monoclonal antibody and CHOP chemotherapy. J Clin Oncol 1999;17:268–76.

69. Larson RA, Boogaerts M, Estey E, et al. Antibody-targeted chemotherapy of older patients with acute myeloid leukemia in first relapse using Mylotarg (gemtuzumab ozogamicin). Leukemia 2002;16: 1627–36.

70. Marty M, Cognetti F, Maraninchi D, et al. Randomized phase II trial of the efficacy and safety of trastuzumab combined with docetaxel in patients with human epidermal growth factor receptor 2-positive metastatic breast cancer administered as first-line treatment: the M77001 study group. J Clin Oncol 2005;23:4265–74.

71. Shin DM, Donato NJ, Perez-Soler R, et al. Epidermal growth factor receptor-targeted therapy with C225 and cisplatin in patients with head and neck cancer. Clin Cancer Res 2001;7:1204–13.

72. Smith I, Procter M, Gelber RD, et al. 2-year follow-up of trastuzumab after adjuvant chemotherapy in HER2-positive breast cancer: a randomised controlled trial. Lancet 2007;369:29–36.

73. Graeven U, Kremer B, Sudhoff T, et al. Phase I study of the humanised anti-EGFR monoclonal antibody matuzumab (EMD 72000) combined with gemcitabine in advanced pancreatic cancer. Br J Cancer 2006;94:1293–9.

74. Xiong HQ, Rosenberg A, LoBuglio A, et al. Cetuximab, a monoclonal antibody targeting the epidermal growth factor receptor, in combination with gemcitabine for advanced pancreatic cancer: a multicenter phase II trial. J Clin Oncol 2004;22:2610–6.

75. Orlando L, Cardillo A, Ghisini R, et al. Trastuzumab in combination with metronomic cyclophosphamide and methotrexate in patients with HER-2 positive metastatic breast cancer. BMC Cancer 2006;6:225.

76. Baselga J, Trigo JM, Bourhis J, et al. Phase II multicenter study of the antiepidermal growth factor receptor monoclonal antibody cetuximab in combination with platinum-based chemotherapy in patients with platinum-refractory metastatic and/or recurrent squamous cell carcinoma of the head and neck. J Clin Oncol 2005;23:5568–77.

77. Slamon DJ, Leyland-Jones B, Shak S, et al. Use of chemotherapy plus a monoclonal antibody against HER2 for metastatic breast cancer that overexpresses HER2. N Engl J Med 2001;344: 783–92.

78. Antonia SJ, Mirza N, Fricke I, et al. Combination of p53 cancer vaccine with chemotherapy in patients with extensive stage small cell lung cancer. Clin Cancer Res 2006;12:878–87.

79. Arlen PM, Gulley JL, Parker C, et al. A randomized phase II study of concurrent docetaxel plus vaccine versus vaccine alone in metastatic androgen-independent prostate cancer. Clin Cancer Res 2006; 12:1260–9.

80. Harrop R, Drury N, Shingler W, et al. Vaccination of colorectal cancer patients with TroVax given alongside chemotherapy (5-fluorouracil, leukovorin and irinotecan) is safe and induces potent immune responses. Cancer Immunol Immunother 2008;57: 977–86.

81. Harrop R, Drury N, Shingler W, et al. Vaccination of colorectal cancer patients with modified vaccinia ankara encoding the tumor antigen 5T4 (TroVax) given alongside chemotherapy induces potent immune responses. Clin Cancer Res 2007;13: 4487–94.

82. Noguchi M, Itoh K, Yao A, et al. Immunological evaluation of individualized peptide vaccination with a low dose of estramustine for HLA-A24+ HRPC patients. Prostate 2005;63:1–12.

83. Sato Y, Fujiwara T, Mine T, et al. Immunological evaluation of personalized peptide vaccination in combination with a 5-fluorouracil derivative (TS-1) for advanced gastric or colorectal carcinoma patients. Cancer Sci 2007;98:1113–9.

84. Wheeler CJ, Das A, Liu G, et al. Clinical responsiveness of glioblastoma multiforme to chemotherapy after vaccination. Clin Cancer Res 2004;10: 5316–26.

85. Yanagimoto H, Mine T, Yamamoto K, et al. Immunological evaluation of personalized peptide vaccination with gemcitabine for pancreatic cancer. Cancer Sci 2007;98:605–11.

86. Appay V, Voelter V, Rufer N, et al. Combination of transient lymphodepletion with busulfan and fludarabine and peptide vaccination in a phase I clinical trial for patients with advanced melanoma. J Immunother 2007;30:240–50.

87. Dudley ME, Wunderlich JR, Robbins PF, et al. Cancer regression and autoimmunity in patients after clonal repopulation with antitumor lymphocytes. Science 2002;298:850–4.

88. Dudley ME, Wunderlich JR, Yang JC, et al. A phase I study of nonmyeloablative chemotherapy and adoptive transfer of autologous tumor antigen-specific T-lymphocytes in patients with metastatic melanoma. J Immunother 2002;25:243–51.

89. Dudley ME, Wunderlich JR, Yang JC, et al. Adoptive cell transfer therapy following nonmyeloablative but lymphodepleting chemotherapy for the treatment of patients with refractory metastatic melanoma. J Clin Oncol 2005;23:2346–57.

90. Rosenberg SA, Dudley ME. Cancer regression in patients with metastatic melanoma after the transfer of autologous antitumor lymphocytes. Proc Natl Acad Sci U S A 2004;101(Suppl 2): 14639–45.

91. Peres E, Wood GW, Poulik J, et al. High-dose chemotherapy and adoptive immunotherapy in the treatment of recurrent pediatric brain tumors. Neuropediatrics 2008;39:151–6.

# Monitoring Immune Responses After Glioma Vaccine Immunotherapy

Brian Jian, MD, PhD, Isaac Yang, MD*,
Andrew T. Parsa, MD, PhD

**KEYWORDS**
- Immunomonitoring • Immune response
- Antigen • Clinical trials

Glial tumors are the most common type of primary brain tumor, and malignant gliomas are the most common glial tumors. Furthermore, malignant gliomas are refractive to current therapeutic approaches including surgery, radiotherapy, and chemotherapy. The current median survival of patient with glioblastoma multiforme with today's standard therapy including radiation and temozolomide is 14 months.[1,2] Given their complex biology, and invasive spread along white matter tracts, an alternative treatment strategy is needed. Surgical resection cannot completely remove the numerous infiltrating neoplastic cells, and radiation subjects non-neoplastic tissues to toxic and collateral damage. Modulation of the immune system, or immunotherapy, provides the ideal candidate of therapeutic attack as it allows for specific targeting of cancer cells.[3–15] In recent years, several candidates have been identified as reasonable approaches to combating malignant gliomas.

The recent expansion of knowledge regarding tumor immunobiology and the clinical application of this knowledge has led to a need for immune monitoring technology to identify successful and unsuccessful therapies. Immunomonitoring could provide more information about the immunologic state and overall effectiveness of the intervention than the current practices of serial radiologic imaging. Given the multimodal therapies that exist, it is not surprising that there are multiple means of monitoring immune system function. This article gives a broad overview of standard approaches used to examine current immunotherapies and their clinical potential in monitoring immunotherapy for malignant gliomas.

## T-CELL MEDIATED RESPONSES AND T-CELL FUNCTION ASSAYS

Based on the current understanding of the immune response to cancerous cells, gliomas create a tumor microenvironment that suppresses immune function and allows the tumor to evade the host, cell-mediated, killing pathways. In the past, cellular immune responses were detected by measuring cytotoxicity, proliferation, or the release of cellular mediators such as cytokines. These laboratory tests typically involved in vitro preincubation of antigens with cultured cells. These analyses, however, were limited in their ability to estimate the quantity of cells that existed in a given population. The advent of the enzyme-linked immunosorbent spot (ELISPOT), Tetramer, cytokine flow cytometry, and chromium-release assays provide the capability of measuring clonal expansion of populations of antigen-responsive T cells.

A study by Galon and colleagues[16] demonstrated that T-cell presence in colorectal cancer tissue is predictive of overall prognosis. Furthermore, data has demonstrated that T-regulatory cell activity increases in patients with known malignant gliomas.[17] These cells are thought to

Department of Neurological Surgery, University of California, San Francisco, 505 Parnassus Avenue, M779, San Francisco, CA 94143-0112, USA
* Corresponding author.
*E-mail address:* yangi@neurosurg.ucsf.edu (I. Yang).

Neurosurg Clin N Am 21 (2010) 195–199
doi:10.1016/j.nec.2009.09.004
1042-3680/09/$ – see front matter © 2010 Elsevier Inc. All rights reserved.

later suppress cytotoxic T-cell activity and reduce the systemic response to tumor burden. Current clinical trials are monitoring systemic T-cell responses after vaccinations.

## ENZYME-LINKED IMMUNOSORBENT ASSAY

Proteins that are secreted into the extracellular space, by tumor cells or neighboring host immune cells, can be monitored to identify multiple variables. These agents can identify if the host is amounting an attack on the tumor cells. It can also identify if the tumor is actively evading immune surveillance. Therefore, understanding the composition of circulating proteins in the intercellular space of tumor and self tissue provides valuable therapeutic and prognostic implications. The enzyme-linked immunosorbent assay (ELISA) was first developed in 1983 by Czerinkinsky and colleagues for the purpose of identifying and quantifying antibody secreting cells. It was later also used for quantifying antigens. The assay involves the administration of a known antibody to a solution of unquantified antibody or antigen. The known antibody is tagged with a known signal that is used for analysis and identification. It is common practice to add a second antibody to bind to the first administered antibody, to amplify the signal that is produced.

ELISAs are highly sensitive, reliable, and accurate tests.[18] This method of analysis will prove invaluable in different methods of monitoring the immune response for various different therapies due to its accuracy and wide applicability in protein analysis.

## ELISPOT

The ELISPOT assay is a modified version of the ELISA immunoassay. ELISPOT assays were originally developed to quantify B cells secreting antigen-specific antibodies. They were later used to quantify the agents that were secreted by these cells, such as cytokines.[19] The ELISPOT assay provides both qualitative (type of immune protein) and quantitative (number of responding cells) information. The ELISPOT assay is exceptionally sensitive, capable of detecting cells that secrete 100 molecules of a given protein.[19] This exceptional sensitivity is because the protein of interest is rapidly captured around the secreting cell, before it is either diluted in the supernatant, captured by receptors of adjacent cells, or degraded. There is growing interest in increased use of ELISPOT as a measure for cytotoxic T lymphocytes (CTL) responses, in large part because it is reliable and highly sensitive. Results

from various clinical trials, including peptide and whole tumor cell vaccination and cytokine treatment, are now available and show the suitability of the ELISPOT assay for monitoring T-cell responses. The ELISPOT technique allows for quantification of tumor-specific T lymphocytes from peripheral blood by detecting antigen-induced cytokine secretion.

## TETRAMER ANALYSIS

A tetramer assay is used to detect the presence of antigen-specific T cells. In order for a T cell to detect the peptide to which it is specific, it must both recognize the peptide and the major histocompatibility complex (MHC) at the surface of a cell as it contacts it. Because the binding affinity of a T-cell receptor (TCR) to MHC complexed with a peptide is so low, creating a sensitive assay was historically difficult. This problem was solved by creating a tetramer of MHC molecules in which all four molecules present an identical peptide. In this manner, the avidity of the binding of the T cell of interest was increased. The resulting mechanism of the assay involves adding the MHC-peptide tetramer to an unknown quantity of T cells. The tetramer is then bound to the T cells that recognize the peptide sequence of interest. The tetramer is then stained typically by fluorescence labeling and bound T cells are measured using flow-cytometry.

Currently tetramer analysis has been used successfully in several phase I and II clinical trials for advanced staged melanoma vaccine trials and malignant gliomas.[14,15] When combined with functional analyses such as staining for specific cytokines, tetramer analysis can provide valuable information about T cells and their activation state.

## CHROMIUM RELEASE ASSAY

The chromium release assay was developed by Brunner and colleagues[20] and quantifies CTL activity by measuring target cell lysis. The process involves bathing target cells with chromium. These labeled cells are then mixed with various amounts of effector T cells. The killing of these labeled cells causes a release of chromium into the supernatant after cell lysis. The accumulated chromium is quantified and compared with spontaneous release rates, to quantify functional CTL activity. Results are typically reported in lytic units.

This assay is dependent on the binding of CTL to target cells via TCR-binding and other accessory adhesion molecules. The crosslinking and binding of the TCR-receptor complex initiates the T-cell lytic process. The lytic process can occur over several minutes to several hours, and variations in any of the above-mentioned processes can alter results. Consequently, the chromium release assay is not a good assay to examine slow-acting mediators of cytotoxicity. Furthermore, the development of tetramer staining of MHC class I complexes has provided a more rapid and sensitive method of quantifying antigen-specific CD8 T cells.

## DISCUSSION

Given the multimodal nature of immunologic therapy regimens today. Monitoring the immune response to immunotherapy covers a number of technological modalities and a broad understanding of current practices in immunotherapy. As these therapies continue to take a foothold in current clinical practice, a basic understanding of the principles, techniques, and weaknesses of these assays should be understood. Of the above-mentioned assays, the ELISPOT has been used the most frequently for monitoring of vaccination trials. Its frequent use is a direct result of its highly sensitive capabilities in detecting and quantifying antigen-reactive T cells.[21]

Several pitfalls of immune monitoring have been noted and often provide some difficulty in analyzing gathered data. A great potential source of variability lies in the heterogenous nature of the tumors being evaluated. It is commonly understood that features that make tumors highly aggressive make them also highly variable in their genetic and pathologic phenotype. In malignant gliomas alone, the location of the tissue and the medical comorbidities of the patients can also affect findings. Many of these patients have undergone, and are still being treated with other previous therapies that could affect immune function. The frequent use of dexamethasone in combating brain edema and the use of Temodar, and more recently Avastin, have unknown effects on current immune monitoring practices.

### Correlation with Clinical Outcome

The ultimate question that remains, does immunologic monitoring provide any prognostic significance? Although little data exists in the field of immunotherapy of gliomas, data gathered from systemic cancers suggests that immunologic response may be important to prognosis.[22]

One reason for the lack of correlation between immunologic response and clinical outcome may be the complexity of the responses required for an anti-tumor response. For example, cytokine production, usually interferon gamma, by T cells in vitro, in response to antigen-specific or polyclonal stimuli, is measured in an attempt to demonstrate type 1 helper T cells cellular responses.[13]

Moreover, it has been clearly shown that the presence of a high number of circulating effector-type T cells is not enough to induce clinical efficacy.[23–27]

### Reliability of Assays

Many of these assays are currently used at the benchside for accurate and reliable measurements of the presence and quantity of antibody or antigen. The highly controlled nature and systematic controls offered with lab work may not be practically or financially feasible for clinical use. Significant work in producing clinically accessible assays is still left to be fully explored and developed.

### Standardization of Immunological Monitoring

Harmonization of methods for monitoring the induction of antigen-specific T-cell responses in clinical vaccination trials has been identified as a key area of development within the field. The purpose of monitoring immunologic outcomes in response to immunotherapeutic treatments is fourfold:

1. To determine the effectiveness of a vaccine to elicit the correct type of immune response. This will further aid in understanding the nature and dynamics of the response elicited by a particular modality and provide proof-of-principle for ensuring trials.
2. Determination of elements of the immune response that correlate with clinical response. This is vital to understanding the dynamics and magnitude of immune responses that are required to elicit clinical responses.
3. Armed with such knowledge, immunologic responses may be uses as surrogate markers for clinical responses, which may ultimately be useful, if validated, as end-points in the later clinical trials.
4. There is an increasing recognition of the importance of obtaining immunologic data that are comparable between different clinical trials.

This area has been identified as highly important in developing to help move the field forward. Therefore, several consortiums have been created to address this issue, including the Immunoassay Proficiency Panel (organized by the Cancer Vaccine Consortium) and the Cancer Immunotherapy Monitoring Panel.

### The future of immune monitoring

It is become increasingly clear that monitoring T-cell function in the patient with malignant cancer will be one of the mainstays of clinical oncologic practice. The ultimate goal for immunomonitoring in immunotherapy is to provide enough information to influence decision-making for later therapy or therapies.

## REFERENCES

1. Pardoll D, Allison J. Cancer immunotherapy: breaking the barriers to harvest the crop. Nat Med 2004;10:887–92.

2. Stupp R, Mason WP, van den Bent MJ, et al. Radiotherapy plus concomitant and adjuvant temozolomide for glioblastoma. N Engl J Med 2005;352(10):987–96.

3. Heimberger AB, Archer GE, Crotty LE, et al. Dendritic cells pulsed with a tumor-specific peptide induce long-lasting immunity and are effective against murine intracerebral melanoma. Neurosurgery 2002;50(1):158–64 [discussion: 164–6].

4. Heimberger AB, Crotty LE, Archer GE, et al. Epidermal growth factor receptor VIII peptide vaccination is efficacious against established intracerebral tumors. Clin Cancer Res 2003;9(11):4247–54.

5. Liau L, Black K, Prins R, et al. Treatment of intracranial gliomas with bone marrow-derived dendritic cells pulsed with tumor antigens. J Neurosurg 1999;90(6):1115–24.

6. Liau L, Fakhrai H, Black K. Prolonged survival of rats with intracranial C6 gliomas by treatment with TGF-beta antisense gene. Neurol Res 1998;20(8):742–7.

7. Liau LM, Jensen ER, Kremen TJ, et al. Tumor immunity within the central nervous system stimulated by recombinant Listeria monocytogenes vaccination. Cancer Res 2002;62(8):2287–93.

8. Liau LM, Prins RM, Kiertscher SM, et al. Dendritic cell vaccination in glioblastoma patients induces systemic and intracranial T-cell responses modulated by the local central nervous system tumor microenvironment. Clin Cancer Res 2005;11(15):5515–25.

9. Parsa AT, Waldron JS, Panner A, et al. Loss of tumor suppressor PTEN function increases B7-H1 expression and immunoresistance in glioma. Nat Med 2007;13(1):84–8.

10. Prins RM, Graf MR, Merchant RE. Cytotoxic T cells infiltrating a glioma express an aberrant phenotype that is associated with decreased function and apoptosis. Cancer Immunol Immunother 2001;50(6):285–92.

11. Sampson JH, Akabani G, Archer GE, et al. Progress report of a Phase I study of the intracerebral microinfusion of a recombinant chimeric protein composed of transforming growth factor (TGF)-alpha and a mutated form of the Pseudomonas exotoxin termed PE-38 (TP-38) for the treatment of malignant brain tumors. J Neurooncol 2003;65(1):27–35.

12. Sampson JH, Crotty LE, Lee S, et al. Unarmed, tumor-specific monoclonal antibody effectively treats brain tumors. Proc Natl Acad Sci U S A 2000;97(13):7503–8.

13. Yang I, Kremen TJ, Giovannone AJ, et al. Modulation of major histocompatibility complex Class I molecules and major histocompatibility complex-bound immunogenic peptides induced by interferon-alpha and interferon-gamma treatment of human glioblastoma multiforme. J Neurosurg 2004;100(2):310–9.

14. Yu JS, Liu G, Ying H, et al. Vaccination with tumor lysate-pulsed dendritic cells elicits antigen-specific, cytotoxic T-cells in patients with malignant glioma. Cancer Res 2004;64(14):4973–9.

15. Yu JS, Wheeler CJ, Zeltzer PM, et al. Vaccination of malignant glioma patients with peptide-pulsed dendritic cells elicits systemic cytotoxicity and intracranial T-cell infiltration. Cancer Res 2001;61(3):842–7.

16. Galon J, Costes A, Sanchez-Cabo F, et al. Type, density, and location of immune cells within human colorectal tumors predict clinical outcome. Science 2006;313(5795):1960–4.

17. Fecci PE, Mitchell DA, Whitesides JF, et al. Increased regulatory T-cell fraction amidst a diminished CD4 compartment explains cellular immune defects in patients with malignant glioma. Cancer Res 2006;66(6):3294–302.

18. Janetzki S, Panageas KS, Ben-Porat L, et al. Results and harmonization guidelines from two large-scale international Elispot proficiency panels conducted by the Cancer Vaccine Consortium (CVC/SVI). Cancer Immunol Immunother 2008;57(3):303–15.

19. Klinman DM, Nutman TB. ELISPOT assay to detect cytokine-secreting murine and human cells. Curr Protoc Immunol 2001. Chapter 6: p. Unit 6 19.

20. Brunner KT, Mauel J, Cerottini JC, et al. Quantitative assay of the lytic action of immune lymphoid cells on 51-Cr-labelled allogeneic target cells in vitro; inhibition by isoantibody and by drugs. Immunology 1968;14(2):181–96.

21. Schmittel A, Keilholz U, Thiel E, et al. Quantification of tumor-specific T lymphocytes with the ELISPOT assay. J Immunother 2000;23(3):289–95.

22. Korangy F, Ormandy LA, Bleck JS, et al. Spontaneous tumor-specific humoral and cellular immune responses to NY-ESO-1 in hepatocellular carcinoma. Clin Cancer Res 2004;10(13):4332–41.

23. Speiser DE. Immunological techniques: ex vivo characterization of T cell-mediated immune

responses in cancer. Curr Opin Immunol 2005;17(4):419–22.

24. Speiser DE, Cerottini JC, Romero P. Tumor cell recognition efficiency by T cells. PLoS Med 2005;2(3):e77, author reply e95.

25. Speiser DE, Romero P. Toward improved immunocompetence of adoptively transferred CD8+ T cells. J Clin Invest 2005;115(6):1467–9.

26. Dannull J, Su Z, Rizzieri D, et al. Enhancement of vaccine-mediated antitumor immunity in cancer patients after depletion of regulatory T cells. J Clin Invest 2005;115(12):3623–33.

27. Dannull J, Nair S, Su Z, et al. Enhancing the immunostimulatory function of dendritic cells by transfection with mRNA encoding OX40 ligand. Blood 2005;105(8):3206–13.

# Challenges in Clinical Design of Immunotherapy Trials for Malignant Glioma

Cleo E. Rolle, PhD, Sadhak Sengupta, PhD, Maciej S. Lesniak, MD*

**KEYWORDS**
- Glioblastoma multiforme (GBM) • Immunotherapy
- Clinical trials • Brain tumors • Vaccines
- Dendritic cells • Cytokines

Glioblastoma multiforme (GBM) is the most common and lethal primary malignant brain tumor, with an incidence of 5 to 8 per 100,000 population, and a median survival of 14 months.[1] The current standard of care for newly diagnosed GBM patients is a tripartite regimen of surgery, radiotherapy, and chemotherapy. The most meaningful improvement for the treatment of GBM has been the efficacy of temozolomide (TMZ). According to the study conducted by Stupp and colleagues,[1] the median survival rate with radiotherapy alone was 12.1 months compared with 14.6 months with radiotherapy plus TMZ. In addition to the efficacy of TMZ, improvements in delivery have also greatly enhanced the treatment of GBM, including local delivery of chemotherapeutics to tumor cells and convection enhanced delivery (reviewed by Sampson).[2]

A major limitation in the treatment of GBM is its location within the brain and the blood-brain barrier (BBB). Evidence of immune surveillance within the central nervous system (CNS) and a role of T cells within glioma have led recently to the development of novel immunotherapeutic strategies.[3–6] Immunotherapy seeks to exploit the immune system's ability to specifically recognize and mount a response against the tumor cells, while leaving the normal brain tissue intact. The success of immunotherapy is fueled by the growing understanding of the immune mechanisms in play within the CNS and glioma immunobiology. These immunotherapeutic strategies fall into 3 categories: immune priming, immunomodulation, and adoptive immune therapy. In addition, antibodies or immune peptides fused to toxins have also been used to treat GBM.

The emergence of novel immunotherapeutic strategies has cultivated a renewed optimism for the treatment of GBM. Most of these strategies are focused on the induction of specific immune responses against tumor associated antigens (TAA). At present 2 of these targeted TAA, EGFRvIII (NCT00458601) and IL-13Rα2 (NCT00089427), are in clinical trials and are discussed here in further detail. Another major immunotherapeutic strategy that has gathered a lot of attention is dendritic cell (DC) vaccination, albeit only demonstrating modest success in clinical trials.

Despite the fact that there are several immunotherapeutic strategies currently in clinical trials (**Table 1**), which were successful in animal models of glioma, convincing evidence of their efficacy remains unclear in patients. It has been difficult to study novel immunotherapeutic strategies in clinical trials because of the rarity of GBM in the population. Moreover, the design of clinical trials is often flawed, especially with regard to patient enrollment in targeted treatment studies. The eligibility criteria should include a screening to assess

The University of Chicago Brain Tumor Center, The University of Chicago, 5841 South Maryland Avenue, MC 3026, Chicago, IL 60637, USA
* Corresponding author.
*E-mail address:* mlesniak@surgery.bsd.uchicago.edu (M.S. Lesniak).

Neurosurg Clin N Am 21 (2010) 201–214
doi:10.1016/j.nec.2009.08.002

**Table 1**
**Current clinical trials for patients with malignant glioma**

| Protocol ID | Immunotherapeutic Strategy | Phase | Treatment Strategy |
|---|---|---|---|
| NCT00089427 | IL-13-*Pseudomonas* exotoxin fusion protein (IL13-PE38QQR) | 1 | Specifically targets IL-13R overexpression on tumor cells to deliver an immunotoxin |
| NCT00509301 | Radiolabeled antibody | 1 | Utilizes an antibody to deliver a radioactive drug specifically to tumor cells |
| NCT00576641 | Peptide-pulsed PBMC | 1 | Autologous PBMC are loaded with autologous tumor peptides in vitro and used to activate the patient's immune cells |
| NCT00694330 | Irradiated tumor cells plus GM-CSF secreting cells | 1 | GM-CSF matures dendritic cells that present autologous tumor antigens to activate the patient's immune cells |
| NCT00639639 | Tumor lysate-pulsed PBMC and anti-CD3 activated lymphocytes | 1/2 | In vitro activation of patient's T cells and autologous tumor antigen presentation by PBMC specifically stimulates tumor antigen-specific T cells |
| NCT00293423 | Gp96-tumor peptide vaccination | 1/2 | Gp96 is associated with multiple peptide antigens in tumor cells and stimulates tumor antigen-specific immune cells |
| NCT00766753 | Tumor peptide-pulsed DC vaccination | 1/2 | Autologous DC are loaded with autologous tumor peptides in vitro and used to activate the patient's immune cells |
| NCT00797940 | IL-4-*Pseudomonas* exotoxin fusion protein (IL-4(38-37)-PE38KDEL) | 2 | Specifically targets IL-4R overexpression on tumor cells to deliver an immunotoxin |
| NCT00045698 | Tumor peptide-pulsed DC vaccination (DCVax) | 2 | Autologous dendritic cells are loaded with autologous tumor peptides in vitro and used to activate the patient's immune cells |
| NCT00458601 | EGFRvIII (CDX-110) | 2 | Specifically targets EGFRvIII overexpression on tumor cells |
| NCT00814593 | LAK cells infusion | 2 | Autologous lymphocytes activated/stimulated in vitro with IL-2 |
| NCT00068510 | Tumor lysate-pulsed PBMC | 2 | Autologous PBMC are loaded with autologous tumor lysate in vitro and used to activate the patient's immune cells to multiple tumor antigens |
| NCT00431561 | Phosphorothioate antisense human TGF-β2 mRNA (AP 12009) | 2b | Inhibits the expression of TGF-β2, thus relieving tumor cell mediated immunosuppression |

*Abbreviations:* DC, dendritic cells; GM-CSF, granulocyte macrophage colony stimulating factor; IL, interleukin; LAK, lymphokine activated killer; PBMC, peripheral blood mononuclear cells; TGF, transforming growth factor.

the expression of target molecules before enrollment. The emergence of better imaging protocols, end-point analyses, and substantial improvements in protocol design should further aid in the development of clinical trials to assess the efficacy of targeted tumor therapies.

## TARGET IDENTIFICATION
### EGFRvIII

The epidermal growth factor receptor (EGFR) is frequently overexpressed in solid tumors. Glioma cells often express a mutated form of EGFR, referred to as EGFR variant III, which has an in-frame deletion from the extracellular domain of the EGFR (**Fig. 1**).[7–15] This mutation results in increased tumorigenicity and migration, and confers radiation and chemotherapeutic resistance to tumor cells.[16–24] A retrospective analysis of Japanese patients with GBM enrolled in clinical trials determined that EGFR amplification was a negative prognostic factor, and in cases where EGFR amplification occurred with EGFRvIII, the prognosis was even worse.[25] The restriction of EGFRvIII expression to tumors makes it an ideal target for antitumor immunotherapy.

In experimental animal models, EGFRvIII-expressing cell lines or an EGFRvIII-specific 14-amino acid peptide (PEPvIII) chemically conjugated to keyhole limpet hemocyanin (KLH)

(PEPvIII-KLH) have been used for the generation of EGFRvIII-specific antibodies and the induction of cellular immune responses.[26–36] EGFRvIII vaccination in mouse models of established intracerebral glioma showed tumor regression compared with controls.[27] EGFRvIII has also been shown to be immunogenic in humans.[37,38] Purev and colleagues[37] determined that patients with EGFRvIII-expressing breast adenocarcinomas and malignant gliomas developed EGFRvIII-specific antibodies.[38] These investigators also observed weak cytotoxic T-lymphocyte (CTL) epitopes restricted by major histocompatibility complex (MHC) Class I and Class II motifs, which were sufficient to induce EGFRvIII-specific lymphocyte proliferation and cytokine production.

According to Heimberger and colleagues,[27] EGFRvIII peptide vaccination in animal models of intracerebral and subcutaneous glioma demonstrated significant efficacy over controls. In phase 2 trials, patients were administered the EGFRvIII peptide vaccine along with temozolomide and radiation, following a complete surgical resection. This study demonstrated efficacy over historical controls. The observed time to progression was 12.8 months and the overall median survival was 18 months or longer. A peptide vaccine directed against EGFRvIII is currently in phase 2 trials (NCT00458601). Tumor-specific mutation is targeted currently under a phase 1 (conducted at Duke University,

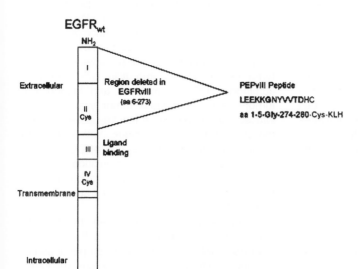

**Fig. 1.** Diagram of epidermal growth factor receptor (EGFR) wild-type protein showing the area of in-frame deletion that forms EGFRvIII. During the deletion amino acids 6 and 273 are split, forming a novel glycine at the junction of amino acids 5 and 274. PEPvIII is a 13 amino acid peptide with a terminal cysteine added to facilitate conjugation to KLH. (*Reprinted from* Sampson JH, Archer GE, Mitchell DA. Tumor-specific immunotherapy targeting the EGFRvIII mutation in patients with malignant glioma. Semin Immunol 2008;20(5):267–75; with permission.)

PI: John H. Sampson) and one multi-institutional phase 2 immunotherapy trial (conducted at Duke University, PI: John H. Sampson; and the University of Texas, M.D. Anderson Cancer Center, PI: Amy B. Heimberger), demonstrating that vaccines targeting EGFRvIII are capable of inducing potent T- and B-cell immunity.[38] The investigators surmise that the vaccine approach has been highly successful at eliminating tumor cells expressing EGFRvIII, very similar to the experimental animal model studies, without any evidence of toxicity.[10,38]

The limitations of clinical studies to evaluate the efficacy of peptide vaccines include patient selection and immune editing. First, expression of EGFRvIII should be confirmed before patient selection for efficacy studies. Second, immune editing was observed in 20 of 23 patients with recurrent tumor, as the tumor biopsies failed to express EGFRvIII (unpublished data from CDX-110 clinical trials). Therefore, based on glioma-restricted expression of EGFRvIII and mechanism of action in glioma, future trials should focus on EGFRvIII targeting in primary glioma patients to assess efficacy. Moreover, to circumvent immune editing in recurrent glioma, initial treatments should target multiple TAA using either whole tumor lysates or personalized peptide vaccines.

### Interleukin-13Rα2

Similar to EGFR, interleukin (IL)-13Rα2 is highly expressed in glioma cells, but not normal brain cells, making it a suitable target for immune cell activation.[39] Despite the overexpression of IL-13Rα2 in glioma cells, its role in glioma cells remains undefined. According to a preclinical study conducted by Okano and colleagues,[40] the IL-13Rα2 protein contains an antigenic peptide that activates CD8[+] T cells to secrete interferon (IFN)-γ and lyse IL-13Rα2[+] tumor cells. This finding deserves further analysis to determine the benefits of IL-13Rα2 targeting in vivo. Furthermore, a fusion protein composed of human IL-13 and *Pseudomonas* exotoxin A (IL13-PE38QQR) showed limited efficacy in 50 patients that received localized intracerebral administration. Moreover, a phase 3 study in which the IL-13Rα2 fusion peptide was compared with carmustime wafers was completed and showed no significant benefits (NCT00076986). As is the case with EGFRvIII studies, the major challenge facing IL-13Rα2 studies is prospective identification of patients that are likely to respond, based on the expression of IL-13Rα2.

### Interleukin-4R

IL-4R is overexpressed in primary tumor specimens and cell lines in a variety of human malignancies, including glioma.[41–46] According to Joshi and colleagues,[42] IL-4 signals via the heterodimeric IL-4Rα and IL-13Rα1 receptor in tumor cells. Therapeutic strategies aimed at specifically targeting tumor cells have used IL-4R over-expression using IL-4 fused to *Pseudomonas* exotoxin (IL4(38-37)-PE38KDEL). In vitro studies using glioma cell lines found IL4(38-37)-PE38KDEL caused glioma cell death, similar to IL13-PE38QQR.[42] Furthermore, in animal models of glioma using human tumors, IL4(38-37)-PE38KDEL was toxic to glioma cells, but largely spared normal brain parenchyma. Phase 1 trials revealed that IL4(38-37)-PE38KDEL was well tolerated, with no incipient drug related toxicity. The most notable finding from the related dose-escalation study was a long-term survival of 3 years in a patient with recurrent malignant glioma treated with a single intratumoral dose of IL4(38-37)-PE38KDEL. The findings of these earlier trials were promising and as such, IL4(38-37)-PE38KDEL is under further consideration (NCT00797940).

### Dendritic Cell Vaccination

Dendritic cells (DC) are hematopoietically derived cells that act as antigen-presenting cells (APCs) to activate innate and adaptive immune responses. DC-based vaccination strategies seek to exploit the potent APC activity of these cells. The potential to generate large numbers of mature DC in vitro from patient blood or bone marrow has resulted in an abundance of DC based vaccination strategies. These studies have used DC pulsed with either tumor peptides eluted from tumor cells or whole tumor lysates.[26–50] In short, autologous DC are matured and loaded with tumor-specific peptides or tumor lysate and then infused into the patient. A few key issues underlie the use of DC cell vaccines, which must be resolved before the routine use of DC vaccines to treat GBM. These issues include the best source of DC, the in vitro maturation protocol, the route and dose of DC administration, and the source of antigen.

In an early study conducted by Yu and colleagues,[48] 4 out of 7 patients that received DC pulsed with eluted MHC class I peptides had developed cytotoxic responses against the tumor, and at the time of reoperation, 2 out of those 4 patients had effector and memory CD8[+] T-cell infiltrates in the tumor. In this study, DC vaccination was not associated with any adverse side effects. In a phase 1 trial, 16 patients with malignant glioma were immunized intradermally with autologous DC pulsed with KLH conjugated to EGFRvIII peptides.[38] This study showed promising results based on the increased time to progression and median survival time. Stable disease was observed in 2 out of 3 grade III patients. The mean time to progression was 46.9 weeks and the median survival was 110.8 weeks. A similar study conducted by Liau and colleagues in 12 GBM patients showed that intradermal infusion of peptide-pulsed DC improved survival compared with historical controls. The median time to progression was 15.5 months and the median survival was 23.4 months.[49] In addition, 100% survival was observed at 6 months, 75% at 1 year, and 50% at 2 years, with 2 patients surviving long term (≥4 years). The administration of DC intradermally presumably allowed the DC to traffic to the lymph nodes, where they are able to activate tumor antigen-specific T cells.

One of the largest DC vaccine studies to date, the HGG-Immuno study conducted by De Vleeschouwer and colleagues,[51] assessed 56 patients with recurrent GBM. The patients were separated into 3 groups and treated with autologous DC pulsed with autologous tumor lysate, followed by tumor lysate boosts every 4 weeks. The clinical response was minimal, with a median progression-free survival of 3 months and overall median survival of 24 to 36 months. Overall, this treatment strategy was not significantly better than historical controls. Despite disappointing results from these clinical trials, multiple other clinical trials are underway.

A large, multi-institutional randomized placebo control study is currently being sponsored by Northwest Biotherapeutics (DCVax-Brain, phase 2, NCT00045968). DCVax-Brain is a personalized (autologous) DC-based vaccine. The vaccine is prepared from peripheral blood mononuclear cells (PBMC) obtained from the patient and are then loaded with tumor lysate from surgically resected tumor tissue. According to the sponsors, in phase 1 trials 8 of 19 GBM patients treated with DCVax-Brain, in addition to the standard of care for GBM, were still alive with stable disease. The median overall survival was 33.6 months. The median time to progression was 18.1 months. In this study, 90% of the patients surpassed the standard of care median time to disease progression of 8.1 months and median overall survival time of 17.0 months. The 2-year survival rate is 68%, and 42% of the patients have survived longer than 4 years (reviewed by Wheeler and colleagues).[52]

Parajuli and colleagues[53] investigated the best protocol for antigen preparation for DC vaccination strategies. DC were isolated and matured from patient-derived PBMC. The 4 conditions evaluated were: DC fused with glioma cells; DC pulsed with apoptotic tumor cells; DC pulsed with total tumor RNA; and DC pulsed with tumor lysate. All 4 conditions produced similar amounts of mature DC; however, DC pulsed with apoptotic tumor cells or total tumor RNA were the best at inducing CTL. Furthermore, DC pulsed with apoptotic tumor cells were also able to induce natural killer T-cell activation. These data collectively suggest that DC pulsed with apoptotic cells are the best preparation for autologous DC vaccination strategies.

### Heat Shock Proteins Tumor Peptide Vaccination

Heat shock proteins (HSP) are chaperone proteins that are localized to the endoplasmic reticulum, which aid in nascent protein folding and also play a role in antigen presentation via MHC Class I (reviewed by Srivastava and colleagues).[54] Recent studies have shown that at least 2 HSP, Gp96 and HSP70, have antigenic properties and are able to generate immune responses directed against the proteins to which they are associated.[55,56] The benefit of using HSP-peptide complexes for vaccination is the potential to limit immune editing, because HSP are associated with a broad range of the tumor peptide repertoire. Furthermore, HSP have been identified as potent activators of APCs, making them ideal candidates for tumor immunotherapy.[57]

Gp96 has been shown to induce immunity specifically against antigens found in the cells from which it has been isolated, and this has been exploited in the case of tumor cells to generate antitumor immune responses. According to Binder and colleagues,[58] one potential mechanism by which this may occur is through cross-presentation by DC via Gp96 binding CD91 expressed on DC. In a study of 12 patients with recurrent high-grade glioma, patients received 4 injections over 2 to 4 weeks. Seven of 8 patients had a survival time of 10.5 months compared with the historical survival time of 6.5 months.[59] More importantly, Gp96 vaccination has garnered success in the treatment of malignant melanoma and renal cell carcinoma, and it is hoped that similar success will be obtained with malignant glioma.[15,60–62] The Gp96-tumor peptide vaccination strategy is currently in phase 1/2 clinical trials (NCT00293423).

### IMMUNOMODULATION
#### Cytokines

The cytokine milieu of the CNS ensures that primarily humoral immune responses are generated to prevent damage due to inflammation. The normal humoral response is further skewed in glioblastoma patients.[63,64] In addition, immuno-suppressive cytokines, such as transforming growth factor (TGF)-β2 and IL-10, are highly expressed in glioma cell lines and patient specimens.[65–68] These cytokines suppress T-cell proliferation and IL-2 production, and also support glioma cell growth. To alter the cytokine milieu of glioma, studies have focused on supplementing the immunoactivating cytokine IL-2, or conversely, inhibiting the immunosuppressive cytokine TGF-β.

IL-2 is the cytokine most often associated with T-cell activation and expansion. Recent studies have shown that IL-2 is required for differentiation of naïve T cells into cytokine producing effector cells. According to a study conducted by Colombo and colleagues,[69] IL-2 was administered as a transgene in combination with herpes simplex virus tyrosine kinase in a retroviral vector to 12 patients with recurrent GBM. Two out of the 12 patients had a partial response, 4 had a minor response, 4 had stable disease, and 2 had progressive disease. In another study, 5 patients with recurrent glioma were infused with IL-2 in combination with cytotoxic T cells.[70] Although 2 patients with GBM died, the other patients showed no evidence of tumor at least 28 weeks post treatment. These studies suggest that IL-2, either in combination with effectors cells or alone, may be beneficial in the treatment of glioma. However, of note is that these studies were small, and lacked adequate randomization or controls.

TGF-β2 was originally named for its ability to suppress T-cell growth and IL-2 production, and was isolated and cloned from glioblastoma cell lines.[67,71] The expression of TGF-β1 and -β2 in 2 glioblastoma cell lines and newly isolated patient samples was confirmed at the mRNA level.[65] However, only TGF-β2 was detected in the supernatant of glioma cell lines and in the cerebral spinal fluid of patients with malignant glioma.[66] Primary glioma cells treated with antisense TGF-β2 (Antisense Pharma, AP 12009) showed a significant reduction in TGF-β2 expression from 73% positive cells to 49% positive cells, and glioma cell proliferation.[72] According to a phase 1/2 trial (NCT00844064), Hau and colleagues[72] reported promising results in 24 patients with malignant glioma treated with antisense oligonucleotides (AP 12009). A complete remission was observed in 2 patients with anaplastic astrocytoma (AA), and the overall survival in AA (146.6 weeks) and GBM (44 weeks) patients was increased relative to historical controls. The 2-year survival for the treatment group was 80%. This immunotherapeutic strategy is designed to improve the immune system's ability to mount antitumor immune responses, and is currently in phase 3 trials (NCT00761280).

Interferons are normally expressed in response to altered cells. In animal models, IFN-α and -β inhibit glioma growth. On this basis, IFN has been investigated in multiple clinical trials for the treatment of malignant glioma. A phase 1 trial using IFN-α in combination with carmustine (BCNU), as an initial treatment modality for high-grade glioma, found that 5 of 9 patients had a partial response and a median survival of 4 years.[73] In a phase 2 trial of 21 patients with recurrent high-grade glioma, 7 patients had partial response and 6 patients maintained stable disease following treatment with IFN-α and BCNU.[74] In contrast to these earlier trials, a phase 3 trial of 214 eligible patients with high-grade glioma, in which patients received BCNU in combination with IFN-α, the response was no better than in patients that received BCNU alone with regard to time to disease progression or overall survival.[75] A few caveats of the early studies involved patient selection and inconsistent end-point analysis. Of note is that in addition to being ineffective for the treatment of glioma, systemic IFN administration also causes severe adverse reactions, including neurocortical effects, fever, chills, and myalgias.

## Depletion of Regulatory T Cells

Regulatory T cells (Tregs; CD4$^+$CD25$^+$FOXP3$^+$) are a fraction of the T-cell population that suppress immune activation and thereby maintain homeostasis and tolerance to self-antigens. Functional deletion of Tregs induces autoimmunity, facilitates transplantation tolerance, and also increases immunity to tumors.[3,76,77] A lack of immune rejection of neoplastic cells is believed to be maintained by Tregs in many malignancies including colorectal, esophageal, pancreatic, breast, lung, ovarian, and brain tumors.[3,78–81] An increased fraction of regulatory T cells has been reported to infiltrate glioma, contributing to the immunosuppressive status associated with glioma.[3–5,82,83] It is therefore very important to understand the biology and function of Tregs for their potential therapeutic potential.

The precise mechanism(s) by which Tregs suppress effector T-cell–mediated immune response have not been definitively characterized. Some studies highlight the importance of cytokines in the regulation, and others cell-to-cell contact with effector T cells, in which case membrane-bound TGF-β and cytotoxic T-lymphocyte protein (CTLA-4) plays an important role.[84–86] Heme oxygenase-1 (HO-1), a rate-limiting enzyme in heme metabolism, also plays a role in Treg-mediated immune suppression. HO-1 is constitutively expressed in human Tregs and is induced by FoxP3 expression.[87,88] It is suggested that HO-1 suppresses effector T cells by carbon monoxide production.[89,90]

In 2006, the authors' group demonstrated tumor infiltration of Tregs in GBM patients.[4] The expression of FoxP3[+] Tregs was significantly higher in patients with GBM than in controls, whereas these cells were absent from control brain specimens. Higher levels of FoxP3 expression were observed in regulatory T cells isolated from the tumor tissue in comparison to autologous patient blood and blood from control individuals. In an in vitro suppression assay, Tregs inhibited T-cell proliferation in a dose-dependent manner. Among various markers analyzed, the expression of CD62L and CTLA-4 was elevated in the glioma-infiltrating Tregs in comparison with that of the controls. The authors showed improved survival of mice with experimental brain tumors, following the depletion of Tregs with anti-CD25 monoclonal antibody (PC61).[3]

A prominent population of Tregs and a corresponding lack of effector/activated T cells was demonstrated in GBM patient specimens.[82] Absolute counts of both CD4[+] T cells and FoxP3[+]CD45RO[+] Tregs were greatly diminished in the peripheral pool of patients with malignant glioma, but the Tregs fraction was increased in the remaining CD4 compartment in 5 out of the 8 patients evaluated.[5] The proportion of Tregs in the peripheral blood of patients with GBM was 2.63 times higher than that found in the blood of normal volunteers. The patients with an elevated Tregs fraction showed significant CD4[+] T-cell lymphopenia, whereas the patients without Tregs elevation possessed normally proliferating CD4[+] T-cell levels. T cells from the patients bearing malignant gliomas regained their function after Tregs depletion in vitro, and proliferated to levels equivalent to those of normal controls.

The depletion of Tregs is normally achieved using anti-CD25 antibodies, which may also deplete activated T cells that express CD25. Curtin and colleagues[91] demonstrated the efficacy of immunotherapy using anti-CD25 depleting antibodies (PC61) in an experimental animal of glioma. Of note, the efficacy of Tregs depletion was time dependent and greatly influenced by tumor burden. Systemic depletion of Tregs 15 days after tumor implantation improved long-term survival, but Tregs depleted 24 days after tumor implantation showed no improvement in survival. Of importance is that this observation suggests immunotherapy alone may not be the fail-safe

therapeutic strategy. Moreover, Tregs depletion should be performed before immunotherapy to limit depletion of effector cells along with Tregs following the administration of anti-CD25 antibodies.

## Small Molecule Inhibitors of STAT-3

Signal transducer and activator of transcription-3 (STAT-3) is a convergence point of several signaling pathways in multiple malignancies including glioblastoma, breast, lung, ovarian, pancreatic, skin, and prostate cancer.[92,93] STAT-3 has recently emerged as a potential target for glioma immunotherapy. The binding of STAT-3 to its target genes affects proliferation, survival, differentiation, and development. Receptor engagement by members of the IL-6 cytokine family such as IL-6, oncostatin M, and leukemia inhibitory factor, or growth factors such as platelet-derived growth factor (PDGF), fibroblast growth factor (FGF), and epithelial growth factor (EGF), activate STAT-3. The activation of STAT-3 requires the activation of receptor-associated kinases like Janus kinase (JAK) family members, FHFR, EGFR, PDGFR, or nonreceptor-associated kinases like Ret, Src, or Bcl-Abl. STAT-3 activity is attenuated by suppressors of cytokine signaling (SOCS) by downregulating its upstream kinase activity, whereas protein inhibitors of activated STAT (PIAS) and protein tyrosine phosphatases target STAT-3 directly.[94–96] Other than promoting oncogenesis, active STAT-3 also enables tumor growth by suppressing tumor recognition by the immune system.[97] STAT-3 promotes tumor immune evasion by inhibiting proinflammatory cytokine signaling and amplifying Tregs. STAT-3 activity in cancers other than glioblastoma has been targeted in several different therapeutic strategies. STAT-3 inhibition has been approached from 2 fronts: through RNA interference or chemical inhibitors, or through modulation of endogenous regulators such as PIAS3 and SOCS-3 (**Fig. 2**).

Several compounds block STAT-3 signaling by directly targeting the STAT-3 protein. Platinum compounds such as CPA-1 and CPA-7 have been successfully used to block STAT-3 activity and induce apoptosis in breast, lung, and prostate cancer cell lines.[98] More recently, Zhang and colleagues[99] used CPA-7 to successfully block STAT-3 activation in glioma-associated microglia. Decoy oligonucleotides such as G-quartets or transcription factor decoy (TFD) oligodeoxynucleotides, and inhibitors such as S31-201 have been used by researchers for directly blocking STAT-3 signal transduction in human cancer

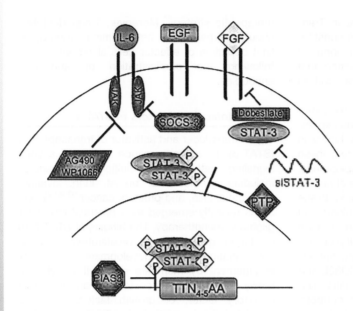

**Fig. 2.** Inhibition of STAT-3 signal transduction. A variety of endogenous and pharmacologic inhibitors can attenuate STAT-3 signaling. SOCS-3, PIAS3, and various protein tyrosine phosphatases (PTP) inhibit STAT-3 activity endogenously. STAT-3–specific siRNA degrades STAT-3 mRNA. Pharmacologic inhibition of JAK activity by AG490 and WP1066 dampens the signals that result in STAT-3 activation. Attenuation of FGF signaling by dobesilate also inhibits STAT-3–mediated gene expression by attenuating kinase signals upstream of STAT-3 activation. (*Reprinted from* Brantley EC, Benveniste EN. Signal transducer and Activator of Transcription-3: a molecular hub for signaling pathways in gliomas. Mol Cancer Res 2008;6(5):675–84; with permission.)

cells.[100–103] Furthermore, the knockdown of STAT-3 in human glioma cell lines by STAT-3 siRNA induced apoptosis and inhibited survival.[104,105] STAT-3 decoy oligodeoxynucleotide treatment in U251 and A172 glioma cell lines blocked STAT-3 signaling and inhibited glioma proliferation by inducing apoptosis and cell cycle arrest.[103]

The pharmacologic inhibitors of growth factor receptors and upstream tyrosine kinases have also been very successful at blocking STAT-3 activity. Inhibitors of JAK and Src showed potential STAT-3 inhibition and are in early stages of experimental testing.[106,107] Preliminary in vivo studies showed that WP1066, a JAK inhibitor, has the potential to cross the BBB, which is very important for glioma patients. WP1066 abrogated immune tolerance in glioblastoma patients and stimulated T-cell proliferation by upregulating secretion of costimulatory molecules and T-cell effector cytokines, and improved immunogenic responses.[108] In an independent experiment, growth of glioma xenografts was restricted by decreased STAT-3–mediated expression of Bcl-xL, Mcl-1, and c-Myc when STAT-3 was inhibited with WP1066.[109] The effects were also tumor specific, as normal astrocytoma cells were not affected. Attenuation of upstream FGF signaling pathway by dobesilate, a vasoactive drug, in C6 glioma cells, triggered apoptosis and growth arrest by inhibiting STAT-3 activation.[110] These observations illustrate a possible relationship between STAT-3 and glioblastoma. Pharmacologic inhibitors of individual kinases that are in command upstream of STAT-3 inhibitors therefore might be an ideal candidate for potential therapeutic intervention of glioma progression.

## ACTIVE IMMUNOTHERAPY
### Lymphokine Activated Killer Cells

In vitro studies using tumor cells from a variety of malignancies, including glioma, showed lymphokine activated killer (LAK) cell lysis.[111,112] Human studies conducted by Rosenberg and colleagues,[113] showed therapeutic benefits of LAK cells in multiple types of tumor cells, and they were largely inefficient at lysing normal tissues. A phase 1 study evaluated 10 patients with recurrent GBM following surgical resection and intratumoral injection of LAK and IL-2.[114] In this study, steroids were restricted during treatment, unless required for the treatment of acute symptoms of IL-2 toxicity (edema and confusion). The therapeutic efficacy of LAK cells was characterized by a median survival of 53 weeks, with 53% of the patients still being alive after 1 year, compared with a median survival of 25.5 weeks for the chemotherapy alone group.[115] This study highlighted the potential benefits of LAK cell infusion for the treatment of glioma. To date, the mechanism of action of LAK cells remains unclear, thereby limiting their use in immunotherapy. Furthermore, LAK cells must be administered locally at the tumor site because they fail to effectively home to tumor lesions. In light of these factors, immunotherapeutic strategies have moved from LAK cells toward T cells. Moreover, T cells have been to be more lytic than LAK cells, on a per cell basis.

### Effector T Cells

Adoptive immunotherapy has emerged as a novel treatment modality for multiple cancers. The use of tumor-specific T cells was based on the belief that tumor antigen-specific T cells could traffic to tumor lesions and preferentially target tumor cells, over nontumor cells. In many of these studies, autologous T cells are primed against tumor antigens and expanded in vitro before reinfusion. Using an animal model of glioma, adoptively transferred CTLs were shown to effectively home to and reject tumors following intravenous administration.[116] According to Yamasaki and colleagues, the mean survival time following intravenous administration of in vitro expanded CTLs was over 15 weeks (except for one animal that died at 10 weeks), compared with approximately 3.3 weeks in vehicle only or in vivo primed CTLs isolated from the draining lymph nodes (3.6 weeks) and spleen (2.0 weeks). Further analysis revealed that the CTL activity of the adoptively transferred cells was specific for tumor cells and not nonglia tumor cells. The ability to generate and maintain tumor-specific T cells was a major advantage compared with LAK cells, and propelled it to prominence in adoptive immunotherapy.

In one such study, Kitahara and colleagues[117] generated CTLs in vitro from the blood of 5 malignant glioma patients. In brief, the peripheral blood lymphocytes were cultured with autologous tumor cells plus IL-2 to generate CTL, which were later administered intracranially. The results from this study were largely poor. One patient showed a transient regression for 20 weeks before recurrence and one patient had a complete regression to at least 104 weeks. Three other patients progressed quickly and died of recurrent tumor. This study underscored the potential benefits of this treatment modality and served as a building block for future trials.

The use of autologous tumor cells to sensitize CTLs in vitro requires the isolation and maintenance of tumor cells. Furthermore, to increase the amount of T cells harvested from peripheral blood, recent studies used bacillus Calmette-Guérin vaccination in combination with granulocyte macrophage colony stimulating factor and IL-2 infusion. In an attempt to circumvent these issues, a more recent study of 9 high-grade glioma patients used anti-CD3 for polyclonal T-cell activation in combination with IL-2.[118] Two patients with grade III disease had complete tumor regression to at least 5 years, and one patient had a partial regression. This treatment strategy was not effective in the GBM patients. Plautz and colleagues[119] obtained encouraging results using autologous CTLs. Patients were infused with GM-CSF and T cells were isolated from the draining lymph nodes. Two patients showed tumor regression and one patient did not observe tumor growth out to 17 months, whereas the remaining 7 patients had progressive disease. Overall, all patients with GBM survived at least a year. Although polyclonal stimulation with anti-CD3 stimulates a large pool of T cells, which may include tumor-specific T cells, the frequency of these cells may be relatively low in the entire T-cell pool, thus minimizing their therapeutic efficacy.

More recent studies sought to isolate and expand tumor-infiltrating lymphocytes (TIL); however, no clear therapeutic benefits were observed. According to Quattrocchi and colleagues,[120] 6 patients with high-grade glioma were treated with autologous TIL plus IL-2 in the tumor cavity following surgical resection. Cerebral edema was the only adverse side effect noted. One in 6 patients demonstrated tumor regression and was tumor free at 45 months. A limitation of this study was that the TIL were simply reinfused without depleting suppressor cells, which have been seen to be highly suppressive and abundant in TIL. Future trials should seek to deplete Tregs before reinfusion, and may consider ex vivo activation and expansion to increase the cytotoxic function of TIL.

## SUMMARY

Novel immunotherapeutic strategies have emerged as the understanding of CNS immunobiology and gliomas has progressed. The anatomic location of glioma within the CNS is beneficial for tumor progression, and limits the success of many treatment modalities. Multiple groups, including the authors', have demonstrated the therapeutic efficacy of immunotherapy in preclinical models of glioma, but these have yet to show clinical efficacy. The authors suggest that the observed deficiencies of many of these treatment modalities are linked to the poor design of many of the clinical trials. In addition, large randomized studies are often difficult to conduct because GBM is rare. Moreover, many preclinical trials are conducted in immune comprised animals, making extrapolation to immune competent hosts difficult.

To truly realize the promise of immunotherapy modalities, there need to be improvements in study design. To date, EGFRvIII has emerged as the key molecule for tumor targeting. As is the case with other targeted therapies, EGFRvIII vaccination has seen minimal successes in the clinic due to poor patient selection. Further, better end-point analyses are required to determine treatment efficacy. In brief, the induction of an immune response does not always correlate with improved time to tumor progression or overall survival. Therefore, studies should clearly define enrollment criteria and result interpretation before study initiation, so that the therapeutic efficacy of immunotherapy can be truly realized.

## ACKNOWLEDGMENTS

This work was supported in part by the National Cancer Institute (RO1-CA138587).

## REFERENCES

1. Stupp R, Mason WP, van den Bent MJ, et al. Radiotherapy plus concomitant and adjuvant temozolomide for glioblastoma. N Engl J Med 2005; 352(10):987–96.

2. Sampson JH, Brady ML, Petry NA, et al. Antisynthetic peptide antibody reacting at the fusion junction of deletion-mutant epidermal growth factor receptors in human glioblastoma. Neurosurgery 2007;60(2 Suppl 1):ONS89–98 [discussion: ONS98–89].

3. El Andaloussi A, Han Y, Lesniak MS. Prolongation of survival following depletion of CD4+CD25+ regulatory T cells in mice with experimental brain tumors. J Neurosurg 2006;105(3):430–7.

4. El Andaloussi A, Lesniak MS. An increase in CD4+CD25+FOXP3+ regulatory T cells in tumor-infiltrating lymphocytes of human glioblastoma multiforme. Neuro Oncol 2006;8(3):234–43.

5. Fecci PE, Mitchell DA, Whitesides JF, et al. Increased regulatory T-cell fraction amidst a diminished CD4 compartment explains cellular immune defects in patients with malignant glioma. Cancer Res 2006;66(6):3294–302.

6. Abou-Ghazal M, Yang DS, Qiao W, et al. The incidence, correlation with tumor-infiltrating inflammation, and prognosis of phosphorylated STAT3 expression in human gliomas. Clin Cancer Res 2008;14(24):8228–35.

7. Libermann TA, Nusbaum HR, Razon N, et al. Amplification, enhanced expression and possible rearrangement of EGF receptor gene in primary human brain tumours of glial origin. Nature 1985; 313(5998):144–7.

8. Bigner SH, Humphrey PA, Wong AJ, et al. Characterization of the epidermal growth factor receptor in human glioma cell lines and xenografts. Cancer Res 1990;50(24):8017–22.

9. Sonabend AM, Dana K, Lesniak MS. Targeting epidermal growth factor receptor variant III: a novel strategy for the therapy of malignant glioma. Expert Rev Anticancer Ther 2007;7(Suppl 12):S45–50.

10. Heimberger AB, Sun W, Hussain SF, et al. Immunological responses in a patient with glioblastoma multiforme treated with sequential courses of temozolomide and immunotherapy: case study. Neuro Oncol 2008;10(1):98–103.

11. Frederick L, Wang XY, Eley G, et al. Diversity and frequency of epidermal growth factor receptor mutations in human glioblastomas. Cancer Res 2000;60(5):1383–7.

12. Heimberger AB, Hlatky R, Suki D, et al. Prognostic effect of epidermal growth factor receptor and EGFRvIII in glioblastoma multiforme patients. Clin Cancer Res 2005;11(4):1462–6.

13. Sok JC, Coppelli FM, Thomas SM, et al. Mutant epidermal growth factor receptor (EGFRvIII) contributes to head and neck cancer growth and resistance to EGFR targeting. Clin Cancer Res 2006;12(17):5064–73.

14. Okamoto I, Kenyon LC, Emlet DR, et al. Expression of constitutively activated EGFRvIII in non-small cell lung cancer. Cancer Sci 2003;94(1):50–6.

15. Belli F, Testori A, Rivoltini L, et al. Vaccination of metastatic melanoma patients with autologous tumor-derived heat shock protein gp96-peptide complexes: clinical and immunologic findings. J Clin Oncol 2002;20(20):4169–80.

16. Batra SK, Castelino-Prabhu S, Wikstrand CJ, et al. Epidermal growth factor ligand-independent, unregulated, cell-transforming potential of a naturally occurring human mutant EGFRvIII gene. Cell Growth Differ 1995;6(10):1251–9.

17. Huang HS, Nagane M, Klingbeil CK, et al. The enhanced tumorigenic activity of a mutant epidermal growth factor receptor common in human cancers is mediated by threshold levels of constitutive tyrosine phosphorylation and unattenuated signaling. J Biol Chem 1997;272(5):2927–35.

18. Boockvar JA, Kapitonov D, Kapoor G, et al. Constitutive EGFR signaling confers a motile phenotype to neural stem cells. Mol Cell Neurosci 2003; 24(4):1116–30.

19. Pedersen MW, Tkach V, Pedersen N, et al. Expression of a naturally occurring constitutively active variant of the epidermal growth factor receptor in mouse fibroblasts increases motility. Int J Cancer 2004;108(5):643–53.

20. Lammering G, Hewit TH, Holmes M, et al. Inhibition of the type III epidermal growth factor receptor variant mutant receptor by dominant-negative EGFR-CD533 enhances malignant glioma cell radiosensitivity. Clin Cancer Res 2004;10(19): 6732–43.

21. Nagane M, Coufal F, Lin H, et al. A common mutant epidermal growth factor receptor confers enhanced tumorigenicity on human glioblastoma cells by increasing proliferation and reducing apoptosis. Cancer Res 1996;56(21):5079–86.

22. Montgomery RB, Guzman J, O'Rourke DM, et al. Expression of oncogenic epidermal growth factor receptor family kinases induces paclitaxel

resistance and alters beta-tubulin isotype expression. J Biol Chem 2000;275(23):17358–63.

23. Lammering G, Hewit TH, Valerie K, et al. EGFRvIII-mediated radioresistance through a strong cytoprotective response. Oncogene 2003;22(36): 5545–53.

24. Akasaki Y, Liu G, Chung NH, et al. Induction of a CD4+ T regulatory type 1 response by cyclooxygenase-2-overexpressing glioma. J Immunol 2004; 173(7):4352–9.

25. Shinojima N, Tada K, Shiraishi S, et al. Prognostic value of epidermal growth factor receptor in patients with glioblastoma multiforme. Cancer Res 2003;63(20):6962–70.

26. Heimberger AB, Archer GE, Crotty LE, et al. Dendritic cells pulsed with a tumor-specific peptide induce long-lasting immunity and are effective against murine intracerebral melanoma. Neurosurgery 2002;50(1):158–64 [discussion: 164–6].

27. Heimberger AB, Crotty LE, Archer GE, et al. Epidermal growth factor receptor VIII peptide vaccination is efficacious against established intracerebral tumors. Clin Cancer Res 2003;9(11): 4247–54.

28. Humphrey PA, Wong AJ, Vogelstein B, et al. Antisynthetic peptide antibody reacting at the fusion junction of deletion-mutant epidermal growth factor receptors in human glioblastoma. Proc Natl Acad Sci U S A 1990;87(11):4207–11.

29. Johns TG, Stockert E, Ritter G, et al. Novel monoclonal antibody specific for the de2-7 epidermal growth factor receptor (EGFR) that also recognizes the EGFR expressed in cells containing amplification of the EGFR gene. Int J Cancer 2002;98(3): 398–408.

30. Jungbluth AA, Stockert E, Huang HJ, et al. A monoclonal antibody recognizing human cancers with amplification/overexpression of the human epidermal growth factor receptor. Proc Natl Acad Sci U S A 2003;100(2):639–44.

31. Kuan CT, Wikstrand CJ, Archer G, et al. Increased binding affinity enhances targeting of glioma xenografts by EGFRvIII-specific scFv. Int J Cancer 2000;88(6):962–9.

32. Perera RM, Narita Y, Furnari FB, et al. Treatment of human tumor xenografts with monoclonal antibody 806 in combination with a prototypical epidermal growth factor receptor-specific antibody generates enhanced antitumor activity. Clin Cancer Res 2005; 11(17):6390–9.

33. Sampson JH, Crotty LE, Lee S, et al. Unarmed, tumor-specific monoclonal antibody effectively treats brain tumors. Proc Natl Acad Sci U S A 2000;97(13):7503–8.

34. Wikstrand CJ, Stanley SD, Humphrey PA, et al. Investigation of a synthetic peptide as immunogen for a variant epidermal growth factor receptor associated with gliomas. J Neuroimmunol 1993;46(1–2): 165–73.

35. Ochiai H, Archer GE, Herndon JE 2nd, et al. EGFRvIII-targeted immunotoxin induces antitumor immunity that is inhibited in the absence of CD4+ and CD8+ T cells. Cancer Immunol Immunother 2008; 57(1):115–21.

36. Wu AH, Xiao J, Anker L, et al. Identification of EGFRvIII-derived CTL epitopes restricted by HLA A0201 for dendritic cell based immunotherapy of gliomas. J Neurooncol 2006;76(1):23–30.

37. Purev E, Cai D, Miller E, et al. Immune responses of breast cancer patients to mutated epidermal growth factor receptor (EGF-RvIII, Delta EGF-R, and de2-7 EGF-R). J Immunol 2004;173(10): 6472–80.

38. Sampson JH, Archer GE, Mitchell DA, et al. Tumor-specific immunotherapy targeting the EGFRvIII mutation in patients with malignant glioma. Semin Immunol 2008;20(5):267–75.

39. Eguchi J, Hatano M, Nishimura F, et al. Identification of interleukin-13 receptor alpha2 peptide analogues capable of inducing improved antiglioma CTL responses. Cancer Res 2006;66(11): 5883–91.

40. Okano F, Storkus WJ, Chambers WH, et al. Identification of a novel HLA-A*0201-restricted, cytotoxic T lymphocyte epitope in a human glioma-associated antigen, interleukin 13 receptor alpha2 chain. Clin Cancer Res 2002;8(9):2851–5.

41. Joshi BH, Leland P, Asher A, et al. In situ expression of interleukin-4 (IL-4) receptors in human brain tumors and cytotoxicity of a recombinant IL-4 cytotoxin in primary glioblastoma cell cultures. Cancer Res 2001;61(22):8058–61.

42. Joshi BH, Leland P, Silber J, et al. IL-4 receptors on human medulloblastoma tumours serve as a sensitive target for a circular permuted IL-4-*Pseudomonas* exotoxin fusion protein. Br J Cancer 2002; 86(2):285–91.

43. Kawakami K, Leland P, Puri RK. Structure, function, and targeting of interleukin 4 receptors on human head and neck cancer cells. Cancer Res 2000; 60(11):2981–7.

44. Obiri NI, Hillman GG, Haas GP, et al. Expression of high affinity interleukin-4 receptors on human renal cell carcinoma cells and inhibition of tumor cell growth in vitro by interleukin-4. J Clin Invest 1993; 91(1):88–93.

45. Obiri NI, Siegel JP, Varricchio F, et al. Expression of high-affinity IL-4 receptors on human melanoma, ovarian and breast carcinoma cells. Clin Exp Immunol 1994;95(1):148–55.

46. Puri RK, Leland P, Kreitman RJ, et al. Human neurological cancer cells express interleukin-4 (IL-4) receptors which are targets for the toxic effects of

IL4-*Pseudomonas* exotoxin chimeric protein. Int J Cancer 1994;58(4):574–81.

47. Wheeler CJ, Das A, Liu G, et al. Clinical responsiveness of glioblastoma multiforme to chemotherapy after vaccination. Clin Cancer Res 2004; 10(16):5316–26.

48. Yu JS, Liu G, Ying H, et al. Vaccination with tumor lysate-pulsed dendritic cells elicits antigen-specific, cytotoxic T-cells in patients with malignant glioma. Cancer Res 2004;64(14):4973–9.

49. Liau LM, Black KL, Martin NA, et al. Treatment of a patient by vaccination with autologous dendritic cells pulsed with allogeneic major histocompatibility complex class I-matched tumor peptides. Case report. Neurosurg Focus 2000;9(6):e8.

50. Heimberger AB, Crotty LE, Archer GE, et al. Bone marrow-derived dendritic cells pulsed with tumor homogenate induce immunity against syngeneic intracerebral glioma. J Neuroimmunol 2000; 103(1):16–25.

51. de Vleeschouwer S, Rapp M, Sorg RV, et al. Dendritic cell vaccination in patients with malignant gliomas: current status and future directions. Neurosurgery 2006;59(5):988–99 [discussioin: 999–1000].

52. Wheeler CJ, Black KL. DCVax-Brain and DC vaccines in the treatment of GBM. Expert Opin Investig Drugs 2009;18(4):509–19.

53. Parajuli P, Mathupala S, Sloan AE. Systematic comparison of dendritic cell-based immunotherapeutic strategies for malignant gliomas: in vitro induction of cytolytic and natural killerlike T cells. Neurosurgery 2004;55(5):1194–204.

54. Srivastava PK, Maki RG. Stress-induced proteins in immune response to cancer. Curr Top Microbiol Immunol 1991;167:109–23.

55. Udono H, Srivastava PK. Heat shock protein 70-associated peptides elicit specific cancer immunity. J Exp Med 1993;178(4):1391–6.

56. Udono H, Srivastava PK. Comparison of tumor-specific immunogenicities of stress-induced proteins gp96, hsp90, and hsp70. J Immunol 1994;152(11):5398–403.

57. Bethke K, Staib F, Distler M, et al. Different efficiency of heat shock proteins (HSP) to activate human monocytes and dendritic cells: superiority of HSP60. J Immunol 2002;169(11):6141–8.

58. Binder RJ, Harris ML, Menoret A, et al. Saturation, competition, and specificity in interaction of heat shock proteins (hsp) gp96, hsp90, and hsp70 with CD11b+ cells. J Immunol 2000;165(5): 2582–7.

59. Parsa A, Crane C, Wilson S, et al. Autologous tumor derived gp96 evokes a tumor specific immune response in recurrent glioma patients that correlates with clinical response to therapy. Paper presented at: AACR-NCI-EORTC International Conference Molecular Targets and Cancer Therapeutics (C274). San Francisco (CA), October 22–26, 2007.

60. Cohen L, de Moor C, Parker PA, et al. Quality of life in patients with metastatic renal cell carcinoma participating in a phase I trial of an autologous tumor-derived vaccine. Urol Oncol 2002;7(3): 119–24.

61. Cohen L, Parker PA, Sterner J, et al. Quality of life in patients with malignant melanoma participating in a phase I trial of an autologous tumour-derived vaccine. Melanoma Res 2002;12(5):505–11.

62. Pilla L, Patuzzo R, Rivoltini L, et al. A phase II trial of vaccination with autologous, tumor-derived heat-shock protein peptide complexes Gp96, in combination with GM-CSF and interferon-alpha in metastatic melanoma patients. Cancer Immunol Immunother 2006;55(8):958–68.

63. Li G, Hu YS, Li XG, et al. Expression and switching of TH1/TH2 type cytokines gene in human gliomas. Chin Med Sci J 2005;20(4):268–72.

64. Roussel E, Gingras MC, Grimm EA, et al. Predominance of a type 2 intratumoural immune response in fresh tumour-infiltrating lymphocytes from human gliomas. Clin Exp Immunol 1996;105(2):344–52.

65. Bodmer S, Strommer K, Frei K, et al. Immunosuppression and transforming growth factor-beta in glioblastoma. Preferential production of transforming growth factor-beta 2. J Immunol 1989;143(10): 3222–9.

66. Tada T, Yabu K, Kobayashi S. Detection of active form of transforming growth factor-beta in cerebrospinal fluid of patients with glioma. Jpn J Cancer Res 1993;84(5):544–8.

67. de Martin R, Haendler B, Hofer-Warbinek R, et al. Complementary DNA for human glioblastoma-derived T cell suppressor factor, a novel member of the transforming growth factor-beta gene family. EMBO J 1987;6(12):3673–7.

68. Huettner C, Paulus W, Roggendorf W. Messenger RNA expression of the immunosuppressive cytokine IL-10 in human gliomas. Am J Pathol 1995; 146(2):317–22.

69. Colombo F, Barzon L, Franchin E, et al. Combined HSV-TK/IL-2 gene therapy in patients with recurrent glioblastoma multiforme: biological and clinical results. Cancer Gene Ther 2005; 12(10):835–48.

70. Kruse CA, Cepeda L, Owens B, et al. Treatment of recurrent glioma with intracavitary alloreactive cytotoxic T lymphocytes and interleukin-2. Cancer Immunol Immunother 1997;45(2):77–87.

71. Wrann M, Bodmer S, de Martin R, et al. T cell suppressor factor from human glioblastoma cells is a 12.5-kd protein closely related to transforming growth factor-beta. EMBO J 1987;6(6):1633–6.

72. Hau P, Jachimczak P, Schlingensiepen R, et al. Inhibition of TGF-beta2 with AP 12009 in recurrent malignant gliomas: from preclinical to phase I/II studies. Oligonucleotides 2007;17(2):201–12.

73. Olson JJ, McKenzie E, Skurski-Martin M, et al. Phase I analysis of BCNU-impregnated biodegradable polymer wafers followed by systemic interferon alfa-2b in adults with recurrent glioblastoma multiforme. J Neurooncol 2008;90(3): 293–9.

74. Buckner JC, Brown LD, Kugler JW, et al. Phase II evaluation of recombinant interferon alpha and BCNU in recurrent glioma. J Neurosurg 1995; 82(3):430–5.

75. Buckner JC, Schomberg PJ, McGinnis WL, et al. A phase III study of radiation therapy plus carmustine with or without recombinant interferon-alpha in the treatment of patients with newly diagnosed high-grade glioma. Cancer 2001;92(2):420–33.

76. Yong Z, Chang L, Mei YX, et al. Role and mechanisms of CD4+CD25+ regulatory T cells in the induction and maintenance of transplantation tolerance. Transpl Immunol 2007;17(2):120–9.

77. Brusko TM, Putnam AL, Bluestone JA. Human regulatory T cells: role in autoimmune disease and therapeutic opportunities. Immunol Rev 2008; 223:371–90.

78. Bayer AL, Yu A, Malek TR. Function of the IL-2R for thymic and peripheral CD4+CD25+ Foxp3+ T regulatory cells. J Immunol 2007;178(7):4062–71.

79. Ichihara F, Kono K, Takahashi A, et al. Increased populations of regulatory T cells in peripheral blood and tumor-infiltrating lymphocytes in patients with gastric and esophageal cancers. Clin Cancer Res 2003;9(12):4404–8.

80. Liyanage UK, Moore TT, Joo HG, et al. Prevalence of regulatory T cells is increased in peripheral blood and tumor microenvironment of patients with pancreas or breast adenocarcinoma. J Immunol 2002;169(5):2756–61.

81. Okita R, Saeki T, Takashima S, et al. CD4+CD25+ regulatory T cells in the peripheral blood of patients with breast cancer and non-small cell lung cancer. Oncol Rep 2005;14(5):1269–73.

82. Hussain SF, Yang D, Suki D, et al. The role of human glioma-infiltrating microglia/macrophages in mediating antitumor immune responses. Neuro Oncol 2006;8(3):261–79.

83. Grauer OM, Nierkens S, Bennink E, et al. CD4+FoxP3+ regulatory T cells gradually accumulate in gliomas during tumor growth and efficiently suppress antiglioma immune responses in vivo. Int J Cancer 2007;121(1):95–105.

84. Takahashi Y, Onda M, Tanaka N, et al. Establishment and characterization of two new rectal neuroendocrine cell carcinoma cell lines. Digestion 2000; 62(4):262–70.

85. Manzotti CN, Tipping H, Perry LC, et al. Inhibition of human T cell proliferation by CTLA-4 utilizes CD80 and requires CD25+ regulatory T cells. Eur J Immunol 2002;32(10):2888–96.

86. Tang Q, Boden EK, Henriksen KJ, et al. Distinct roles of CTLA-4 and TGF-beta in CD4+CD25+ regulatory T cell function. Eur J Immunol 2004; 34(11):2996–3005.

87. Pae HO, Oh GS, Choi BM, et al. Differential expressions of heme oxygenase-1 gene in CD25- and CD25+ subsets of human CD4+ T cells. Biochem Biophys Res Commun 2003;306(3):701–5.

88. Choi BM, Pae HO, Jeong YR, et al. Critical role of heme oxygenase-1 in Foxp3-mediated immune suppression. Biochem Biophys Res Commun 2005;327(4):1066–71.

89. Choi BM, Pae HO, Jeong YR, et al. Overexpression of heme oxygenase (HO)-1 renders Jurkat T cells resistant to fas-mediated apoptosis: involvement of iron released by HO-1. Free Radic Biol Med 2004;36(7):858–71.

90. Song R, Zhou Z, Kim PK, et al. Carbon monoxide promotes Fas/CD95-induced apoptosis in Jurkat cells. J Biol Chem 2004;279(43):44327–34.

91. Curtin JF, Candolfi M, Fakhouri TM, et al. Treg depletion inhibits efficacy of cancer immunotherapy: implications for clinical trials. PLoS One 2008;3(4):e1983.

92. Bromberg J. Stat proteins and oncogenesis. J Clin Invest 2002;109(9):1139–42.

93. Brantley EC, Benveniste EN. Signal transducer and activator of transcription-3: a molecular hub for signaling pathways in gliomas. Mol Cancer Res 2008;6(5):675–84.

94. Chung CD, Liao J, Liu B, et al. Specific inhibition of Stat3 signal transduction by PIAS3. Science 1997; 278(5344):1803–5.

95. Rakesh K, Agrawal DK. Controlling cytokine signaling by constitutive inhibitors. Biochem Pharmacol 2005;70(5):649–57.

96. Pillemer BB, Xu H, Oriss TB, et al. Deficient SOCS3 expression in CD4+CD25+FoxP3+ regulatory T cells and SOCS3-mediated suppression of Treg function. Eur J Immunol 2007;37(8):2082–9.

97. Yu H, Kortylewski M, Pardoll D. Crosstalk between cancer and immune cells: role of STAT3 in the tumour microenvironment. Nat Rev Immunol 2007; 7(1):41–51.

98. Turkson J, Zhang S, Palmer J, et al. Inhibition of constitutive signal transducer and activator of transcription 3 activation by novel platinum complexes with potent antitumor activity. Mol Cancer Ther 2004;3(12):1533–42.

99. Zhang L, Alizadeh D, Van Handel M, et al. Stat3 inhibition activates tumor macrophages and abrogates glioma growth in mice. Glia 2009;57: 1458–67.

100. Jing N, Li Y, Xu X, et al. Targeting Stat3 with G-quartet oligodeoxynucleotides in human cancer cells. DNA Cell Biol 2003;22(11):685–96.

101. Leong PL, Andrews GA, Johnson DE, et al. Targeted inhibition of Stat3 with a decoy oligonucleotide abrogates head and neck cancer cell growth. Proc Natl Acad Sci U S A 2003;100(7):4138–43.

102. Siddiquee K, Zhang S, Guida WC, et al. Selective chemical probe inhibitor of Stat3, identified through structure-based virtual screening, induces antitumor activity. Proc Natl Acad Sci U S A 2007;104(18):7391–6.

103. Gu J, Li G, Sun T, et al. Blockage of the STAT3 signaling pathway with a decoy oligonucleotide suppresses growth of human malignant glioma cells. J Neurooncol 2008;89(1):9–17.

104. Konnikova L, Kotecki M, Kruger MM, et al. Knockdown of STAT3 expression by RNAi induces apoptosis in astrocytoma cells. BMC Cancer 2003;3:23.

105. Ren W, Duan Y, Yang Y, et al. Down-regulation of Stat3 induces apoptosis of human glioma cell: a potential method to treat brain cancer. Neurol Res 2008;30(3):297–301.

106. Rahaman SO, Harbor PC, Chernova O, et al. Inhibition of constitutively active Stat3 suppresses proliferation and induces apoptosis in glioblastoma multiforme cells. Oncogene 2002;21(55):8404–13.

107. Blaskovich MA, Sun J, Cantor A, et al. Discovery of JSI-124 (cucurbitacin I), a selective Janus kinase/signal transducer and activator of transcription 3 signaling pathway inhibitor with potent antitumor activity against human and murine cancer cells in mice. Cancer Res 2003;63(6):1270–9.

108. Hussain SF, Kong LY, Jordan J, et al. A novel small molecule inhibitor of signal transducers and activators of transcription 3 reverses immune tolerance in malignant glioma patients. Cancer Res 2007;67(20):9630–6.

109. Iwamaru A, Szymanski S, Iwado E, et al. A novel inhibitor of the STAT3 pathway induces apoptosis in malignant glioma cells both in vitro and in vivo. Oncogene 2007;26(17):2435–44.

110. Cuevas P, Diaz-Gonzalez D, Gimenez-Gallego G, et al. Dihydroxy-2,5 benzenesulphonate (dobesilate) elicits growth arrest and apoptosis in glioma cells. Neurol Res 2005;27(8):797–800.

111. Rayner AV, O'Brien JG, Schoenbachler B. Behavior disorders of dementia: recognition and treatment. Am Fam Physician 2006;73(4):647–52.

112. Iwasaki K, Kikuchi H, Miyatake S, et al. Clonal analysis in the ultrastructure of cell-to-cell interaction between a human glioma cell line and autologous tumor-specific cytotoxic T lymphocytes. Cell Immunol 1990;126(1):164–75.

113. Rosenberg SA, Lotze MT, Muul LM, et al. Observations on the systemic administration of autologous lymphokine-activated killer cells and recombinant interleukin-2 to patients with metastatic cancer. N Engl J Med 1985;313(23):1485–92.

114. Jacobs SK, Wilson DJ, Kornblith PL, et al. Interleukin-2 or autologous lymphokine-activated killer cell treatment of malignant glioma: phase I trial. Cancer Res 1986;46(4 Pt 2):2101–4.

115. Hayes RL, Koslow M, Hiesiger EM, et al. Improved long term survival after intracavitary interleukin-2 and lymphokine-activated killer cells for adults with recurrent malignant glioma. Cancer 1995;76(5):840–52.

116. Yamasaki T, Kikuchi H. An experimental approach to specific adoptive immunotherapy for malignant brain tumors. Nippon Geka Hokan 1989;58(6):485–92.

117. Kitahara T, Watanabe O, Yamaura A, et al. Establishment of interleukin 2 dependent cytotoxic T lymphocyte cell line specific for autologous brain tumor and its intracranial administration for therapy of the tumor. J Neurooncol 1987;4(4):329–36.

118. Tsurushima H, Liu SQ, Tuboi K, et al. Reduction of end-stage malignant glioma by injection with autologous cytotoxic T lymphocytes. Jpn J Cancer Res 1999;90(5):536–45.

119. Plautz GE, Miller DW, Barnett GH, et al. T cell adoptive immunotherapy of newly diagnosed gliomas. Clin Cancer Res 2000;6(6):2209–18.

120. Quattrocchi KB, Miller CH, Cush S, et al. Pilot study of local autologous tumor infiltrating lymphocytes for the treatment of recurrent malignant gliomas. J Neurooncol 1999;45(2):141–57.

# Index

*Note:* Page numbers of article titles are in **boldface** type.

# Moving?

## Make sure your subscription moves with you!

To notify us of your new address, find your **Clinics Account Number** (located on your mailing label above your name), and contact customer service at:

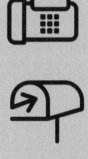

**Email: journalscustomerservice-usa@elsevier.com**

**800-654-2452** (subscribers in the U.S. & Canada)
**314-447-8871** (subscribers outside of the U.S. & Canada)

**Fax number: 314-447-8029**

**Elsevier Health Sciences Division**
**Subscription Customer Service**
**3251 Riverport Lane**
**Maryland Heights, MO 63043**

ELSEVIER

Printed and bound by CPI Group (UK) Ltd, Croydon, CR0 4YY

03/10/2024

01040361-0007